PRINCIPLES OF BIOCHEMISTRY

(For Home Science / Nursing)

PRINCIPLES OF
BIOCHEMISTRY

(For Home Science / Nursing)

S.P. Singh Ph.D., F.A.C.B.I.
Former WHO Fellow, Texas A&M University, Texas, U.S.A.
Nominated by Govt. of India for
Commonwealth Medical Fellowship, 1983
Professor & Head, Deptt. of Biochemistry,
MLB Medical College, Jhansi - 284 128 (U.P.)
and
Chief Consultant in Biochemistry,
MLB Medical College Associated Hospital, Jhansi

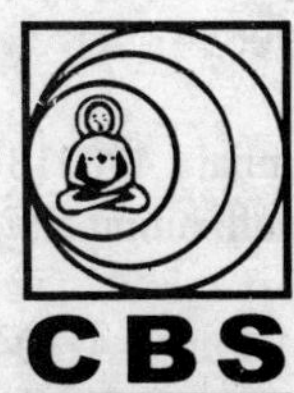

CBS PUBLISHERS & DISTRIBUTORS PVT. LTD.
New Delhi • Bengaluru • Chennai • Kochi • Mumbai • Pune

ISBN: 81-239-1322-2

First Edition: 2006
Reprint: 2007, 2008, 2010, 2011, 2015

Published by:
Satish Kumar Jain for CBS Publishers & Distributors Pvt. Ltd.,
CBS Plaza, 4819/XI Prahlad Street, 24 Ansari Road,
Daryaganj, New Delhi – 110002, India
delhi@cbspd.com, cbspubs@airtelmail.in • www.cbspd.com
Ph.: 23289259, 23266861, 23266867 • Fax: 011-23243014

Branches:

- ***Bengaluru:*** Seema House, 2975, 17th Cross, K.R. Road,
  Bansankari 2nd Stage, Bengaluru - 560070
  Ph: +91-80-26771678/79 • Fax: +91-80-26771680
  E-mail: cbsbng@gmail.com, bangalore@cbspd.com
- ***Chennai:*** No. 7, Subbaraya Street, Shenoy Nagar, Chennai - 600030
  Ph: +91-44-26681266, 26680620 • Fax: +91-44-42032115
  E-mail: chennai@cbspd.com
- ***Kochi:*** 36/14, Kalluvilakam, Lissie Hospital Road, Kochi - 682018
  Ph: +91-484-4059061-65 • Fax: +91-484-4059065
  E-mail: cochin@cbspd.com
- ***Mumbai:*** 83-C, Dr. E. Moses Road, Worli, Mumbai - 400018
  Ph: +91-9833017933, 022-24902340/41 • E-mail: mumbai@cbspd.com
- ***Pune:*** Bhuruk Prestige, Sr. No. 52/12/2+1+3/2,
  Narhe, Haveli (Near Katraj-Dehu Road Bypass), Pune - 411041
  Ph: +91-20-64704058/59, 32342277 • E-mail: pune@cbspd.com

Printed at :
J.S. Offset Printers, Delhi

PREFACE TO THE FIRST EDITION

It gives me immense pleasure to bring out 1st edition of text book of **'Biochemistry'** for **Home-Science & Nursing students of B.Sc. and M.Sc. classes** of Indian Universities. The syllabus of this book has been kept after consulting syllabi of such courses of various Indian Universities. I was feeling to write such a book for B.Sc. & M.Sc. students of these classes for long as there was no such small book for such courses; either the books available in the market for such courses are too voluminous or the chapter of **'Nutrition', a very important and meaningful chapter for them was not up to the mark,** therefore, I decided to write such a cozy book keeping in view all the optimum necessities of them in mind. The inspirer of this book are **Dr. (Smt) Meenakshi Singh,** Head of the department of Home- Science, Bundelkhand University, Jhansi (U.P.) and Dr. (Smt.) Pratibha Arya, Lecturer of the same department; Dr. Ajay Bhargava, Reader & Head Biochemistry department, Maharana Pratap Dental College, Gwalior and Dr. Harshvardhan Singh, Lecturer in Biochemistry, Santosh Medical College, Ghaziabad (U.P.)

I am sure this book shall serve the purpose of the students of such courses, however, I earnestly appeal to the students, the readers and the learned teachers to feed me their valuable suggestions/ ideas to improve it further for the cause of students and as a whole the **'academy'. Let us work open heartedly together for the betterment of 'Education' in India or elsewhere. No work is greater than EDUCATION.**

1st January, 2006
(New year's day)

- S.P. Singh

ACKNOWLEDGEMENT

First of all, I express my deep gratitude to my family members i.e., **wife Dr. (Smt) Manju Singh, Reader, History Department, Bundelkhand Postgraduate College, Jhansi; sons Er. Vikrant Singh and Er. Vijyant Singh, daughter-in-law Smt. Charu Singh, pets Pasha and Gini who all always not only inspired me but also encouraged me from time to time for this gigantic work as writing of a book paralyses one's social and family life.**

I shall fail in my duties if I do not express my gratitude to my well wishers i.e.; Lt. Colonel (Retd) A.R.N. Setalvad, Secretary, Medical Council of India (a thorough gentleman who speaks little and says everything from eyes); Dr. Narendra Kumar Jain, Joint Secretary, University Grants Commission, New Delhi (inspirer for me for writing work); Dr. R.K. Srivastava, Director - General, Ministry of Health and Family Welfare, Govt of India, New Delhi (who acts as a **'lamp'** for me), Dr. A.K. Gupta, Principal & Dean, M.L.B. Medical College, Jhansi, Professor (Smt) Mridula Kapur, Professor R.K. Gandhi, Professor Bhakt Prakash Mathur, Dr. K.P. Singh, Prof. V.N. Pandey, Principal, Bundelkhand Postgraduate College, Jhansi; Sri M.P. Gupta, Senior Advocate, Jhansi; Prof. R.K. Bhatia, History Department, BKD College, Jhansi; Er. S.S. Chaturvedi, Er. V.N. Pathak, Sri K.V. Srivastava, Sri Bishan Lal, Sri S.A. Siddiqui, Sri S.S. Shukla, Sri Ashok Kumar Srivastava, Sri Chintamani, Sri Khalak Singh, Sri Vinod Kumar - all of M.L.B. Medical College, Jhansi.

I am also indebted to my well wishers i.e., Sri Satish Kumar Jain, Sri Vinod Kumar Jain, Sri Sonu Jain, Sri B.M. Singh, Sri B.M. Sharma, Sri Dharam Veer, Sri Nayar- all of M/s CBS Publishers, New Delhi; and Dr. D.P. Singh Maurya (Meerut) who all always guided me for creative works from time to time.

I am also really indebted to **Mr. Prakash Sahu**, Compositor, 390, Sadar Bazar, Jhansi and **Mr. Sunil Sharma,** Artist, Nagra, Jhansi for preparing beautiful figures of this book in such a short period.

1st January, 2006 **- S.P. Singh**
(New year's day)

By
the grace and kind blessings
of
***Sri Rawatpura Sarkar ji,** a great saint*
*(a very pious recognised place in **district Bhind, Madhya Pradesh)***
who himself illiterate is untiringly working round the clock for the upliftment and spread of
'Education' in India and opening colleges/universities in India at his own

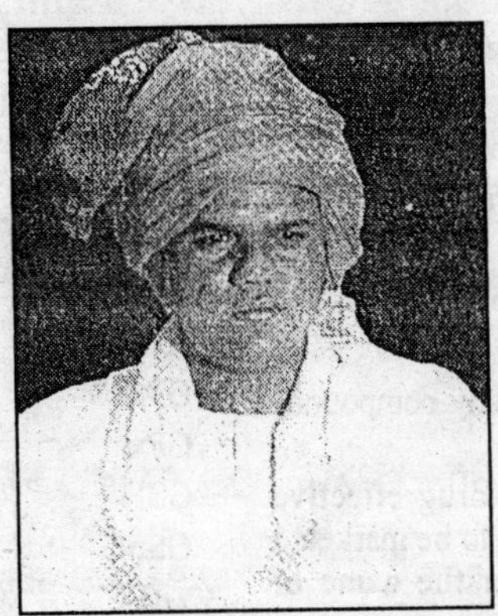

Dedicated
To
Honourable Sri Mulayam Singh Ji
Chief Minister, Uttar Pradesh
and
Sri Vinod Kumar Singh Ji Urf Pandit Singh Ji
State Minister for Medical Education (Independent Charge), U.P.
Upright honest, dynamic and very enthusiastic persons who are solely responsible for the upliftment of medical education in U.P., the largest state of our country.

and

Dr. R. K. Baslas
Ph.D., D.Sc., PDF (Germany)
Director, Higher Education, Uttar Pradesh, Allahabad
an upright, kind hearted, peace-loving and literary illuminary of our country who is whole heartedly dedicated to the upgradation of education in degree and postgraduate colleges of U.P.

BIOCHEMICAL ABBREVIATIONS

Ac : Acetate
Ac CoA : Acyl coenzyme A
A : Adenine
ACD bottle : Acid citrate dextrose bottle
ALD : Aldolase
AIDS : Acquired immune deficiency syndrome
AMP : Adenosine monophosphate (adenylic acid)
ADP : Adenosine diphosphate
ACE : Angiotensin converting enzyme
ACP : Acid phosphatase
ALT : Alanine transaminase (previously GPT)
AST : Aspartate transaminase (previously GOT)
ATP : Adenosine triphosphate
ADPR : Adenosine diphosphate ribose
ATPase : Adenosine triphosphatase
AT-10 : Dehydrotachysterol (antitetany compound-10)
AZT : Azidothymidine the only drug effective against AIDs, this is going to be marketed in India by 'Cipla' under the name of 'Zidovir'
BCG : Bacillus Calmette and Guerin
BMR : Basal metabolic rate
CF : Citrovorum factor (folinic acid)
CoA : Coenzyme A
CoA SH : Coenzyme A reduced
C : Cytosine
CMP : Cytosine monophosphate (cytidylic acid)
CDP : Cytosine diphosphate
cDNA : Complementary DNA
CT : Computed tomography
CTP : Cytosine triphosphate
cTnT : Cardiac troponin T
Cal : Calorie, large (kilocalorie)
ChE : Choline esterase
CPK : Creatine phosphokinase
DAP : Dihydroxyacetone phosphate
DFP : Diisopropyl fluorophosphate
1,25 DHCC : 1,25 dihydroxy cholecalciferol
DMD : Duchenne muscular dystrophy
DNP : 2, 4 - dinitrophenol
DPN^+ : Diphosphopyridine nucleotide, oxidized
$DPNH_2$: Diphosphopyridine nucleotide, reduced
DNA : Deoxyribonucleic acid
DOC : Deoxycorticosterone
DOPA : Dioxyphenylalanine or Dihydroxyphenylalanine
EDTA : Ethylene diamine tetra acetic acid
EAA : Essential amino acids
EFA : Essential fatty acids
FA : Folic Acid
FAD : Flavin adenine dinucleotide
FDP : Fructose 1, 6-diphosphate
FH_2 : Dihydro folic acid
FH_4 : Tetrahydro folic acid
FMN : Flavin mono nucleotide
FAO : Food and Agriculture Organization
GC-MS : Gas Chromatograph-Mass spectrometer
GA : Glyceraldehyde
GPx : Glutathione peroxidase
GSH : Glutathione (reduced form)
GSSG : Glutathione (oxidized form)
γ-GT : γ- glutamyl transferase
G : Guanine
GMP : Guanosine monophosphate (guanylic acid)
GDP : Guanosine diphosphate
GTP : Guanosine triphosphate
GDH : Glucose dehydrogenase
GLDH : Glutamate dehydrogenase
GnRH : Gonadotropin- releasing hormone
HbCO : Carboxy(Carbon monoxy) hemoglobin
HBsAG : Hepatitis B surface antigen i.e., Australia antigen
HBV : Hepatitis B virus
HPLC : High performance liquid chromatography
HIV : Human immuno-deficiency virus
IAA : Iodoacetate
I : Inosine
ICD : Isocitrate dehydrogenase
IMP : Inosine monophosphate (Inosinic Acid)
IDP : Inosine diphosphate
ITP : Inosine triphosphate
KG : α- Ketoglutarate
LTs : Leukotrienes
Mb : Myoglobin

MB : Methylene blue
MRI : Magnetic resonance imaging
NMN : Nicotinamide mononucleotide
NAD^+ : Nicotinamide adenine dinucleotide (older name is DPN^+, also known as Co I)
$NADP^+$: Nicotinamide adenine dinucleotide phosphate (older name is TPN^+, also known as Co II)
NPN : Non protein nitrogen
OAA : Oxaloacetate
OD : Optical density
PABA : Para amino benzoic acid
PBI : Protein bound iodine
PEP : Phosphoenolpyruvate
3-PGA : 3- Phosphoglyceric acid
PGE_2 : Prostaglandin E_2
Pi : Inorganic phosphate
PP : Pyrophosphate
PKU : Phenylketonuria
POMC : Pro-opio melanocortin
PSA : Prostate specific antigen (semenogelase)
RNA : Ribonucleic acid
RNAse : Ribonuclease
R-5-P : Ribose-5-Phosphate
R.Q. : Respiratory Quotient
SOD : Superoxide dismutase
SRP : Signal recognition particle
STH : Somatotropic hormone
TCA : Trichloroacetic acid
THAM : Tris (hydroxymethyl) aminoethane
TPP : Thiamine pyrophosphate
TPN^+ : Triphosphopyridine nucleotide (oxidized form)
$TPNH_2$: Triphosphopyridine nucleotide (reduced form)
U : Uracil residue
UMP : Uridine monophosphate (uridylic acid)
UDP : Uridine diphosphate
UTP : Uridine triphosphate
UDPG : Uridine diphosphoglucose
UDPGal : Uridine diphosphogalactose
USP : United States Pharmacopoeia
WHO : World Health Organization
XMP : Xanthosine monophosphate
Xyl : Xylose
Xul : Xylulose

AMINO ACIDS

Ala : Alanine
Arg : Arginine
Val : Valine
His : Histidine
Leu : Leucine
Ile : Isoleucine
Met : Methionine
Pro : Proline
Phe : Phenylalanine
Trp : Tryptophan
Asp : Aspartic acid
Asn : Asparagine
Gln : Glutamine
Glu : Glutamic acid
Gly : Glycine
Ser : Serine
Thr : Threonine
Thx : Thyroxine
Tyr : Tyrosine
Cys-SH : Cysteine
Cys-S- : 1/2 Cystine
Lys : Lysine

HORMONES

ACTH : Adrenocorticotrophic hormone
FSH : Follicle stimulating hormone
GH : Growth hormone
HCG : Human chorionic gonadotropin
ICSH : Interistitial cell stimulating hormone
LH : Luteinizing hormone
LTH : Leuteotrophic hormone
MSH : Melanocyte stimulating hormone
PTH : Parathyroid hormone
TSH : Thyroid stimulating hormone
T_3 : Triiodothyronine
T_4 : Tetraiodothyronine (thyroxine)

MISCELLANEOUS

AHG : Antihemophilic globulin
BAL : British anti- lewisite
IR : Infrared
PRPP : Phosphoribosyl pyrophosphate
UV : Ultraviolet
VDM : Vasodepressor material
HRP : Horseradish peroxidase

TMB : Tetra methyl benzidine
Eukaryotes : Mammalian cells
Prokaryotes : Bacteria
NEPH : Nephelometry
REP : Radio electrophoresis
RU : Radio uptake
CC : Column Chromatography
RIA : Radio-immunoassay
CLIA : Chemiluminescence immunoassay
ELISA : Enzyme linked Immunosorbent assay
HAA : Haem agglutination assay
ABP : Androgen- binding protein
ACAT : Acyl-CoA: cholesterol acyltransferase
ADH : Alcohol dehydrogenase
ADH : Antidiuretic hormone, vasopressin
AFP : α_1-Fetoprotein
AIP : Aldosterone-induced protein
ALA : Aminolevulinic acid
BDGF : Bone-derived growth factor
BMP : Bone morphogenic protein
CaBP : Calcium- binding protein
CBG : Corticosteroid- binding globulin
CCK : Cholecystokinin
COMT : Catechol-O-methyltransferase
CRBP : Cellular retinol-binding protein
CRH : Corticotropin-releasing hormone
D : Dopamine receptor
DA : Dopamine
DES : Diethylstilbestrol
DHEA : Dehydroepiandrosterone
DHT : Dihydrotestosterone
DIT : Diiodotyrosine
DPG : Diphosphoglycerate
dsRNA : Double-stranded RNA
E : Epinephrine
EGF : Epidermal Growth Factor
Enz : Enzyme (Also E)
Figlu : Formiminoglutamic acid
GIP : Gastric inhibitory polypeptide
HAL : Hepatic acylglycerol lipase
HMG-CoA : β-Hydroxy-β-methylglutaryl-CoA
HMM : Heavy meromyosin
HSL : Hormone-sensitive lipase
I : Isoproterenol
IGF : Insulin-like growth factor
IL : Interleukin
kat : Katal
kJ : Kilojoule
LATS : Long- acting thyroid stimulator
LMM : Light meromyosin
LPH : Lipotropic hormone
LPL : Lipoprotein lipase
MCR : Metabolic clearance rate
MDR : Minimum daily requirement
MIT : Monoiodotyrosine
MJ : Megajoule
NE : Norepinephrine
NGF : Nerve growth factor
NSN : Nicotine-sensitive neurophysin
PAF : Platelet-activating factor
PAPS : Phosphoadenosine-phosphosulfate
PGI : Prostacyclin
RDA : Recommended daily (dietary) allowance
SAM : S - Adenosylmethionine
SC : Secretory component
SDS : Sodium dodecyl sulfate
SMP : Submitochondrial particle
TG : Thyroglobulin
TMP : Thiamine monophosphate
TPA : Tissue plasminogen activator
VIP : Vasoactive intestinal polypeptide
VMA : Vanillylmandelic acid

CONTENTS

CHAPTER 1

BIOCHEMISTRY : IMPORTANCE AND APPLICATIONS

Biochemistry, these days is treated to be the most important subject of life-sciences whether medical sciences or plant-sciences. Nearly 70 years ago, this subject was in infancy but now it is deep rooted and possesses an unique position because it is said to be the foundation of the modern medicine on which it is erected.

The word 'Biochemistry' is very broad in its meaning which may be defined as the study of different chemical processes going on in the body at molecular level, no matter it's a plant or animal body.

Besides, it also deals with the nature of the chemical constituents of the living organisms; the functions and transformations of such chemical entities in the biological systems and also with the chemical and energetic changes associated with such transformations during the course of activity.

Day by day, its applicability in the field of life sciences is going on increasing and it is being utilized for the benefit of mankind and plant kingdom as well.

The history of biochemistry as it is in the present form is not very old. Most of the work in the field of biochemistry has been carried out in the last half-century. In this period of development, it is being increasingly recognized as an essential discipline among the life-sciences. In some of the advanced Western countries, there are full fledged independent institutes of biochemistry but unfortunately there is even not a single separate full fledged independent institute of Biochemistry in India because of the want of which our country is lagging behind as far as *biochemical sciences* are concerned. Unfortunately our country has neither got a separate *'Institute of Biochemistry'* nor *'Biochemical Engineering'*; whereas now the time is fully mature to establish such an independent institute in India, so that we could keep pace with the Western world. Although, we have some good institutes of Science and Technology like **Central Drug Research Institute at Lucknow; Industrial Toxicology Research Centre at Lucknow; National Institute of Immunology at New Delhi; National Institute of Nutrition at Hyderabad; Centre for Food & Technological Research Institute at Mysore; Indian Institute of Science at Bangalore; Centre for Biochemical Technology at New Delhi; National Chemical Laboratory at Pune; Indian Institute of Chemical Technology at**

Hyderabad; Bhabha Atomic Research Centre at Trombay (Mumbai); Tata Institute of Fundamental Research at Mumbai; All India Institute of Medical Sciences at New Delhi; Centre for Cellular and Molecular Biology at Hyderabad, Centre for DNA Finger Printing & Diagnostics at Hyderabad; National Brain Research Centre at Manesar (Haryana); Institute of Genomics & Integrative Biology at New Delhi; International Centre for Genetic Engineering & Biotechnology at New Delhi etc, which have got very good well equipped biochemistry sections. Scientists and doctors are working whole heartedly round the clock at these centres to make 'science' more approachable and meaningful to the mankind. We have some eminent biochemists in India like ***Prof G.P. Talwar, Padam Shree*** *(Ex-Professor & HOD, Department of Biochemistry, AIIMS, New Delhi & ex*-Director, National Institute of Immunology, New Delhi), and at present Director, Talwar Research Foundation, New Delhi, whose team has so far been able to publish wonderful research papers in the field of 'Immunology' in world class journals and still working on several projects like "developing peptide based vaccine for **Plasmodium vivax malaria"** etc; **Dr. Lalji Singh, Director, Centre for Cellular and Molecular Biology, Hyderabad;** whose team is working on several projects related to **DNA finger printing technology,** uses of various biochemical techniques/ applications in forensic sciences, etc., for e.g., in establishing **parentage problems/issues,** etc. ***Prof D.P. Burma,*** Ex-Professor and Head of the Department of Biochemistry, Institute of Medical Sciences, B.H.U., Varanasi, now a days settled at Calcutta is a worker on *Nucleic Acids (Ribosomologist);* ***Prof P.P. Singh,*** Ex-Head of the Department of Biochemistry, R.N.T. Medical College, Udaipur is a worker on ***Urolithiasis; Prof T.N. Pattabiraman,*** Ex-Head of the Department of Biochemistry, Kasturba Medical College, Manipal, is an ***Enzymologist; Prof. B.C. Harinath,*** *Ex-* Head of the Department of Biochemistry, Mahatma Gandhi Institute of Medical Sciences, Sevagram (Wardha, Maharastra), is an ***Immunologist*** of repute and high profile. **Dr. P.M. Bhargava,** Ex- Director, CCMB, Hyderabad is a Biochemist of repute who is working with his team on several projects of National interest.; **Dr. G.K. Khullar,** Professor & Head, Biochemistry Department, P.G.I., Chandigarh is a Biochemist of repute working on **'designing polymer based novel drug carriers for Experimental Tuberculosis; Professor Balaram,** Chairman, Division of Biological Sciences, Indian Institute of Science, Bangalore is a Biochemist of repute working on several projects of human interest; **Dr. K. Taranath Shetty,** Professor and Head Department of Biochemistry, NIMHANS, Bangalore, is a Biochemist of repute working on several projects related to **neurobiochemistry; Dr. V. S. Chauhan,** Director, International Centre for Genetic Engineering & Biotechnology, New Delhi whose team is working on hereditary and allied disorders; **Dr. Samir Brahmachari,** Director, Institute of Genomics & Integrative Biology, New Delhi whose team is working on **'Genome Project'** and allied topics; **Dr. Sandeep Basu,** Director, National Institute of Immunology, New Delhi whose team is working in developing vaccines

CBT	: New Delhi
CDRI	: Lucknow
CFTRI	: Mysore
CCMB	: Hyderabad
ITRC	: Lucknow
ICGEB	: New Delhi
IGIB	: New Delhi
I.I.Sc	: Bangalore
IICT	: Hyderabad
NCL	: Pune
NII	: New Delhi
NIN	: Hyderabad
TIFR	: Mumbai
CDFD	: Hyderabad
NBRC	: Manesar (Haryana)

for various disorders; **Dr. P. N. Tandon,** Director, National Brain Research Centre whose team is working on several projects of brain chemistry and **Dr. Seyed E Hasnain,** Director, Centre for DNA Finger Printing & Diagnostics, Hyderabad whose team is working on several topics of human interest.

We are having **National Institute of Nutrition at Hyderabad,** an institute of its type in whole of Asia which is dedicated towards the inventions of cheaper sources of proteins, vitamins, etc. and also trying to evolve cheaper vegetable/plant substitutes of animal proteins for the vegetarians as in our country quite a sizable population is vegetarian and in the Western world too quite a good number of people conscious to health and obesity are now a days turning to vegetarianism. This institute also attracts young doctors having aptitude for research in medicine; institute is also dedicated in quality research work in bringing out solution of the diseases being caused due to the deficiency of vitamins and hormones, also involved in the search of good cheaper easily available sources of calories so that the poorer around the world may be benefited. Besides, **institute is also doing work as to how sufferers of certain diseases like diabetes mellitus, kwashiorkor, marasmus, protein energy malnutrition (PEM),etc. may get rid of such fierceful diseases/ states.** Institute is also looking after various interests of pregnant and lactating women with special reference to poverty.

CFTRI (Mysore), is also looking after the interest of the good health of the people of the globe with special reference to pure drinking water, beverages, adulterations (trend of adulteration is on increase day by day in some countries like India where the punishment for the adulterators, if at all existing is either of mild nature or nil) etc. Adulteration in edibles/ beverages like sweets, oils, spices, condiments, milk, medicines, flour, and a number of variety of preparations which are used in daily routine by the human beings and the animals has become a common thing now-a-days. **Adulteration is the mother of so many diseases and a perfect sound 'Nation' can not be footed so long the adulterators are alive.** Therefore, the Governments should be very strict in dealing with such adulterators.

C.D.R.I. (Lucknow) is also dedicated towards the search of newer, safer, potent drugs having no or lesser toxicity.

I.T.R.C. (Lucknow) is likewise dedicated in studying various aspects of toxicity to mankind with special reference to pollutants, gases, adulteration of toxic substances like lead, cadmium, cobalt etc. i.e., non-permitted (banned) colours etc, to the edibles. They are also working to see the effect of poisonous gases/ materials etc. on the health of factory/industry workers.

NII (New Delhi) is dedicated towards the synthesis of newer vaccines of certain diseases. They are also doing work towards the synthesis of ***'birth control vaccine';*** it shall be the most revolutionary day in the history of science. It shall be a laurel not only to the Indian Scientists but to the entire scientific community of the world. ***Prof. G.P. Talwar,*** Ex-Head of the Department of Biochemistry, All India Institute of Medical Sciences, New Delhi and at present working in NII as an emeritus scientist is engaged for more than last two decades towards the synthesis of birth control vaccine. One such group from Mumbai, besides some groups from the Western world are also engaged for the same cause. These days, control of the explosion of the population is the ever biggest challenge before the entire scientific community of the world.

A lot of work is being done both on basic and applied fields of biochemistry in order to make it more useful and viable for the benefit of mankind and understanding the secrets of life. The discipline has so far established an unique position in the field of medicine because of the fact that it is forming a **major tool in explaining the development of disorders and diseases in the body;** that is why, one finds sophisticated latest update biochemical instruments like **PCR, gas liquid chromatography, atomic absorption spectrophotometer, autoanalysers, radioisotope laboratory, tissue culture laboratory, etc.** in the well established good departments/sections/units of biochemistry. The knowledge of biochemistry has been able to pinpoint the exact site of the disorder and to give a clue towards the line of treatment in most of the diseases. **The new offshoot of biochemistry i.e. genetic engineering is flourishing like anything in the Western advanced countries like U.S.A., U.K., Germany, France, Japan, etc. which may bring solution of several disorders like those of hereditary disorders and other incurable diseases, the treatment of which is not possible at the moment. Scientists and doctors are working day and night in these countries to synthesize genes responsible for various genetic defects but unfortunately in our own country, this science is still lagging behind. It is a cause of serious concern to the Government of India.**

Hereditary diseases, which are considered to be incurable at present might be easily controlled or treated satisfactorily in the near future by simply changing the nature of the particular gene(s) responsible for the causation of such disease(s). **Attempts are being made to synthesize genes biochemically. Success in this field is bound to bring revolutionary, miraculous changes in the world of life-sciences.** Genes are the carriers of hereditary characters. After the synthesis of newer genes, it might be quite possible to produce off-springs of ones own choice. Suppose, then, if someone wishes a wrestler, or an athlete or a gymnast or a tall fellow, or a very intellectual one, it would be quite possible to have it. This also means that the usage of genes for the betterment of mankind may also be misused by someone, hence, care must be taken for its 'use' and not 'misuse'; therefore the Governments must enact some law(s) in future for the use of **'genes'** and the power of its usage should never be vested in a single hand (single doctor), rather in a board comprising of atleast 5-7 highly qualified specialists of that field.

Dr Har Gobind Khorana, India born Chemist, turned into a Biochemist, now-a-days settled in U.S.A. (a permanent citizen of U.S.A at present) is working for more than a quarter century on DNA and the synthesis of genes for which he was awarded the most prestigious award i.e. ***"Nobel Prize"* in the year 1968.**

The knowledge of biochemistry is also being extensively used in the field of diagnosis of diseases. Estimations of the levels of biogenic compounds and enzymes in the circulating blood/urine have been proved to be of valuable guidance to the Physicians/Surgeons in making the diagnosis of diseases, for instance, blood sugar level gets elevated in diabetes mellitus, blood urea and creatinine levels get raised in nephritis, serum calcium level gets elevated in hyperthyroidism and gets decreased in infantile tetany, serum inorganic phosphorus gets decreased in rickets, serum cholesterol level gets elevated in nephrosis, diabetes mellitus, obstructive jaundice, myxoedema and xanthomatosis and may be decreased in *hyperthyroidism,* level of enzyme acid phosphatase gets increased in the carcinoma of prostate glands, serum glutamic oxaloacetic transaminase (GOT) and creatine phosphokinase (CPK or CK) levels get elevated in myocardial infarction, and so on.

Certain qualitative tests in urine, e.g. for the detection of sugar, protein, bile pigments, bile salts, blood, chyle, etc. are of great importance to the Physicians/Surgeons in making proper diagnosis. Besides qualitative tests, certain quantitative tests in urine like that of the estimation of total proteins in a 24 hrs urine sample is of diagnostic value in cases of nephrotic syndrome.

Estimations of hormones in serum are of equally great diagnostic value, e.g. the estimations of T_3 and T_4 are most reliable means of confirming the diagnosis of hyperthyroidism or hypothyroidism. Highly specific and sensitive radioimmunoassays are used to measure serum T_3 and T_4 concentrations. In thyrotoxic states, serum TSH concentration is almost always low or undetectable. This is of little diagnostic value, since most assays can not distinguish between normal and subnormal values. Measurement of serum TSH is the best means of distinguishing between untreated hypothyroidism of thyroid origin, in which the values are invariably increased, and pituitary or hypothalamic hypothyroidism, in which the values are usually undetectable or within the normal range.

NORMAL RANGE		
T_4	:	4-12 μg/dl
T_3	:	80-100 ng/dl
TSH	:	Less than 5 μU/ml

Certain diseases are merely controlled by using specific enzyme inhibitors or activators. Recent studies have proved that the medicines mostly act by influencing certain enzyme or enzyme systems. The same also holds true for hormones. Structure activity relationships have been established in most of the cases. Such studies are covered in the field of ***biochemical pharmacology***. After ascertaining the site of action and the structure responsible for a particular activity, it has now become possible to synthesize newer medicines having lesser toxicity and greater beneficial effects.

Radioisotopes are of great use in certain types of diseases like malignancies (cancers) of different origin of various organs/tissues. Isotopes of cobalt, iodine, etc. are used satisfactorily with very good results in different types of early diagnosed cancers by the radiophysicists under the guidance/consultation of Physicians/Surgeons treating such patients. In our country, establishment of radioisotope laboratory requires clearance by the *Bhabha Atomic Research Centre* ***(BARC),*** *Trombay as* one must take all kinds of precautions in the handling of radioisotopes. All staff members connected with such a laboratory must be well versed with the ***"Radiation Hazards",*** which are otherwise very fatal and injurious to the humans, many times more fatal than the X-Rays.

Disposal of the used radioactive material is also a cause of great concern. This material must be disposed as per the guidelines and instructions laid down by BARC, Trombay. All kinds of wares i.e: plasticwares/glasswares etc. being used for the estimation purposes or therapy purposes or otherwise should not be used for routine work, hitherto must be disposed safely. **Radioactive material, if handled casually, may otherwise kill the normal healthy cells, may also cause *'mutation'* which may even persist in the off-springs (1-2-3 generations).**

CHAPTER 2

CARBOHYDRATES

We are very important for the human beings as we are the driving force (petrol) for them. We are polyhydroxy aldehydes or ketones or their derivatives. To achieve us is very easy and we are inexpensive but teeth should take care of us, especially the infants and the children. When you eat us like other things and do not brush, we get accumulated in the interspaces of teeth, thus invite bacteria to grow which results in caries, a fierceful disease. We have storehouses in the body like liver, muscles, etc.

INTRODUCTION

The class of substances known as carbohydrates is comprised of a large number of relatively heterogenous compounds. They are especially prominent constituents of plants, but also do occur and serve important functions in animals.

Carbohydrates serve as the chief source of energy in the food of humans and many other animals. As is evident from the name itself, these are generally the compounds of carbon, hydrogen and oxygen but the higher carbohydrates have also been found to possess nitrogen and sulphur in their structures.

Carbohydrates

||

carbon + hydrogen + oxygen

or

carbon + hydrogen + oxygen + nitrogen + sulphur

They are found in abundance in plant kingdom in the form of cellulose and starch; besides are also found in abundance in animal kingdom as well in the form of glucose or glycogen or chondroitin sulphates, etc.

Carbohydrates may be defined as polyhydroxy-aldehydes or polyhydroxy-ketones or their derivatives. Their molecular weight ranges from less than 100 to well over 1 million and in general are, white solids, sparingly soluble in organic solvents but soluble in water except some high molecular weight carbohydrates.

Classification (Table 2.1)

For convenience, carbohydrates may be classified into three major groups namely :

(a) Monosaccharides or simple sugars (mono = single or one; saccharide = sugar moiety i.e. unit).

(b) Oligosaccharides (oligo= a few)

(c) Polysaccharides (poly = many)

(d) Derived carbohydrates; these include :

(i) Oxidation products (ascorbic acid, uronic acids, aldonic acids, saccharic acids, etc.)

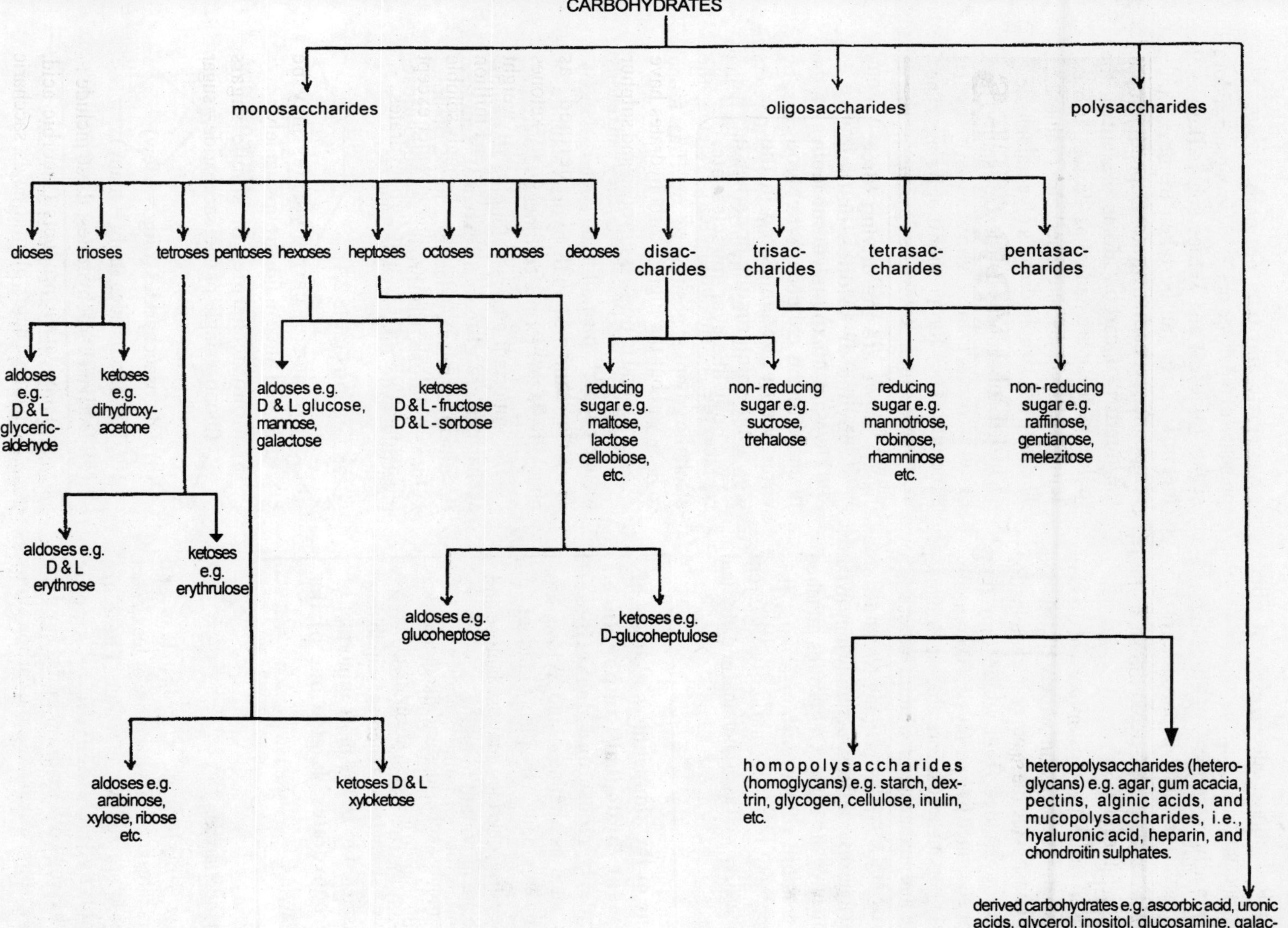

Table 2.1 : Classification of Carbohydrates

(ii) Reduction products (glycerol, ribitol, inositol).

(iii) Aminosugars (glucosamine, galactosamine, mannosamine).

(iv) Deoxysugars (2-deoxyribose, methyl pentoses).

The hexoses are the most important class of monosaccharides and occur widely distributed in nature, either in the free state or in combination with other molecules from which they may usually be separated by hydrolysis. Biologically, the most important hexoses are glucose, fructose, galactose and mannose, of which fructose is a ketohexose and the others are aldohexoses.

The aldohexoses differ structurally only in the arrangement of the H and OH groups attached to one or more of the carbon atoms; this difference may result in markedly different physiological, as well as in chemical and physical properties.

Some of the aldopentoses also are of significant biological importance, particularly ribose and deoxyribose. Others, such as arabinose and xylose, are primarily important in the plant kingdom.

Three disaccharides, maltose lactose and sucrose are important in nature.

The monosaccharides and disaccharides are easily soluble in water, are optically active and have a sweet taste. Glucose, which may be considered to be the most important of the carbohydrates, is also one of the sweetest.

(a) Monosaccharides

These are simple sugars, colourless and crystalline substances having more or less sweet taste. These are soluble in water. **These are either polyhydric aldehydic or ketonic alcohols having both primary and secondary alcoholic groups** which make the carbon atoms asymmetric and thus optically active. The presence of aldehyde or ketone groups i.e. aldose sugars (aldoses) and ketone sugars (ketoses); the suffix- ose can be taken to mean that a compound is a carbohydrate. Depending upon the number of carbon atoms present in the molecule, these are named as 'dioses', 'trioses', 'tetroses', 'pentoses', 'hexoses' etc. (Table 2.2). The simplest carbohydrate is glycolaldehyde.

In the nature mostly 'D' (dextrorotatory) form occurs. Sugars may show mostly cyclic structures. They form either α or β rings. The 6 membered ring is known as "pyranose" ring in which one of the members is oxygen atom, whereas the 5 membered ring is known as "furanose" ring. Again one member of the furanose ring is oxygen atom. The sugars, by virtue of their alcoholic group can form esters with acids, all the free hydroxy groups being replaceable. In the biological systems, the alcoholic groups at position "6" or "1" are found to be most reactive.

Being aldehydes or ketones, they can readily reduce copper*, bismuth** or silver solutions. They can condense with hydroxylamine or phenylhydrazine forming oximes and osazones.

The important sugars belonging to monosaccharides are **glucose (dextrose), fructose (levulose),** mannose, galactose, ribose, ribulose, xylose, xylulose, erythrose, sedoheptulose, glyceraldehyde, dihydroxyacetone etc.

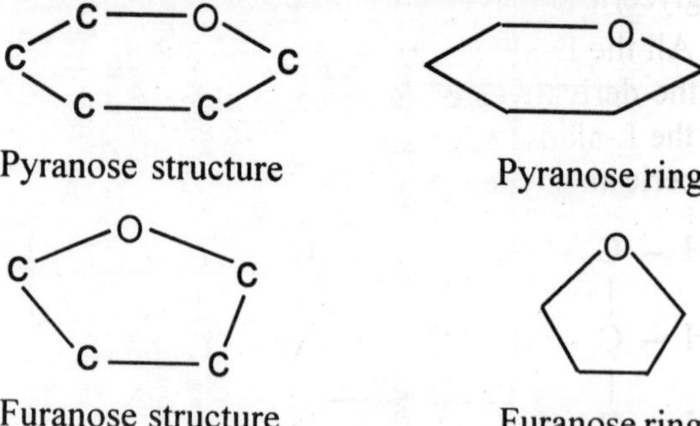

* *Basis of Fehling's test, Barfoed's test and Benedict's test*

** *Basis of Nylander's test*

Table 2.2 : Classification of monosaccharides

General formula $C_n(H_2O)_n$	Aldoses	Ketoses
Dioses, $C_2H_4O_2$	glycolaldehyde	
Trioses, $C_3H_6O_3$	D-&L*-glycerose or glyceric aldehyde	dihydroxyacetone
Tetroses, $C_4H_8O_4$	D-&L-erythrose	erythrulose
	D-&L-threose	
Pentoses, $C_5H_{10}O_5$	D-&L-ribose	D-&L-xyloketose
	D-&L-arabinose	
	D-&L-xylose	
Hexoses, $C_6H_{12}O_6$	D-&L-glucose	D-&L-fructose
	D-&L-mannose	D-&L-sorbose
	D-&L-galactose	
	D-&L-gulose	
Heptoses, $C_7H_{14}O_7$	glucoheptose	D-glucoheptulose
	mannoheptose	L-glucoheptulose

* *Levorotatory*

If the primary alcoholic group of the monosaccharides is oxidized to -COOH; the acid formed is known as " uronic acid" such as glucose forms glucuronic acid, galactose forms galacturonic acid etc. Such uronic acids are found in mucoproteins.

H – C = O
|
H – C –OH
|
CH_2OH

D-glyceric aldehyde

H – C = O
|
HO – C – H
|
CH_2OH

L-glyceric aldehyde

All the D-aldose sugars may be considered as the derivatives of D-glyceric aldehyde and all the L-aldose sugars as the derivatives of L-glyceric aldehyde.

H – C = O
|
H – C –OH
|
H – C –OH
|
CH_2OH

D- erythrose

H – C = O
|
HO – C – H
|
H – C –OH
|
CH_2OH

D-threose

H – C = O
|
H – C –OH
|
H – C –OH
|
H – C –OH
|
CH_2OH

D-ribose

H – C = O
|
HO – C – H
|
H – C –OH
|
H – C –OH
|
CH_2OH

D-arabinose

H – C = O
|
H – C –OH
|
HO– C – H
|
H – C –OH
|
CH_2OH

D-xylose

H – C = O
|
HO – C – H
|
HO – C – H
|
H – C –OH
|
H – C –OH
|
CH_2OH

D-glucose

H – C = O
H – C –OH
HO– C – H
HO– C – H
H – C –OH
CH_2OH
D-galactose

H – C = O
HO – C – H
HO – C – H
H – C –OH
H – C –OH
CH_2OH
D-mannose

H_2 – C = O
C = O
HO– C – H
H – C –OH
H – C –OH
H_2 – C –OH
D-fructose

Some important reactions of monosaccharides are as mentioned below:

1. Reactions of monosaccharides characteristic of the aldehyde and ketone group. Reaction with hydrazines to form hydrazones and osazones:
   Phenylhydrazine and substituted hydrazones react with the monosaccharides and other carbohydrates containing a free sugar group to form hydrazones and osazones. With few exceptions, the hydrazones are soluble and difficult to isolate. On the other hand, osazones of different sugars are relatively insoluble and crystallize in beautiful and characteristic forms.
2. Monosaccharides react with hydrogen cyanide to form cyanhydrins.
3. Monosaccharides react with hydroxylamine to form oximes.
4. Reduction to form sugar alcohols: Both aldoses and ketoses may be reduced to the corresponding polyhydroxy alcohols. This may be accomplished with sodium amalgam, or better, electrolytically or by hydrogen under high pressure in the presence of a catalyst. Thus, the alcohols formed from glucose, mannose and fructose are as follows :

D- glucose ⟶ D - sorbitol
D-mannose ⟶ D - mannitol
D-fructose ⟶ D-mannitol, D-sorbitol

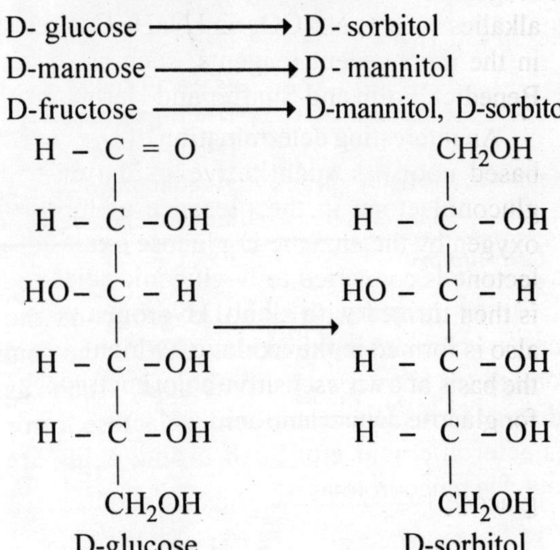

5. Monosaccharides get oxidized to form sugar acids, for example:

D-glucose $\xrightarrow{\text{bromine water}}$ D-gluconic acid

6. Reducing action of sugars in alkaline solution:

Determination of sugars

All the sugars that contain free sugar group undergo enolization and various other changes when placed under alkaline solution. The enediol forms of the sugars are highly reactive and are easily oxidized by oxygen and other oxidizing agents. This means that these sugars in alkaline solution are very powerful reducing agents. They readily reduce oxidising ions such as Ag^+, Hg^{++},

Bi^{+++}, Cu^{++} and $Fe(CN)_6^{---}$ and the sugars are odixized to complex mixture of acids. This reducing action of sugars in alkaline solution is utilized for both the qualitative and quantitative determination of sugars. Reagents containing Cu^{++} ions are most commonly used. These are generally alkaline solutions of cupric sulphate containing sodium potassium tartarate (Rochelle salt) or sodium citrate. Sodium or potassium hydroxide is used as the alkali in the older reagents such as Fehling's solution; but weaker alkalies such as Na_2CO_3 and $NaHCO_3$ are used in the more recent reagents, such as those of Benedict, Folin and Shaffer and Hartmann.

An interesting determination of D-glucose is based upon its quantitative oxidation to D-gluconolactone in the presence of molecular oxygen by the enzyme D-glucose oxidase. The lactone is converted to D-gluconic acid, which is then titrated with alkali. Hydrogen peroxide also is formed in the oxidation which is used as the basis of a very sensitive colorimetric method for glucose determination.

$$\text{glucose} + O_2 \xrightarrow[\text{oxidase}]{\text{glucose}} \text{gluconolactone} + H_2O_2$$

$$\downarrow + H_2O$$

D- gluconic acid

$$H_2O_2 + \text{o} - \text{dianisidine}$$

$$\downarrow \text{peroxidase}$$

yellow compound

(b) Oligosaccharides

The term 'oligosaccharide' is used for compounds made up by the condensation of 2-10 molecules of simple sugars. The important carbohydrates of this group are sucrose, maltose, lactose and raffinose. These are distinguished from each other by nomenclature such as disaccharides, tri, tetra and pentasaccharides. On hydrolysis such saccharides give simple sugars. These may be regarded as the products of condensation of two or more sugars with the elimination of water. These have a general formula $C_n(H_2O)_{n-1}$. In general the reducing disaccharides are less potent as reducing agents than monosaccharides.

Disaccharides: The following tabulation gives the better known disaccharides with their component monosaccharides. Those possessing a free sugar group, are reducing sugars and give reactions characteristic of monosaccharides.

	Disaccharides $C_{12}H_{22}O_{11}$	Constituent Monosaccharides
I	**Reducing sugars**	
	(a) Maltose	glucose+glucose
	(b) Lactose	glucose+galactose
	(c) Cellobiose	glucose+glucose
II	**Non-reducing sugars**	
	(a) Sucrose	glucose+fructose
	(b) Trehalose	glucose+glucose

Of the above, maltose, lactose and sucrose are the most important examples of disaccharides.

Maltose: It is composed of two glucose units (Fig. 2.1) and is formed when the enzyme amylase or diastase hydrolyzes starch. It is a product of the action of salivary amylase (ptyalin) and pancreatic amylase (amylopsin) upon starch during the process of digestion. It is also formed as an intermediate product in the acid hydrolysis of starch and is an important constituent of corn syrups, which are prepared by partial hydrolysis

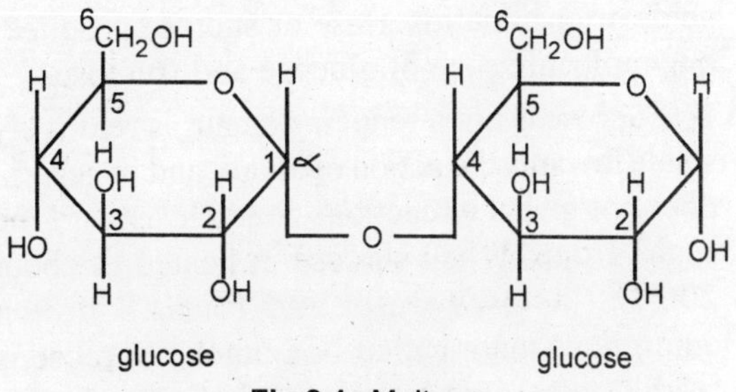

Fig 2.1 : Maltose

of starch with dilute acids. Enzyme maltase hydrolyzes it to glucose.

Lactose : It is formed by the secretory cells of the mammary glands during lactation and occurs to the extent of about 2 - 6 percent in the milk. It is prepared commercially from milk whey. It is hydrolyzed by acids and the **specific enzyme lactase** into its constituent monosaccharides, glucose and galactose. It is a reducing sugar, forms osazones, a cyanhydrin, and an oxime, and is decomposed by alkali. It accordingly contains a free sugar group in its structure (Fig 2.2).

It is of interest to know that the human milk differs from cow's milk in containing, in addition to regular lactose, **other oligosaccharides, such as L-fucosyl lactose.**

Sucrose: It occurs especially in the juices

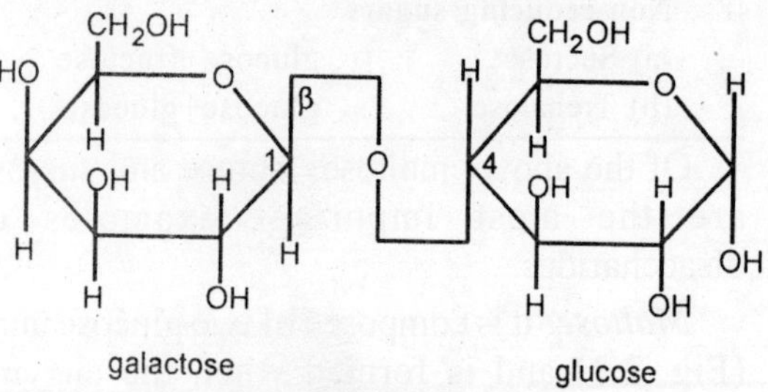

Fig 2.2 : Lactose

of plants such as sugar beets, sugar cane, sorghum, sugar maple and pineapple and in smaller quantities in the juices of many other plants. Ripe fruits are rich in sucrose. It is by far the most abundantly distributed of the sugars.

Hydrolysis of sucrose (Fig. 2.3) by dilute acids or enzyme invertase or sucrase produces one molecule each of glucose and fructose.

Sucrose is not a reducing sugar, is relatively stable towards the action of alkali, and in general does not give the reactions characteristic of the sugar group. When surcose in heated to about 200°C, it loses water and forms a brown amorphous mass called "Caramel". Surcose is readily fermented by yeast. It is first split into glucose and fructose by invertase, and the monosaccharides are then fermented by the zymase system of enzymes.

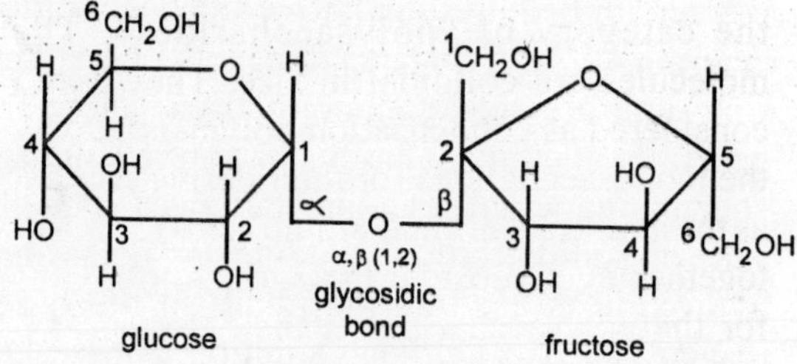

Fig. 2.3 : Surcose

Trisaccharides. Several oligosaccharides containing three monosaccharide units occur in nature. These are given in the following tabulation (Table 2.3) :

Amongst the trisaccharides, the most important of them is raffinose which occurs in sugar beets and is concentrated in sugar beet molasses. Cottonseed meal contains about 7 percent of raffinose. It is also frequently found in higher plants and fungi. It is hydrolyzed by enzymes of the gastrointestinal bacteria of herbivorous animals and serves as food for these animals whereas it is not well utilized as food by the human beings. Raffinose is fermented by yeast.

Table 2.3 : Classification of trisaccharides

Trisaccharides	Constituent monosaccharides with order of linkage
I **Reducing sugars**	
(a) Mannotriose	galactose, galactose, glucose
(b) Robinose	galactose, rhamnose, rhamnose
(c) Rhamninose	galactose,rhamnose, rhamnose
II **Non-reducing sugars**	
(a) Raffinose	fructose, glucose, galactose
(b) Gentianose	fructose, glucose, glucose
(c) Melezitose	glucose, fructose, glucose

(c) Polysaccharides

Carbohydrates composed of ten or more monosaccharide units are generally classified in the category of "polysaccharides". Their molecules are colloidal in size. They may be considered as condensation polymers in which the monosaccharides (or their derivatives such as the amino sugars and uronic acids) are joined together by glycosidic linkages. Another term for the polysaccharides is the "glycans". The polysaccharides such as starches, glycogen and cellulose, which are made up of a single kind of monosaccharide, are called "homoglycans" i.e. homopolysaccharides and the polysaccharides composed of two or more kinds of monosaccharides (or their derivatives), such as the **mucopolysaccharides,** are called as **"heteroglycans"** i.e. heteropolysaccharides made up of mannose and xylose are called as **"mannans"** and **"xylans"** respectively etc.

Some polysaccharides contain units that are derivatives of the monosaccharides, for example, chitin is made up of the amino sugar glucosamine and hyaluronic acid is composed of glucuronic acid and glucosamine.

Since the monosaccharide units of polysaccharides are joined together by glycosidic linkage, the polysaccharides are readily hydrolyzed by mineral acids but are resistant to alkaline hydrolysis.

The polysaccharides are hydrolyzed by the group or enzymes called "polysaccharidases". Important examples of polysaccharides include starch, glycogen, cellulose, dextrins, inulin etc. their molecules are so large that they can't be obtained in the form of true solution. **They give colloidal solutions except cellulose, which is insoluble.** Determination of their molecular weight reveals that a particular type of compound may have different molecular weights and shapes. Polysaccharides such as cellulose, starch, glycogen and dextrins are made up of many D-glucose units. They can be readily hydrolyzed to glucose by boiling with dilute acids except cellulose which is hydrolyzed by strong acids only. The polysaccharide **inulin is a compound made up of fructose units exclusively.**

HOMOPOLYSACCHARIDES

Starches

These occur widespread as reserve carbohydrate in tubers such as potatoes, in grains and seeds, in many fruits and in the rhizomes and pith of plants. Native starches are a mixture of two types of compounds that are separable from each other and are named as amylose and amylopectin.

The enzymes which hydrolyze starch are known as the **'amylases'**. The animal amylases are represented by **ptyalin of saliva and amylopsin of pancreatic juice.**

Starches generally contain 80-90% amylopectin and the remaining i.e. 10-20% amylose. Both the amylose and amylopectin are hydrolyzed by acid to D-glucose. Partial acid hydrolysis gives complex mixtures of dextrins, maltose and glucose.

Amylose

Molecule of amylose consists of many glucose units joined together through α-glycosidic linkage, chiefly as found in maltose. The glucose units of amylose are linked in the unbranched chain. The amylose structure (Fig. 2.4) may be considered as an expanded maltose structure with a free sugar group on one end.

Amylose may be easily hydrolyzed by acids

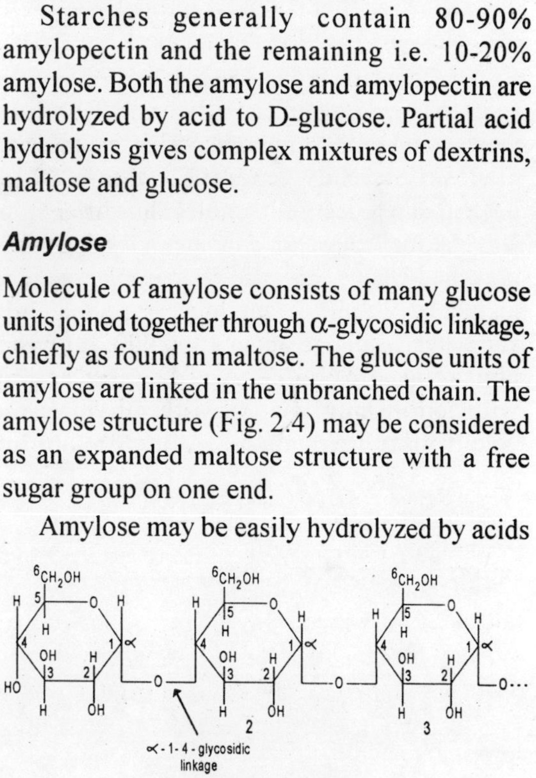

$^6CH_2OH$ $^6CH_2OH$ $^6CH_2OH$

α-1-4-glycosidic linkage

Fig 2.4 : Amylose

to D-glucose. Partial acid hydrolysis gives complex mixtures of dextrins, maltose and glucose. Starches generally contain 10-20 percent amylose, though in a few instances the amylose content is higher. The amylose extracted from starch grains is a mixture of molecules of different sizes. Amylose fractions with molecular weights from 4,000 to 4,00,000 have been obtained. It gives a characteristic colour reaction with iodine. **It produces a blueblack colour with iodine solution.** The colour disappears upon heating the solution and reappears upon cooling.

Amylopectin

Like that of amylose molecule, it too consists of many glucose units joined together through α-glycosidic linkage, chiefly as found in maltose. Its molecule also contains chains of glucose units like that of amylose and also has branches of these glucose chains linked through the 6-OH of glucose in the following manner:(Fig. 2.5).

Amylopectin is also easily hydrolyzed by acids to D-glucose units. Partial acid hydrolysis yields complex mixtures of dextrins, maltose and glucose. Starches generally contain 80-90 percent amylopectin. Its molecules differ from amylose molecules not only in possessing many branched chains, but also in being larger. The molecular weight of amylopectins apparently vary from 50,000 to about 1000,000. **It gives a characteristic violet to red-violet colour with iodine solution. As with amylose, the colour disappears upon heating the solution and reappears upon cooling.**

Fig. 2.5 : Amylopectin

Glycogen

It is the carbohydrate reserve of animals. It is stored chiefly in the liver and muscles. It is also found in the plants which have no chlorophyll content such as fungi and yeast. Its structure is similar to that of amylopectin in that it is a branched molecule. It has been found to have 7 to 12 glucose residues per non- reducing end group and hence it is even more highly branched. Molecular weights ranging from 270,000 to 100 million have been reported. It is readily soluble, **its solution is opalescent and gives a red-brown or red colour with iodine solution.** It yields D-glucose upon complete hydrolysis. Its structure may be represented as shown below (Fig. 2.6), where each bead of chain represents a glucose molecule.

Biochemically, glycogen is one of the most important substances in the body. Liver glycogen is broken down to glucose and passed into the blood stream for use by the tissues. **Muscle glycogen is a source of energy for muscle contraction. Mollusks such as oysters and clams are usually rich in glycogen.**

Amylo- 1-6-glucosidase is involved in the

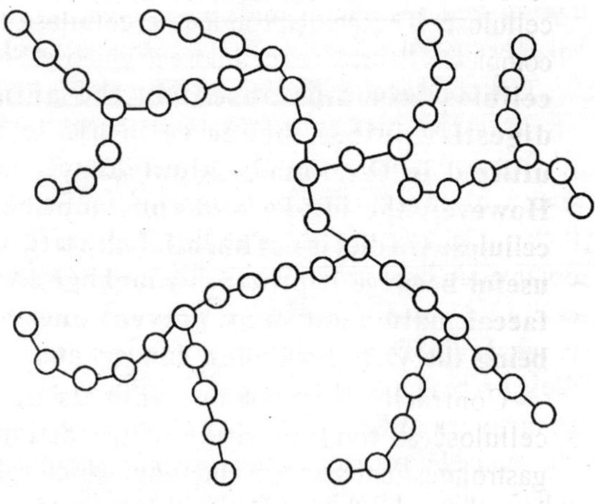

Fig. 2.6 : Model of a glycogen molecule

specific cleavage, by hydrolysis, of the 1,6-branching linkage of glycogen, releasing free glucose. The combined action of the phosphorylase and the amylo 1,6-glucosidase results in the liberation of glucose- 1-phosphate and glucose. Indeed, the ratio of these two defines the extent of branching in a glycogen (or amylopectin) molecule.

Cellulose

Cellulose is the chief constituent of the fibrous parts of the plants and consequently **is the most abundant organic material in nature.** The cellulose content of flax, ramie and cotton amounts **from 97 to 99 percent,** while the content in wood varies from 41 to 53 percent. Cereal straws contain from 30 to 43 percent cellulose. Thus, it is the most abundant **structural polysaccharide of plant kingdom. It does not occur in animal body.**

Although usually considered to be only a plant product, **cellulose (tunicin) is also found in certain marine animals.**

Cellulose yields D-glucose as the final product of hydrolysis. It is resistant to hydrolysis and requires the action of strong acids. Various bacteria and other lower forms possess enzymes **called cellulases**, capable of hydrolyzing cellulose. The snail produces a cellulase that completely hydrolyzes cellulose to glucose. **Since cellulase remains absent in the animal digestive juices, hence cellulose is not utilized in the human alimentary canal. However, the intake and consumption of cellulose via diet is not harmful hitherto very useful because it provides roughage to the faecal matter and may prevent one from being the victim of colon cancer, etc.**

Contrarily, herbivorous animals utilize cellulose as food by virtue of the action of gastrointestinal bacteria and fungi which split it into glucose and other utilizable products.

Partial hydrolysis of cellulose by acids yields a mixture of cellodextrins, various oligosaccharides, cellobiose and glucose.

Studies seem to indicate that cellulose is a linear polysaccharide consisting of β-1,4 linked glucose units. The M.W. of cellulose samples vary from 200,000 to 2,000,000. It is insoluble in water. It does not give characteristic colour with iodine solution.

Cellulose may be nitrated to form nitrocellulose which is of much importance in the manufacture of explosive celluloid and other substances. Cellulose acetates are used in making photographic films, rayon and various plastic materials.

Dextrins

Partial hydrolysis of starch by acids, or α-and β- amylases, produces substances known as "dextrins". These substances consist of a very complex mixture of molecules of different sizes and structures and are known as amylodextrins, erythrodextrins and achrodextrins. **Amylodextrin** gives **blue colour** with iodine, **erythrodextrin** gives **reddish- brown colour** whereas **achrodextrin does not give any colour.** Their reducing property is feeble and they have got faint sweet taste. **They are generally soluble in water and produce sticky solutions and hence are used as adhesives and binders.** All dextrins have free sugar groups and accordingly reduce alkaline copper solutions and give other sugar reactions.

Dextrins occur in the leaves of all starch producing plants, and in honey etc. They are important constituents of various food products such as corn syrups.

$$\text{Starch} \xrightarrow[\text{or acids}]{\text{ptyalin}} \text{amylodextrins} \longrightarrow \text{erythrodextrins} \longrightarrow \text{achrodextrins}$$

Inulin

It is a polysaccharide which exclusively contains **D-fructose units.** It occurs as the reserve carbohydrate in the tubers of chicory, Jerusalem artichoke, dahlia and in the bulbs of onion and garlic. It is a white, more or less crystalline powder. It is very easily hydrolyzed by acids. It is not hydrolyzed by amylase **but is split by inulinase.**

Inulin is used as a source of commercial fructose. It is also administered to animals in the studies of glomerular membrane filtration rates. It is not hydrolyzed by any of the enzymes of the gastrointestinal tract and is not utilized as food.

HETEROPOLYSACCHARIDES (HETEROGLYCANS)

Agar

Agar is a vegetable mucilage obtained from seaweeds. It is a sulfuric acid ester of a complex galactose polysaccharide. It is odourless and tasteless. It swells strongly in cold water but does not dissolve. It gets dissolved in hot water to form a sol which upon cooling sets into a gel. A 1 percent agar gel is fairly rigid, and a 2 percent gel is very rigid. Agar is non-digestible and at times is given to provide bulk to the faeces in the treatment of constipation.

Gum Acacia or Gum Arabic

The vegetable gums are carbohydrate materials containing hexoses or pentoses or both in glycosidic union and a carbohydrate acid group. It is one of the most important and best- known gums. Gum arabic appears to be the salt of a high polymer of arabic acid which upon complete hydrolysis yields galactose, arabinose, rhamnose and glucuronic acid.

Gum arabic is used in the preparation of pharmaceuticals, in confections, and as an adhesive.

Pectins

"Pectin" is the term used to represent the substance or substances which in the presence of sugar and the proper acid concentration causes the formation of jellies. **It occurs in abundance in nature and is found especially in the pulp of citrus fruits, apples, carrots, beets, etc.** Commercial pectin is generally prepared from lemons or apples. When soluble, pectin is boiled with dilute acid, it is slowly hydrolyzed to pectic acid and methyl alcohol.

Large amounts of pectin are used in the fruit conserving industry and for other purposes.

"Pectin" is a group term and a number of different pectins are known today, some of which are insoluble and useless for gelation.

Alginic Acids

Alginic acids consist chiefly of linear polymers of D-mannuronic acid units. Its molecular weights range from 50,000 to 1,85,000. These are found in many marine algae and in giant kelp, which is a commercial source. Large amounts are used as emulsifier and smoothening agents in food industries.

Mucopolysaccharides (Glycosaminoglycans)

These are referred to as the substances which are composed of amino sugar and uronic acid units as the principal components, though some are chiefly made up of amino sugar and monosaccharide unit without the presence of uronic acid. The hexosamine present is generally acetylated.

Mucopolysaccharides are essential components of tissues. **They may be combined with proteins as mucoproteins or mucoids.** Important examples of mucopolysaccharides include hyaluronic acid, heparin and the chondroitin sulphates.

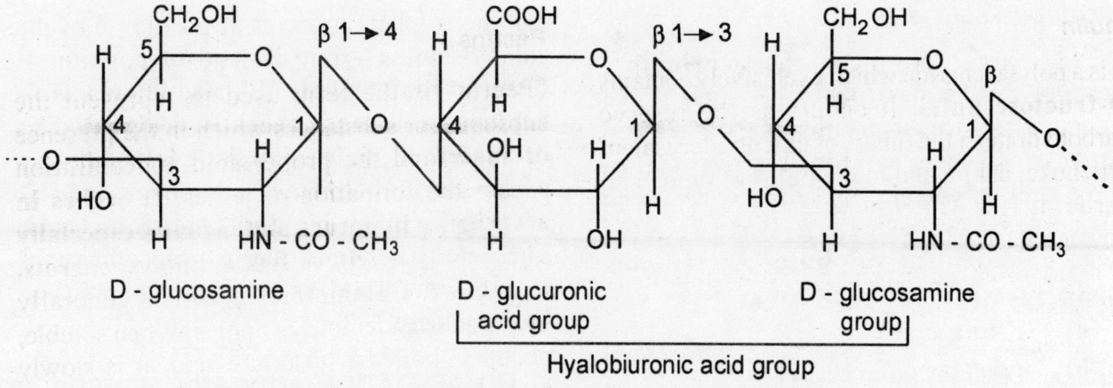

Fig. 2.7 : Repeating units in hyaluronic acid structure

Hyaluronic acid

It is found in vitreous humour, synovial fluid, skin, umbilical cord and other sources. It appears to serve as an integral part of the gel-like ground substance of connective and other tissues and as lubricant and shock absorbent in joints. It acts as an intercellular cement. It is a viscous, high molecular weight (several million) polysaccharide consisting of chains of N-acetylglucosamine and glucuronic acid residues. **Hyaluronidase** is a the enzyme which hydrolyzes it into its constituents, This enzyme is widely distributed in microorganisms and mammalian tissues (Fig 2.7).

Heparin

It is a blood anticoagulant which is found in liver, lung, thymus, spleen and blood. It is a polymer of **D-glucosamine and D-glucuronic acid.** The amino groups and some of the hydroxyl groups remain combined with sulphuric acid. The molecular weight of heparin appears to be in the range of 17,000 to 20,000. **It is strongly acidic due to the presence of sulphuric acid group and readily forms salts. It inhibits the transformation of prothrombin to thrombin, preventing the conversion of fibrinogen to fibrin, which is catalyzed by thrombin. The probable repeating units are as follows (Fig.2.8).**

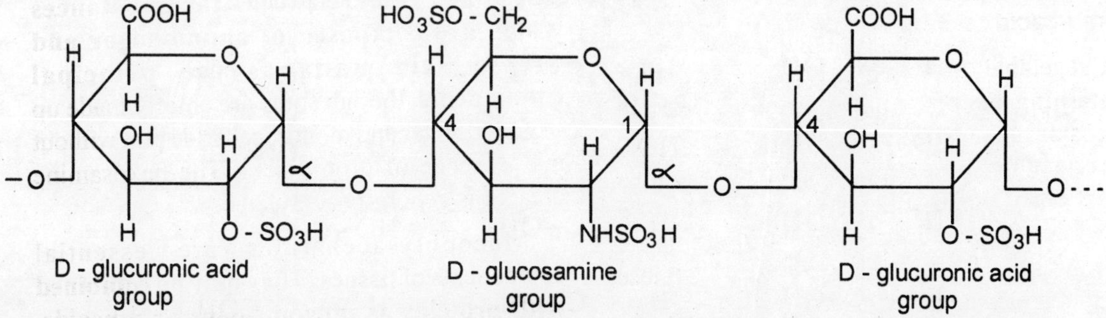

Fig. 2.8 : Repeating units in heparin

Chondroitin sulphates

These are among the principal mucopolysaccharides **(proteoglycans)** in the ground substance of mammalian tissues and cartilage, and occur **combined with proteins.** Three kinds of chondroitin sulphate have been isolated so far and named as A, B and C. Out of them, **chondroitin sulphate 'A' remains chiefly present in the following:**

(a) Cartilage,
(b) Adult bone,
(c) Cornea, etc.

Chondroitin sulphate 'B' remains chiefly present in:

(a) Skin
(b) Heart valves
(c) Tendons, etc.

Chondroitin sulphate 'C' remains chiefly present in:

(a) Cartilage
(b) Tendons, etc.

The basic structure of chondroitin sulphate 'A' consists of repeating unit of **N-acetyl galactosamine** and **glucuronic acid** with esterified sulphate at position 4 of galactosamine. The structure of chondroitin sulphate 'C' is the same as that of chondroitin sulphate 'A' except that the sulphate group is at position 6 of the galactosamine group instead of position 4. **Chondroitin sulphate `B', also known as β-heparin, and more recently designated as dermatan sulphate** (from skin), is the sulphate of a polysaccharide composed of **N-acetylgalactosamine and L-iduronic acid.** These are hydrolyzed to their corresponding units by the mammalian enzyme named as hyaluronidase.

MUTAROTATION, ANOMERS, EPIMERS

The α-and β-forms of glucose spontaneously undergo interconversion (mutarotation) in water (Fig. 2.9). α-D-glucose and β- D- glucose differ only in the conformation of the hydroxyl group on carbon atom number 1. **These and other pairs of sugar molecules that differ only in**

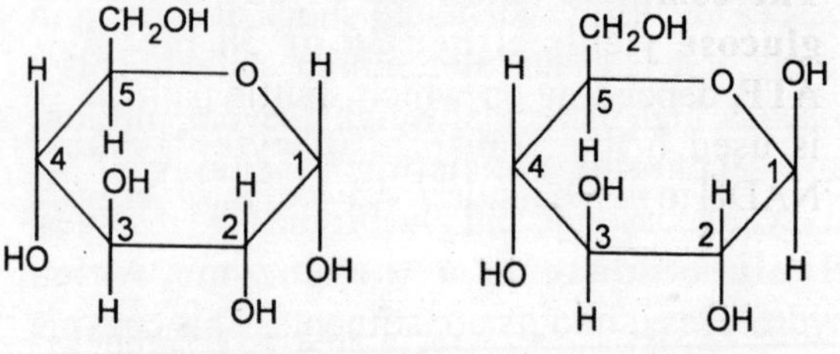

α - D - glucose   β - D - glucose

Fig. 2.9 : Two conformations of D-glucose

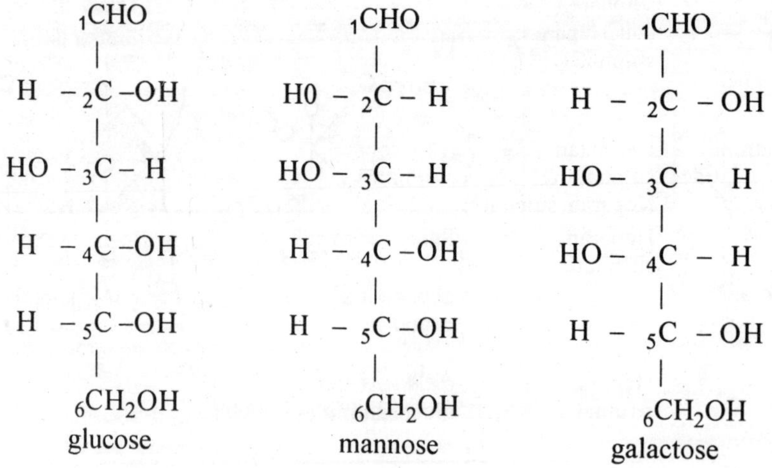

glucose:
$_1CHO$
$H - _2C - OH$
$HO - _3C - H$
$H - _4C - OH$
$H - _5C - OH$
$_6CH_2OH$

mannose:
$_1CHO$
$H0 - _2C - H$
$HO - _3C - H$
$H - _4C - OH$
$H - _5C - OH$
$_6CH_2OH$

galactose:
$_1CHO$
$H - _2C - OH$
$HO - _3C - H$
$HO - _4C - H$
$H - _5C - OH$
$_6CH_2OH$

this respect are termed as anomers.

Such isomers which differ only in the configuration of a single carbon atom are termed as **"epimers"**. Examples of epimeric pairs include those of glucose-mannose and glucose-galactose. Glucose and mannose are epimers with respect to carbon atom 2; whereas glucose and galactose are epimers with respect to carbon atom 4.

Mucopolysaccharidoses (Table 2.4) are the hereditary disorders caused due to the absence/deficiency of certain enzymes of the metabolism of mucopolysaccharides leading to the accumulation of certain mucopolysaccharide(s) in one or the other tissue(s) of the body; there are atleast seven types of such disorders out of which two are of paramount importance, **namely Hurler's syndrome** and **Hunter's syndrome.**

The complete oxidation of one mol. of glucose yields either 36 or 38 mol of ATP, depending on which shuttle pathway is used in the transport of cytoplasmic NADH to mitochondria. A list of the energy-yielding reactions of glucose oxidation is as shown below:

Energy yielding reactions in the complete oxidation of Glucose:

Reaction	Net moles of ATP generated per mole of glucose
Glycolysis	
(phosphoglycerate kinase, pyruvate kinase; 4 ATPs are formed whereas 2 are utilized)	2
NADH shuttle	
glycerol-phosphate shuttle (or malate-aspartate shuttle)	4 (6)
Pyruvate dehydrogenase (NADH)	6
Succinyl CoA synthetase	
(GTP is equivalent to ATP)	2
Succinate dehydrogenase	
(succinate $\longrightarrow$ fumarate + $FADH_2$)	4
Other TCA cycle reactions	
(isocitrate $\longrightarrow$ α-ketoglutarate, α-ketoglutarate $\longrightarrow$ succinyl CoA, malate $\longrightarrow$ oxaloacetate; total of 3NADH generated)	18
Total	36 (38)

Table 2.4 : Different types of Mucopolysaccharidoses

Sl. No.	Name of disorder	Affected compound (s)	Enzyme defect	Clinical manifestations	Age of onset
1.	Hurler's syndrome (Mucopolysaccharidose -I)	Dermatan sulphate (DS) and Heparan sulphate(HS)	α-L-Iduronidase	Corneal opacity, deafness, claw hands, stubby fingers, hepatomegaly, spleenomegaly, severe mental retardation. Urine contains DS & HS.	1 year
2.	Hunter's syndrome (MPS-II)	Dermatan sulphate & Heparan sulphate	L-Iduronate sulphatase	Same as in (1); usually no corneal opacity. Urine contains DS & HS	1 year
3.	MPS-III A Sanfilippo A syndrome	Heparan sulphate	Sulphamidase	Coarse facies, hypertrichosis, HS in urine, mild hepatomegaly, progressive spastic quadriparesis, severe mental retardation	2 - 3 years
4.	MPS-III B Sanfilippo B syndrome	Heparan sulphate	α- N - Acetyl glucosaminidase	HS excreted in urine Rest same as in (3)	2 - 3 years

CHAPTER 3

LIPIDS

> **We do not have affinity with water but have with organic solvents. We make the food palatable and delicious. We are some what costly. We are found in many food oils/ seeds/ pulses and other innumerable eatables. In excess, we make you run to the doctor, hence use us with full precautions. We have store houses in the body like subcutaneous tissue, omentum, adipose tissue, etc. We can disfigure your body if consumed in excess.**

Lipids are the organic compounds that are poorly soluble in water but quite soluble in organic solvents such as the structural components of cell membranes, as storage forms of energy, as metabolic fuel and as emulsifying agents. Surprisingly, four of the vitamins (A, D, E and K) are lipids. In addition, the prostaglandins, substances that stimulate smooth muscle contractions and function in intracellular regulatory processes, are lipid derivatives. The transport of lipids through the blood plasma is an extremely important subject from the standpoint of health, because the abnormalities in these processes are thought to be a major factor in the development of coronary artery diseases which are on the increase throughout the globe. **Obesity results from the storage of excessive amounts of lipids in the body. Such common diseases like diabetes mellitus, obstructive jaundice, pancreatitis, and hypothyroidism have associated plasma lipid transport abnormalities. In addition, there are a number of rare inherited diseases, known as the lipid storage diseases or lipidoses. For instance, Tay-Sach's disease, Niemann-Pick disease, Gaucher's disease, Fabry's disease, Farber's disease, etc.**

To summarize, lipid is a term used to describe a group of fats and fat like substances that constitute a major portion of tissue components and a major foodstuff.

Isolation of lipids from tissue

The chloroform- methanol (2:1) solvent introduced by Folch for lipid extraction has largely replaced the older well-known ethanol- ether (3:1) solvent introduced by Bloor.

Classification of lipids

There is no single internationally accepted system of classification for the lipids. However, generally accepted classification is given in Table 3.1.

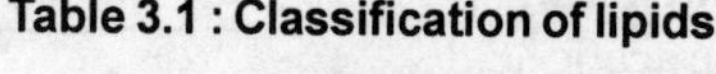

Table 3.1 : Classification of lipids

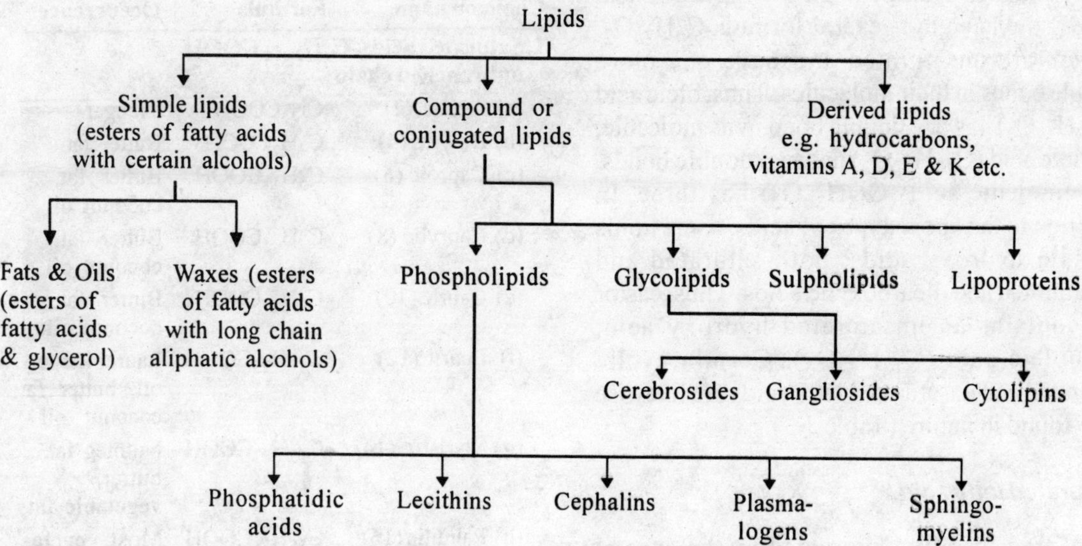

Functions of lipids

There are numerous functions of lipids in the animal body. They play vital functions in the body which may be remembered as given in Table 3.2

Table 3.2 : Functions of lipids

Sl. No.	Lipid	Function(s)
1.	Fatty acids	Metabolic fuel, building blocks for other lipids
2.	Prostaglandins	Intracellular modulators
3.	Glyceryl esters	
	(a) Acylglycerols	Fatty acid storage, metabolic intermediates
	(b) Phospho-glycerides	Membrane structure
4.	Sphingolipids	
	(a) Sphingomyelin	Membrane structure
	(b) Glycosphingo-lipids	Membranes, surface antigens
5.	Sterol derivatives	
	(a) Cholesterol	Membrane and lipoprotein structure
	(b) Cholesterol esters	Storage and transport
	(c) Bile acids	Lipid digestion and absorption
	(d) Steroid hormones	Metabolic regulation
	(e) Vitamin D	Calcium and Phosphorus metabolism
6.	Terpenes	
	(a) Vitamin A	Vision, epithelial integrity
	(b) Vitamin E	Lipid antioxidant
	(c) Vitamin K	Blood coagulation

Simple lipids

These are the esters of fatty acids with certain alcohols. They are usually further classified according to the nature of the alcohols, as follows:

Fats and Oils

These are the esters of fatty acids and glycerol. If they are solid at room temperature, then they are known as fats and if liquid at room temperature, then they are termed as oils.

Fatty acids. Fatty acids found in fats and other lipids are of various types. Some of them, like palmitic acid ($CH_3(CH_2)_{14}.COOH$) and stearic acid ($CH_3(CH_2)_{16}.COOH$) are straight-chain saturated acids belonging to the acetic acid series, and have the general formula $C_nH_{2n}O_2$. Others are unsaturated and have one more double bonds in their molecules. Thus, oleic acid ($C_{18}H_{34}O_2$) has one double bond in its molecule, linoleic acid ($C_{18}H_{32}O_2$) has two double bonds, and linolenic acid ($C_{18}H_{30}O_2$) has three. In addition to the above types of acids, some lipids contain hydroxy acids, both saturated and unsaturated and dicarboxylic acids. Thus, castor oil contains an unsaturated hydroxy acid, ricinoleic acid ($C_{18}H_{32}O_3$). Certain cyclic saturated and unsaturated fatty acids are likewise also found in nature (Table 3.3).

Saturated fatty acids

They are generally represented by the general formula $C_nH_{2n}O_2$ or $C_nH_{2n+1}COOH$. Physical properties of the saturated fatty acids depend upon their molecular weights. Whereas those fatty acids that contain ten carbon atoms or fewer in their molecules are liquids at room temperature, the remainder are solids whose melting points rise with increasing molecular weight. The liquid acids are also known as **volatile fatty acids,** since they may be distilled with steam, whereas the others, the **nonvolatile acids,** are carried over by steam distillation only in traces or not at all. Fatty acids with four carbon atoms or fewer are miscible with water in all proportions. As the length of the carbon chain increases beyond this, the solubility rapidly decreases to zero. The important examples of straight chain **saturated fatty acids** found in nature as constituents of lipid molecules include **butyric, caproic, caprylic, capric, lauric, myristic, palmitic, stearic etc.** (Table 3.3).

Unsaturated fatty acids

These are characterized by the presence of one or more double bonds in the molecule.

Table 3.3 : Classification of the fatty acids

Common name	Formula	Occurrence
1. Saturated acids, C_nH_{2n+1} COOH, unbranched chain		
(a) Acetic (2)*	CH_3COOH	Vinegar
(b) Butyric (4)	C_3H_7COOH	Butter fat
(c) Caproic (6)	$C_5H_{11}COOH$	Butter fat, coconut oil
(d) Caprylic (8)	$C_7H_{15}COOH$	Butter fat, coconut oil
(e) Capric (10)	$C_9H_{19}COOH$	Butter fat, coconut oil
(f) Lauric (12)	$C_{11}H_{23}COOH$	Laurel kernel oil, butter fat, coconut oil
(g) Myristic (14)	$C_{13}H_{27}COOH$	Nutmeg fat, butter, vegetable fats
(h) Palmitic (16)	$C_{15}H_{31}COOH$	Most vegetable & animal fats
(i) Stearic (18)	$C_{17}H_{35}COOH$	Most vegetable & animal fats
(j) Arachidic acid (20)	$C_{19}H_{39}COOH$	Peanut oil
(k) Behenic acid (22)	$C_{21}H_{43}COOH$	Rapeseed oil, peanut oil
(l) Lignoceric acid (24)	$C_{23}H_{47}COOH$	Cerebrosides, sphingomyelin, peanut oil
II, Unsaturated fatty acids		
A. **Monoethenic,** $C_nH_{2n-1}COOH$, one double bond (Monounsaturated)		
(a) **Paimitoleic,** Δ^9 (16)	$C_{15}H_{29}COOH$	Animal and vegetable fats
(b) **Oleic acid,** Δ^9 (18)	$C_{17}H_{33}COOH$	Animal and vegetable fats
(c) **Erucic acid** Δ^{13}(22)	$C_{21}H_{41}COOH$	Animal and vegetable fats
(d) **Nervonic acid** Δ^{15} (24)	$C_{23}H_{45}COOH$	Animal and vegetable fats
B. **Dienoic,** $C_nH_{2n-3}COOH$, two double bonds (Diunsaturated)		

**number of carbon atoms in the fatty acid molecule*

Linoleic acid, $\Delta^{9,12}$ (18) — $C_{17}H_{31}COOH$ — Linseed oil, animal & plant fats, corn oil, soyabean oil, peanut oil etc.

C. **Trienoic,** $C_nH_{2n-5}COOH$, three double bonds (Triunsaturated)

Linolenic acid, $\Delta^{9,12,15}$ (18) — $C_{17}H_{29}COOH$ — Linseed oil, rapeseed oil soyabean oil, liver oil etc.

D. **Polyenoic,** $C_nH_{2n-7}COOH$, more than three double bonds. (Many unsaturations)

Arachidonic acid, $\Delta^{5,8,11,14}$ (20) — $C_{19}H_{31}COOH$ — Fats, phospholipids etc.

III. Branched-chain acids

(a) Isobutyric acid (4)	C_3H_7COOH	Waxes
(b) Tuberculo-stearic acid (19)	$C_{18}H_{37}COOH$	Wax of tubercle bacillus

IV. Hydroxy acids

(a) Cerebronic acid (24)	$C_{23}H_{46}(OH)COOH$	Animal and vegetable fats
(b) Ricinoleic acid (18)	$C_{17}H_{32}(OH)COOH$	
(c) Hydroxy-nervonic Acids (24)	$C_{23}H_{44}(OH)COOH$	

V. Cyclic acids

(a) Chaulmoogric acid	*R-$(CH_2)_{12}$-COOH	seed oils
(b) Hydnocarpic acid	*R-$(CH_2)_{10}$-COOH	seed oils

* Where R is

$$\begin{array}{l} CH=CH \diagdown \quad H \\ | \qquad\qquad\quad > C- \\ CH_2-CH_2 \diagup \end{array}$$

They have been classified in accordance with the number of double bonds and named by reference to the parent hydrocarbon, the position of the double bond or bonds in the chain being indicated by a number referred to the carboxyl carbon atom as number one.

Nomenclature of fatty acids

Carbon atoms are numbered from the carboxyl carbon (carbon No. 1). The carbon atom adjacent to the carboxyl carbon (No.2) is also known as α- carbon. Carbon atom No.3 is the β-carbon, and the end methyl carbon is known as a ω-carbon or n- carbon. Various conventions are in use for indicating the number and position of the double bonds; for e.g., Δ^9 indicates a double bond between carbon atoms 9 and 10 of the fatty acid. The ω- 9 indicates a double bond on the 9th carbon counting from the ω-carbon atom. Widely used conventions to indicate the number of carbon atoms, the number of the double bonds, and the positions of the double bonds are prevalent. To cite an example, see the structure of oleic acid.

Oleic (C'$_{18}$) $C_{18}H_{34}O_2$

18 : 1; 9 or Δ^9 18 : 1

$$\overset{18}{CH_3}-\overset{17}{CH_2}-\overset{16}{CH_2}-\overset{15}{CH_2}-\overset{14}{CH_2}-\overset{13}{CH_2}-\overset{12}{CH_2}-\overset{11}{CH_2}-\overset{10}{CH}$$

$$=\overset{9}{C}H(CH_2)_7\overset{1}{C}OOH$$

OR

$$\underset{n}{\overset{\omega}{CH_3}}-\overset{2}{CH_2}-\overset{3}{CH_2}-\overset{4}{CH_2}-\overset{5}{CH_2}-\overset{6}{CH_2}-\overset{7}{CH_2}-\overset{8}{CH_2}-\overset{9}{CH_2}$$

$$=\overset{10}{C}H(CH_2)_7\overset{18}{C}OOH$$

In animals, additional double bonds are introduced only between the existing double bonds e.g., ω9, ω6, or ω3 and the carboxyl carbon, leading to three series of fatty acids known as the ω9, ω6 and ω3 families, respectively.

Some unsaturated fatty acids of physiologic and nutritional importance are as given below:

Number of carbon atoms and position of double bonds	*Series*	*Common name*
Monoenoic acids (one double bond)		
16 : 1; 9	ω 7	Palmitoleic
18 : 1; 9	ω 9	Oleic
22 : 1; 13	ω 9	Erucic

Dienoic acids (2 double bonds)		
18 : 2 ; 9, 12	ω 6	Linoleic
Trienoic acids (3 double bonds)		
18 : 3; 6, 9, 12	ω 6	γ - Linolenic
18 : 3; 9, 12, 15	ω 3	α - Linolenic
Tetraenoic acids (4 double bonds)		
20 : 4; 5, 8, 11, 14	ω 6	Arachidonic

Triglycerides (Neutral fats)

The neutral fats (triglycerides) are important because the bulk (as much as 90 per cent) of the lipid material stored in the adipose tissue of the body is **neutral fat** and represents a concentrated form of energy stored until required for metabolic purposes.
Glycerol reacts with one molecule of fatty acid to form a **monoglyceride,** with two molecules to form a **diglyceride** and with three to form a **triglyceride** as shown below:

$$\begin{array}{c} CH_2OH \\ | \\ CHOH \\ | \\ CH_2OH \\ \text{glycerol} \end{array} + \begin{array}{c} HO.OC.C_3H_7 \\ \\ HO.OC.C_3H_7 \\ \\ HO.OC.C_3H_7 \\ \text{butyric acid} \\ \text{(3 moles)} \end{array} \longrightarrow \begin{array}{c} CH_2.O.CO.C_3H_7 \\ | \\ CH.O.CO.C_3H_7 \\ | \\ CH_2.O.CO.C_3H_7 \\ \text{tributyrin} \\ \text{(a triglyceride)} \end{array} + 3H_2O$$

General formula for a fat is

$$\begin{array}{c} CH_2.O.CO.R_1 \\ | \\ CH.O.CO.R_2 \\ | \\ CH_2.O.CO.R_3 \end{array}$$

where R_1, R_2 and R_3 may be derived form the same or different fatty acids.

1. Phospholipids (Phosphatides)

Lipids which upon hydrolysis, yield fatty acids, phosphoric acid, sometimes, but not always, glycerol and a nitrogenous base. These are subdivided into the following groups:

(A) Phosphatidic acids: Lipids which when hydrolyzed yield one molecule each of glycerol and phosphoric acid and two molecules of fatty acids of which one is probably saturated and the other unsaturated.

(B) Lecithins: These are the lipids containing fatty acids, phosphoric acid, glycerol, and the nitrogenous base choline.

The saturated fatty acids present in lecithin molecules include palmitic and stearic acids while the unsaturated fatty acids present include oleic, linoleic, linolenic and arachidonic acids. Lecithins are widely distributed in animal tissues for instance brain, liver, blood, cardiac muscles etc., they are also found in vegetable sources e.g. plant seeds etc.

Lecithins when purified are waxy white substances but soon become brownish when exposed to air and light, owing to autoxidation and decomposition. They are soluble in ordinary

Compound or conjugated lipids

These are the esters of fatty acids which, upon hydrolysis, yield other substances in addition to the fatty acids and an alcohol. Some important members of this group are:

$$
\begin{array}{l}
{}^1CH_2\text{-}O\text{-}CO\text{-}R \quad \text{(saturated fatty acid)} \\
R\text{-}CO\text{-}O\text{-}{}^2CH \quad O \\
\text{(unsaturated fatty acid)} \quad {}^3CH_2\text{-}O\text{-}\overset{\|}{P}\text{-}O\text{-}[CH_2\text{-}CH_2\text{-}\overset{+}{N}\equiv (CH_3)_3] \\
\qquad\qquad OH \qquad\qquad OH^- \\
\qquad\qquad\qquad\qquad \text{choline}
\end{array}
$$

α - Lecithin

fat solvents like ethanol, ether etc. but not in acetone. **Large quantities of soyabean lecithins are used these days as emulsifying and smoothening agents in the food industry.**

Lecithins are hydrolyzed by boiling with alkalies and dilute mineral acids and also by the corresponding enzymes i.e. **lecithinases (phospholipases).** The nature of hydrolysis depends upon the kind of phospholipase acting. Scientist **'Hanahan' has shown that lecithinase A (phospholipase A) found in certain snake venoms (cobra, cotton mouth moccasin, vipers), poisons of scorpions and bees,and various mammalian tissues, specifically hydrolyzes off the fatty acid (unsaturated) present at C_2 of α- lecithin molecule to form lysolecithins. The lysolecithins so formed are very powerful haemolytic agents which rapidly haemolyze blood erythrocytes, and are considered to be responsible for harmful physiological effects of venoms containing phospholipase A.**

$$
\begin{array}{l}
H_2{}^1C - O - CO - R \\
HO - {}^2C - H \\
H_2{}^3C - O - \overset{O}{\overset{\|}{P}} - O - CH_2.CH_2.\overset{+}{N}\equiv (CH_3)_3 \\
\qquad\qquad\quad O \qquad\qquad\qquad OH^-
\end{array}
$$

L-α-Lysolecithin

Four kinds of lecithinases i.e. A, B, C and D are known today which are very specific in nature. These are found in different vegetables, mammalian tissues and microorganisms.

(C) Cephalins. Lipids which upon hydrolysis yield fatty acids, glycerol, phosphoric acid, and either the nitrogenous base ethanolamine (colamine) or the amino acid serine. Lipids of uncertain structures which contain inositol, fatty acids, phosphoric acid, ethanolamine, and possibly galactose and tartaric acid have also been included in this class.

$$
\begin{array}{l}
{}^1CH_2 - O - CO - R \\
R - CO - O - {}^2CH \\
{}^3CH_2 - O - \overset{O}{\overset{\|}{P}} - O \ [-CH_2.CH_2.NH_2] \\
\qquad\qquad\quad OH \qquad \text{ethanolamine}
\end{array}
$$

α-Cephalin (L-α-Phosphatidyl ethanolamine)

Cephalins contain the saturated fatty acid called stearic acid and the unsaturated fatty acids, **oleic, linoleic** and **arachidonic acids.** They are found in various animal tissues e.g. brain, liver, egg yolk, erythrocytes and cardiac muscles and are also found to be present in various plant sources i.e. plant seeds etc. Cephalins, like lecithins, are hygroscopic solids and are decomposed on exposure to air. These are insoluble in alcohol and acetone, but soluble in ether.

The cephalins are hydrolyzed by boiling with alkalies and dilute mineral acids. Lecithinase A from snake venom hydrolyzes cephalins to form lysocephalins which are similar to the lysolecithins formed from lecithins.

(D) Plasmalogens. These on hydrolysis yield one molecule each of aliphatic aldehyde, fatty acid, glycerol, phosphoric acid, and a nitrogen containing base (ethanolamine or choline). These contribute to an appreciable proportion (about 10 percent) of the phospholipids of muscles and brain. Cardiac muscles and erythrocytes also contain plasmalogens.

(E) Sphingomyelins. These on hydrolysis yield a nitrogenous base sphingosine, a single fatty acid molecule, phosphoric acid, and choline, but no glycerol. These are soluble in hot ethanol, but not in ether, acetone or cold ethanol. They are found in brain, liver, blood, cardiac muscles etc.

2. *Glycolipids*

As the name indicates, these are the complex lipids containing carbohydrate in combination with long chain aliphatic acids or alcohols.

(A) Cerebrosides. Lipids which contain carbohydrate (galactose or glucose), one fatty acid, and sphingosine, but no phosphoric acid or glycerol. The fatty acids of the cerebrosides chiefly are lignoceric, behenic, and palmitic acids.

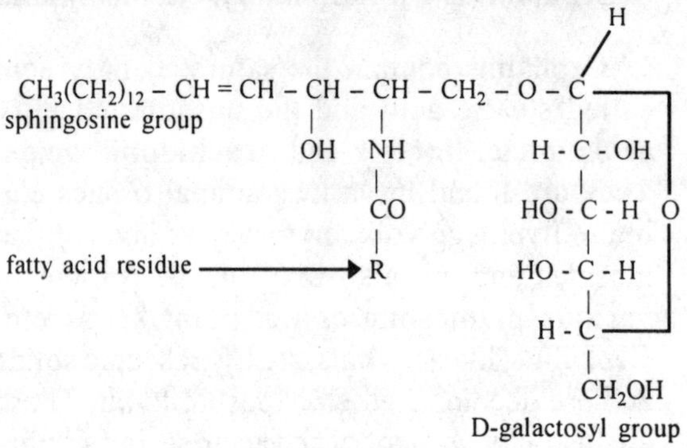

```
                                                          H
                                                         /
CH3(CH2)12 – CH = CH – CH – CH – CH2 – O – C ─────┐
sphingosine group      |    |                 |        |
                       OH   NH            H - C - OH   |
                            |                 |        |
                            CO           HO - C - H    O
                            |                 |        |
fatty acid residue ───────► R            HO - C - H    |
                                              |        |
                                          H - C ───────┘
                                              |
                                             CH2OH
                                      D-galactosyl group
```

Cerebroside

Various cerebrosides have been obtained from brain and nerves which are differentiated from each other by the presence of other fatty acids they possess. Such fatty acids are cerebronic acid, lignoceric acid, nervonic acid, and oxynervonic acid.

These are found in large amounts in the white matter of brain and in the myelin sheaths of nerves. In smaller quantities, they appear to be very widely distributed in animal tissues. **Large amounts of the cerebrosides accumulate in the liver and spleen in Gaucher's disease- a rare hereditary disease of lipid metabolism. This disease was for the first time noticed by the scientist Gaucher in a patient in whom the splenic pulp was replaced entirely by large pale cells, which now are known after his name as "Gaucher Cells". These cells are found particularly in spleen, brain, and bone marrow.**

(B) Gangliosides. These arc related to the cerebrosides and contain sphingosine, long-chain fatty acids, hexoses (usually galactose or glucose) and neuraminic acid (sialic acid). These are rich in carbohydrates. Brain gangliosides are known to be complex one.

Gangliosides have been isolated from nerve cells, spleen and red blood cell stroma. Large amounts of it are found in the brain in cases of Tay-Sachs disease and Niemann-Pick disease (diseases of lipid metabolism).

(C) Cytolipins. These lipids contain fatty acids, sphingosine, glucose and galactose.

3. Sulpholipids

Lipid material containing sulphur has long been known to be present in the tissues, examples being liver, kidney, brain, salivary glands, testicles, tumours etc. It's most abundantly found to be present in the white matter of the brain. In composition, these are similar to the cerebrosides except for the fact that sulphuric acid is present as cerebronic acid ester.

4. *Lipoproteins*

These compounds found in mammalian plasma are composed of lipid material bound to the proteins. The lipid moiety consists mainly of cholesterol esters and phospholipids containing principally stearic, palmitic and oleic acids although palmitoleic, linoleic and arachidonic acids have also been identified.

A number of proteins in serum are called lipoproteins because their function is to transport lipids; without them, the lipids could not exist in a dissolved state in the blood. The four major classes of lipoproteins are chylomicrons, pre-beta lipoproteins, beta lipoproteins and alpha lipoproteins. This classification is based on paper electrophoresis, which separates the lipoproteins into these four groups. They can also be separated by ultracentrifugation, and, although basically same groups are observed, different names are applied. These alternate names as well as the lipid content of the lipoprotein fractions are summarised in the following Table 3.4 (Also consult chapter on lipid metabolism).

Table 3.4: Lipoproteins

Category based on paper electrophoresis	Category based on ultracentrifugation	Major lipid component
Chylomicrons	Chylomicrons	Triglycerides
Pre-beta lipoproteins	Very low density lipoproteins (VLDL)	Triglycerides
Beta lipoproteins	Low density lipoproteins (LDL)	Cholesterol
Alpha lipoproteins	High density lipoproteins (HDL)	Phospholipid

Lipoproteins not only are named but also measured in terms of the separation provided by electrophoresis or ultracentrifugation. These measurements are carried out principally in cases of increased concentrations of blood lipids (hyperlipidemia), which, of course, mean that the lipoprotein concentrations also must be increased (hyperlipoproteinemia) since they involve the same lipids. Various combinations of lipoproteins can be increased in these disorders; correlation of hyperlipidemia; hyperlipoproteinemia and clinical disorders is under intensive study these days, but no universally acceptable explanation is available so far.

Hyperlipidemia currently is receiving considerable attention of the scientists because it has been positively correlated with atherosclerotic cardiovascular disease, which has a high mortality and morbidity rate.

Derived lipids

Derived lipids are substances formed during the hydrolysis of simple or compound lipids which still retain the properties of this class of compound.

1. **Fatty Acids:** Saturated and unsaturated acids
2. **Alcohols:** Compounds of high molecular weight but not glycerol. These may be classified as follows:
   (A) **Aliphatic alcohols** such as cetyl, stearyl and myricyl alcohols.
   (B) **Sterols** which contain the phenanthrene nucleus (cholesterol, ergosterol, sitosterol and stigmasterol).

Steroids

A large number of compounds found in nature belong to the class of compounds known as steroids. These have the parent nucleus named as perhydrocyclopentanophenanthrene, which consists of three six-membered rings (A, B and C) and a five membered ring (D) which is known as a cyclopentane ring. These rings are joined together as shown in Fig. 3.1 with a total of 17 carbon atoms.

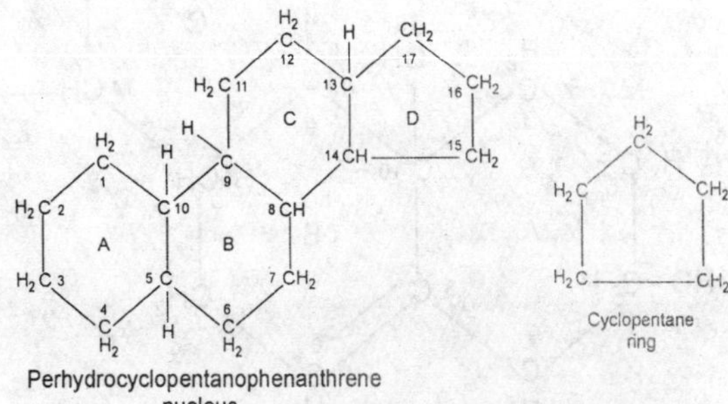

Fig. 3.1 : Structures of perhydrocyclopentanophenanthrene and cyclopentane ring

Steroids may be classified in the following categories:

(a) Sterols
(b) Bile acids
(c) Male sex hormones
(d) Female sex hormones
(e) Adrenal corticosteroids
(f) Vitamins D
(g) Saponins
(h) Cardiac glycosides

Sterols

The best known of the sterols is cholesterol. In the animal kingdom, the most abundant steroid is the sterol called as cholesterol. It remains present in all animal cells and is particularly abundant in nervous tissue. It is not found in vegetables and plant tissues. Because of its abundance, its historical interest, structure and clinical importance to man will be considered in some detail over here.

As early as 1815, **Chevreul** gave the name cholesterine to a white waxy material that could be isolated **from gallstones.** It was later identified as an alcohol stable to boiling with strong alkali. Fatty acid esters of the alcohol were also isolated from certain tissues.

Cholesterol, literally means bile solid-alcohol; derives its name from the fact that it was first isolated from human gallstones, of which it is generally the chief component. The amount of cholesterol in animal tissues varies widely. It is particularly abundant in brain, nerve tissue, adrenal glands and egg yolk. Dry white matter of brain contains about 14 per cent of cholesterol, and spinal cord 10-15 per cent. Scientist Bloor, an authority on lipids gives the percentage values (Table 3.5) for the average cholesterol content of dry tissues.

Cholesterol is usually accompanied by dihydrocholesterol and 7-dehydrocholesterol. It has the structure as shown in Fig. 3.2.

Cholesterol generally crystallizes as white,shining rhombic plates. It melts at 149°-150°C. It is tasteless and odourless. It is insoluble in water, acids and alkalies, somewhat soluble in soap solutions and much more soluble in the solution of bile salts. It is readily soluble in ether, benzene, chloroform, petroleum ether, carbon bisulfide and acetone. It is also readily soluble in hot alcohol, but only slightly soluble in cold alcohol. It dissolves readily in oleic acid and liquid

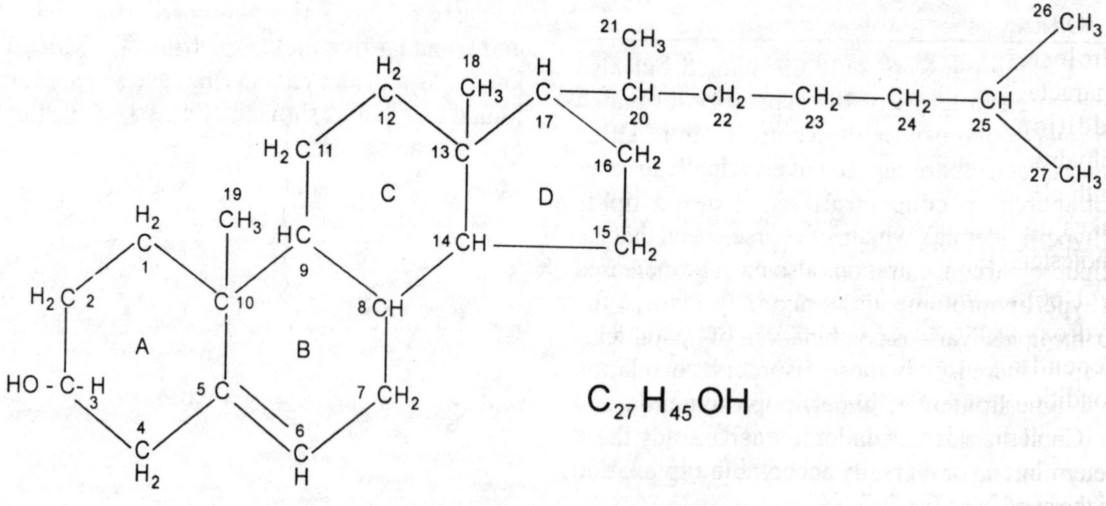

$C_{27}H_{45}OH$

Fig. 3.2 : Structure of cholesterol

Table 3.5 : Percentage of cholesterol in dry tissues

Sl.No.	Tissue	%
1.	White matter of brain	14.00
2.	Gray matter of brain	6.00
3.	Kidney	1.60
4.	Spleen	1.50
5.	Skin	1.30
6.	Liver	0.93
7.	Mammary glands	0.70
8.	Whole blood	0.65
9.	Smooth muscle	0.55
10.	Diaphragm	0.35
11.	Skeletal muscle	0.25

fats. It is commercially produced from the spinal cords of the cattle. It may be readily prepared in the laboratory by extraction from gallstones or brain tissue with the help of organic solvents.

Since cholesterol is a poor conductor of electricity and has a high dielectric value, it's a good insulator against electric discharge. Possibly, as an abundant constituent of brain, nerves and spinal cord, it functions as an insulating covering of impulse generating and transmitting structures. It is well established that brain and nerve impulses are electrical in character.

On account of the presence of a double bond, cholesterol gives the addition reactions characteristic of unsaturated compounds. The addition of hydrogen produces dihydrocholesterol. This substance occurs along with cholesterol in animal tissues. Cholesterol takes up halogens at the double bond to form cholesterol dihalides.

Upon oxidation, it gives various ketones, hydroxy compounds and acids, the products depending upon the oxidizing agents and conditions used.

Cholesterol is the best known and most widely determined lipid and is an important intermediate in the synthesis of steroid hormones. In the blood it occurs both in the free and esterified forms. The latter form is a mixture of many cholesterol esters, each of which has a different fatty acid bound in ester linkage to cholesterol at the OH group. Usually, only the total cholesterol concentration is of clinical interest but occasionally separate estimation of the free and esterified forms is of value to the clinicians. The normal range of cholesterol esters is between 70 and 75% of the total with free cholesterol making up the remaining 25 to 30%. **The normal range of the concentration of cholesterol in the serum is from 150 to 200 mg/dl. In normal infants and children lower values of cholesterol are found in the serum whereas higher values are found in normal older persons. The concentration of total cholesterol gets elevated in several diseases like nephrosis, diabetes mellitus, and hypothyroidism. Low values may be found in hyperthyroidism, malnutrition, Gaucher's disease and acute hepatitis.** However, the increase usually is not clinically diagnostic of these diseases. In some diseases, total cholesterol concentration is affected, while in others only the ester fraction is disturbed. **Jaundice of obstructive type usually is accompanied by an elevated level of total serum cholesterol with a normal ester fraction. Diabetes, hypothyroidism and certain types of kidney diseases are other disorders that may exhibit the same type of cholesterol disturbance.**

Total serum cholesterol concentration may vary markedly in healthy individuals; change in concentration of ± 50 mg/dl over the course of a few hours have been noted.

Since, the liver cells esterify cholesterol, infectious hepatitis cirrhosis and most types of liver damage are accompanied by a decreased percentage of cholesterol esters. Only the ester percentage is significant, not the absolute ester concentration.

In the recent years, interest in lipid metabolism has increased tremendously, primarily as a result of possible relationship between lipid metabolism and atherosclerosis.

Other Animal Sterols: A number of sterols closely related to cholesterol are found in various tissues. 7-dehydrocholesterol is a precursor of vitamin D_3. **Skin is a good source of both Δ^7- cholesterol (lathosterol) and 7 - dehydrocholesterol.** Desmosterol (24-dehydrocholesterol) and several methyl derivatives such as lanosterol and agnosterol have been isolated from skin lipids and are recognised as intermediates in cholesterol biosynthesis. Lanosterol and agnosterol are also present in wool lipids.

7 - Dehydrocholesterol

Δ^7 - Cholesterol, lathosterol

Lanosterol

Agnosterol

Sterols of yeast and fungi: Mycosterols

Important examples of this category are two:

(a) Ergosterol

(b) Zymosterol

Ergosterol. This sterol is the principal sterol of fungi and yeast and is classed as a mycosterol. **Its name derives from the fact that it was first discovered in ergot bodies which are formed on rye and other cereal plants diseased with ergot fungi. It is produced commercially in large quantities from certain strains of yeast.**

It is an important substance because when irradiated with ultraviolet light, a series of substances is formed which even includes calciferol (vitamin D_2) and tachysterol, from which another member of the vitamin D group, dihydrotachysterol is derived.

Sterols of higher plants: Phytosterols

Important examples of this category are the following:

(a) ***Stigmasterol.*** **This sterol occurs especially in calabar and soybean oils. It is of interest because it can be converted in the laboratory into the hormone of the corpus luteum i.e., progesterone.**

(b) ***Sitosterols.*** These are generally found in the oils of higher plants, being especially abundant in wheat germ oil. Seven sterols of this group have been reported.

Sterols and their occurrence

Table 3.6 indicates certain important sterols with their occurrence:

Bile acids

Human bile contains three different bile acids cholic, deoxycholic, and chenodeoxycholic acids.

Table 3.6 : Sterols and their occurrence

Sl.No.	Sterol	Formula	Occurrence
1.	Cholesterol	$C_{27}H_{45}OH$	All animal cells
2.	Dihydro-cholesterol	$C_{27}H_{47}OH$	Accompanies cholesterol
3.	7 -Dehydro-cholesterol	$C_{27}H_{43}OH$	Skin, brain, other tissues
4.	Coprostanol	$C_{27}H_{47}OH$	Faeces
5	β-Equistanol	$C_{30}H_{53}OH$	Urine of pregnancy
6.	Sitosterols	$C_{29}H_{49}OH$	Lipids of higher plants
7.	Stigmasterol	$C_{29}H_{47}OH$	Soya & calabar beans
8.	Brassicasterol	$C_{29}H_{47}OH$	Rapeseed oil
9.	Spinasterol	$C_{27}H_{45}OH$	Spinach, alfalfa
10.	Ergosterol	$C_{28}H_{43}OH$	Ergot, yeast
11.	Zymosterol	$C_{27}H_{43}OH$	Yeast
12.	Fucosterol	$C_{29}H_{47}OH$	Algae

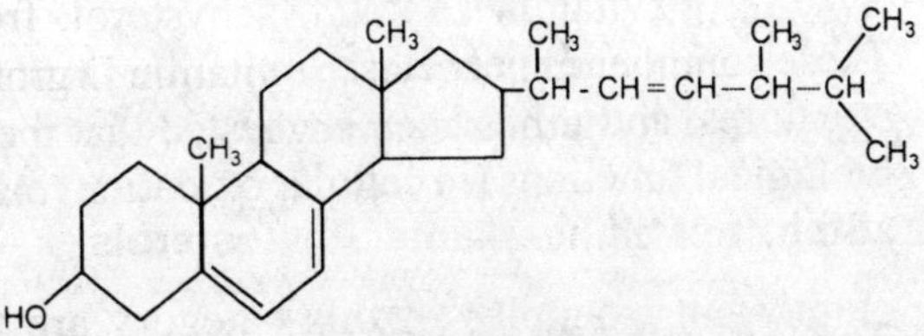

Ergosterol, $C_{28}H_{43}OH$

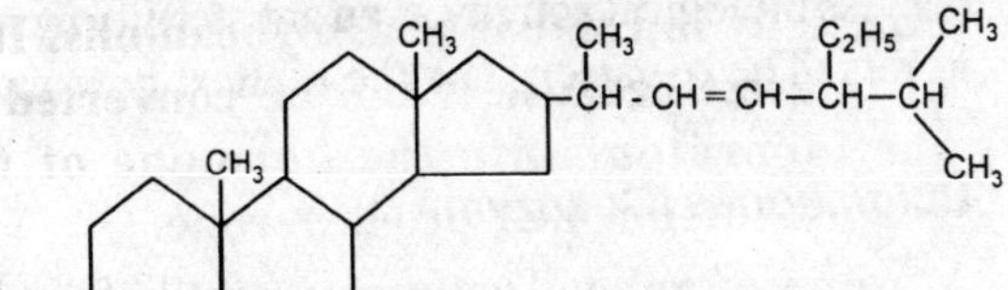

Stigmasterol, $C_{29}H_{47}OH$

Deoxycholic acid is microbial in origin and is absorbed from intestinal contents. The bile acids are present largely as derivatives of glycine and taurine. The bile acids differ from the sterols because of the *trans* relationship of its OH group at the 3- carbon to the angular CH_3 group. Structures of some of the bile acids are as given in Fig. 3.3.

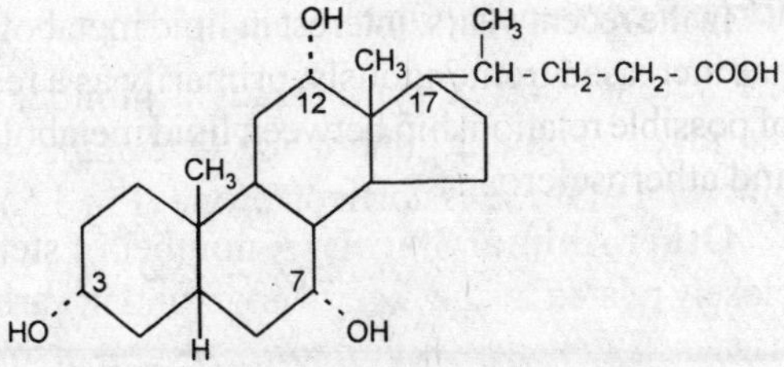

Cholic acid
3,7,12 - Trihydroxycholanic acid

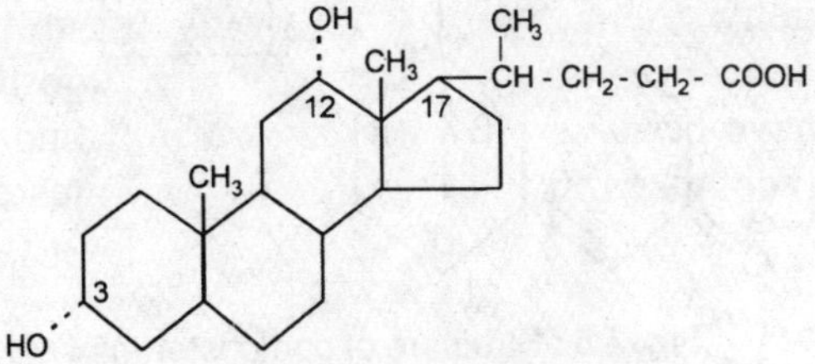

Deoxycholic acid
3,12 - Dihydroxycholanic acid

Fig. 3.3 : Cholic and deoxycholic acids

Sex hormones

The principal hormone of the ovary is estradiol and that of the testis is testosterone. Their structures are as shown in Fig 3.4.

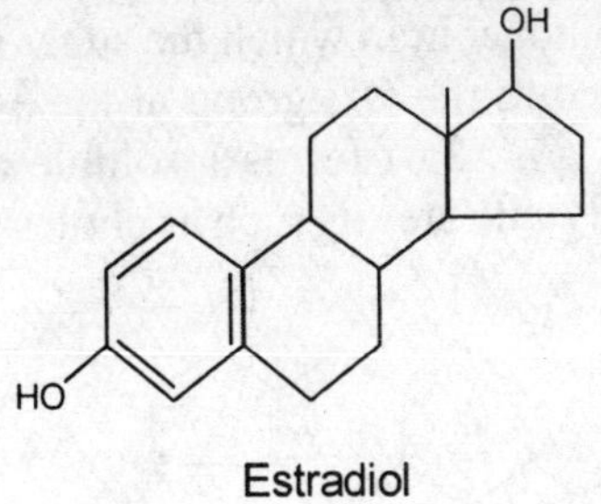

Estradiol

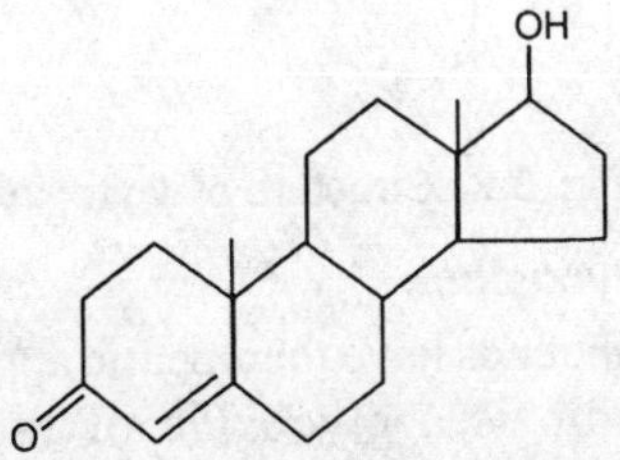

Testosterone

Fig. 3.4 : Estradiol and testosterone

Adrenal corticosteroids

The adrenal cortex synthesizes a number of steroids of metabolic importance. One of the very important of these is corticosterone (Fig 3.5).

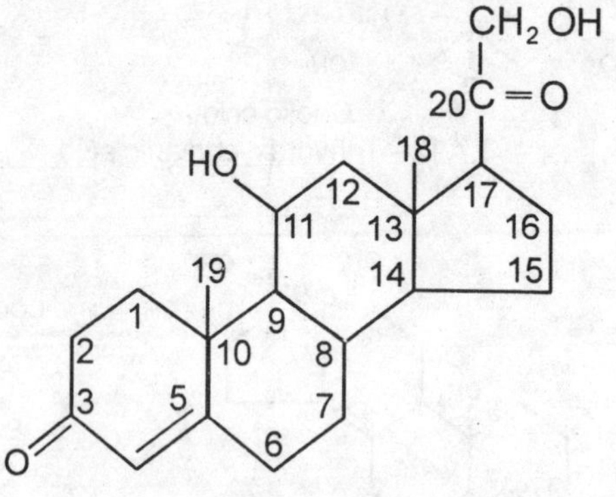

Fig. 3.5 : Structure of corticosterone

***Vitamin* D**

Irradiation with ultraviolet light converts a number of sterols to compounds with vitamin D activity.

Saponins

Digitonin (Fig. 3.6) is a plant glycoside of a steroid-digitogenin in which the sugar residues are attached to the OH group at the 3-carbon. Digitonin (Fig. 3.6) forms insoluble addition compounds with sterols such as cholesterol.

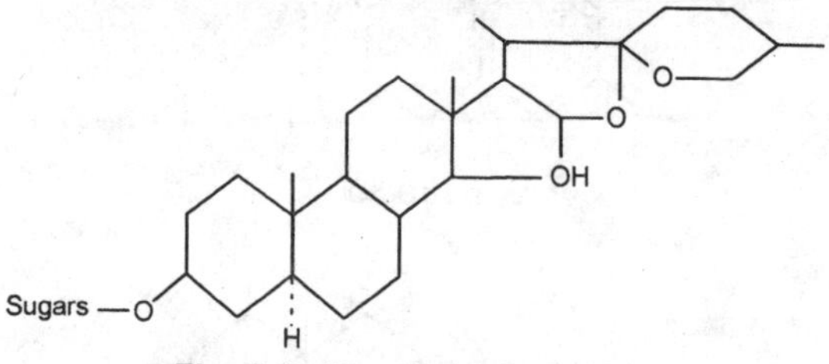

Fig. 3.6 : Structure of digitonin

Cardiac glycosides

These compounds have therapeutic applications. Strophanthin is a glycoside of the steroid strophanthidin.

Carotenoids and Vitamin A

Carotenoids are isoprenoid hydrocarbons of plant origin containing 40 carbon atoms. Because carotenoids have a system of conjugated double bonds, they show strong light absorption and are often brightly coloured. The carotenes have two rings (β-ionone) connected by a chain of repeating isoprene linkages. Because of the double bond arrangement, these compounds are subject to geometrical isomerism.

Closely related to the carotenes chemically, and derived from them biochemically, are the vitamins A, A_1, found in the liver of all land animals and of marine and freshwater fishes; and A_2 found in liver oils from some fresh water fishes. Metabolic intermediates of vitamin A occur in the form of aldehydes - the retinines (for details, consult chapter on vitamins).

Vitamin E and the quinones

These compounds bear close similarities in their structures, and it has been suggested that their biological functions (in cellular oxidation) may also be related.

Tocopherols (Vitamin E)

Several forms of this compound are known to possess biological activity as an antisterility factor in rats. The α-variety has the highest potency.

Ubiquinones (Coenzyme Q)

A group of related quinones with variable number of isoprene residues have been isolated. **Coenzyme 'Q' is found in mitochondria and is a part of the electron transport mechanism.**

Phylloquinones (Vitamin K)

These vitamins display anti-hemorrhagic activity.

Plastoquinone

This quinone is found in the chloroplasts and is not found in the animal kingdom.

CHAPTER 4

CHEMISTRY OF AMINO ACIDS, PROTEINS AND IMMUNOGLOBULINS

We are very complex substances having large molecular weights and are expensive of all the foodstuffs and found in innumerable eatables. We have the wonderful unimaginable properties like involvement in (i) blood clotting (ii) hereditary transmission (iii) transport of O_2 and CO_2 (iv) defence (antibodies) mechanisms (v) enzymes (vi) cementing substances (vii) buffers and many more.

There will come no end in our inventions and our contribution in various physiological/ biochemical/ metabolic processes is everlasting.

Proteins may be defined as extremely complex nitrogen containing organic compounds which are polymers of amino acids and possess high molecular weight. Amino acids present in the protein molecules remain linked to each other with the help of a special linkage known as a peptide linkage (– CO – NH –). In addition to carbon, hydrogen and oxygen, proteins invariably contain nitrogen and generally sulphur also. **Besides, proteins have also been found to contain phosphorus, iron, copper, iodine, manganese, zinc and other elements.**

Consequently, there is a great variety and range of proteins according to their composition, size and shape. They are of utmost importance in biological processes; although some have a purely structural function; however the majority not only plays a static role in living tissues but a very dynamic role. Such proteins include the **enzymes.**

The molecular weight of proteins ranges from **5,734 of human insulin** through the 60, 000 of bovine serum albumin to the 6,00,000 of myosin and even higher. The proportion of various amino acid residues in proteins vary considerably; some such as serum albumin contains all the common amino acids, others for e.g. insulin lacks methionine, tryptophan and cysteine. **Collagen,** the protein of connective tissue contains 33% glycine residues and 12% each of alanine and proline with very low proportion of the other amino acids.

Proteins may be highly insoluble, such as **keratins** of hair and nails or highly soluble such as albumins of the blood plasma.

Chemistry of amino acids

Normally occurring amino acids are those amino acids which contain (i) amino group and (ii) carboxyl group in the carbon atom and are represented by the following general formula:

$$\begin{array}{c} COOH \\ |\,\alpha \\ R - C - NH_2 \\ | \\ H \end{array}$$

α - amino acid

All amino acids (structures as given ahead) found in living systems i.e. plant and animal proteins are L -α - amino acids (derived from L-glyceraldehyde). In nature, glycine is the only amino acid which is optically inactive and cannot be resolved into D - or L - form because of symmetry on the α - carbon atom. Rest amino acids are optically active.

The configuration of L - α - amino acid is as follows :

$$\begin{array}{c} COOH \\ |\,\alpha \\ NH_2 - C - H \\ | \\ R \end{array}$$

L- amino acid

Classification of the amino acids

Amino acids have been classified in many ways. They can either be classified according to the presence of (a) acidic, basic, or neutral groups or due to the presence of (b) polar groups, non-polar groups, sulphur containing groups, aromatic groups, heterocyclic ring, branched chain, etc. in their structures.

It is as metioned ahead in Table 4.1

1. Aliphatic amino acids.

Table 4.1 : Classification of amino acids

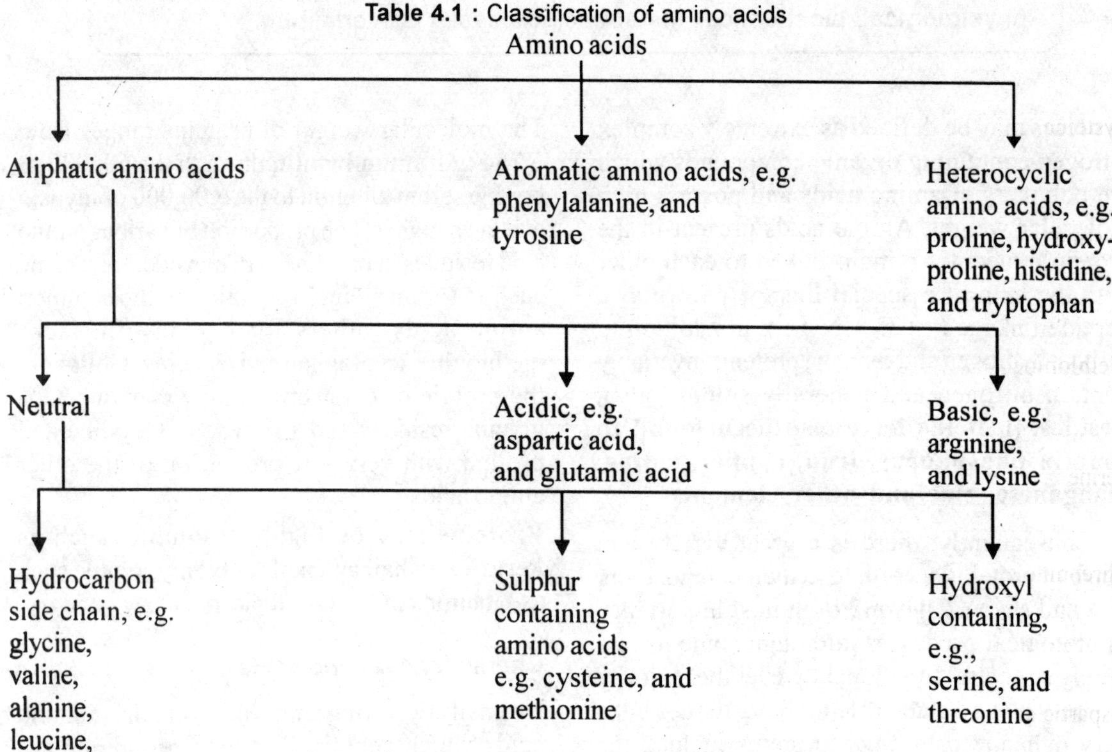

Glycine $H-\underset{H}{\overset{NH_2}{C}}-COOH$

Alanine $H_3C-\overset{NH_2}{CH}-COOH$

Valine $\begin{matrix}H_3C\\ \\ H_3C\end{matrix}>CH-\overset{NH_2}{CH}-COOH$

Leucine $\begin{matrix}H_3C\\ \\ H_3C\end{matrix}>CH-CH_2-\overset{NH_2}{CH}-COOH$

Isoleucine $\begin{matrix}CH_2-CH_3\\ \\ H_3C\end{matrix}>CH-\overset{NH_2}{CH}-COOH$

Cysteine $HS-CH_2-\overset{NH2}{CH}-COOH$

Cystine $(-S-CH_2-\overset{NH_2}{CH}-COOH)_2$

Methionine $H_3C-S-CH_2-\overset{NH_2}{CH}-COOH$

Serine $HO-CH_2-\overset{NH_2}{CH}-COOH$

Threonine $H_3C-\overset{OH}{CH}-\overset{NH_2}{CH}-COOH$

Aspartic acid $HOOC-CH_2-\overset{NH_2}{CH}-COOH$

Glutamic acid $HOOC-CH_2-CH_2-\overset{NH_2}{CH}-COOH$

Arginine $NH_2-\overset{NH}{\overset{\|}{C}}-NH-(CH_2)_4-\overset{NH_2}{CH}-COOH$

Lysine $H_2N-(CH_2)_4-\overset{NH_2}{CH}-COOH$

Phenylalanine $C_6H_5-CH_2-\overset{NH_2}{CH}-COOH$

Tyrosine $HO-C_6H_4-CH_2-\overset{NH_2}{CH}-COOH$

Proline $\begin{array}{ccc}CH_2 & - & CH_2\\ | & & |\\ CH_2 & & CH-COOH\\ & \diagdown N \diagup & \\ & H & \end{array}$

Asparagine $H_2N-\overset{O}{\overset{\|}{C}}-CH_2-\overset{NH_2}{CH}-COOH$

Glutamine $H_2N-\overset{O}{\overset{\|}{C}}-CH_2-CH_2-\overset{NH_2}{\overset{\|}{CH}}-COOH$

Histidine $\begin{array}{l}HC=C-CH_2-\overset{NH_2}{CH}-COOH\\ \ \ |\qquad |\\ \ \ N\quad\ NH\\ \quad \diagdown\!\!\!\!= C \diagup\\ \qquad H\end{array}$

Tryptophan

$$\text{(indole ring)}-C(=CH-NH)-CH_2-C(NH_2)(H)-COOH$$

Ornithine $H_2N-CH_2-CH_2-CH-H-COOH$ (with C–NH_2 branch)

Cirtulline $CH_2-CH_2-CH_2-CH(NH_2)-COOH$, with $NH-C{=}O-NH_2$ on the first CH_2

γ - Amino butyric acid (GABA) $H_2N-CH_2-CH_2-CH_2-COOH$

β - Alanine $H_2N-CH_2-CH_2-COOH$

3-Monoiodotyrosine $HO-C_6H_3(I)-CH_2-CH(NH_2)-COOH$

3,5-Diiodotyrosine $HO-C_6H_2(I)_2-CH_2-CH(NH_2)-COOH$

3,5, 3'- Triiodo-thyronine (T_3) $HO-C_6H_3(I)-O-C_6H_2(I)_2-CH_2-CH(NH_2)-COOH$

3,5,3',5'- Tetraiodo-thyronine (T_4) $HO-C_6H_2(I)_2-O-C_6H_2(I)_2-CH_2-CH(NH_2)-COOH$

2. Aromatic amino acids
3. Heterocyclic amino acids

Besides the regular 20 amino acids, there are number of special amino acids which are found in free or combined form but do not occur in protein molecules, these include triiodothyronine (T_3), tetraiodothyronine (T_4), ornithine, citrulline, β-alanine, γ - aminobutyric acid, etc.

Examples of relatively smaller peptides that possess biological activity include:

(i) glutathione,
(ii) oxytocin, and
(iii) vasopressin, etc.

Out of the above **glutathione is a tripeptide** which consists of glutamic acid, cystine and glycine in its structure and is found in RBCs. **Oxytocin and vasopressin are *octapeptides*** and are secreted by the posterior part of the pituitary gland, each is made up of 8 amino acids. ***Oxytocin* causes contraction of smooth muscles and is used in obstetrics to initiate labour whereas vasopressin increases blood pressure and reduces the formation of urine.**

Functions of of amino acids

Amino acids play very important role in human system and serve as :

(1) **Building blocks of proteins, and**
(2) **As precursors of:**
  (a) **hormones,**
  (b) **purines,**
  (c) **pyrimidines,**
  (d) **porphyrins,**
  (e) **vitamins, etc.**

Essential amino acids (EAA)

EAA are those amino acids which are not synthesized in the body and hence have to be provided in the diet. They are also termed as *indispensable* amino acids and are eight in number. To remember them, there is a formula known as **M A TTVIL Ph Ly in which A is silent;** these are as follows:

(i) Leucine,
(ii) Isoleucine,
(iii) Valine
(iv) Methionine
(v) Tryptophan
(vi) Phenylalanine
(vii) Lysine, and
(viii) Threonine

Histidine is treated under the category of 'Essential' in case of infants, otherwise semiessential.

Sufficient amounts of EAA are required to maintain the proper nitrogen balance. Deficiency of one or more EAA in the diet affects the synthesis of proteins resulting failure in the growth of the child, negative nitrogen balance in the adults and fall in the levels of plasma proteins and hemoglobin.

Semiessential amino acids: Are those amino acids which are required half-heartedly by the body for proper growth and development, these include:

(i) Arginine
(ii) Tyrosine
(iii) Cystine
(iv) Glycine
(v) Serine and
(vi) Histidine

Non-essential Amino Acids

These are not required by the body but are synthesized by the body and include aspartic acid, glutamic acid, proline, hydroxyproline, etc. These are derived from the carbon skeletons of carbohydrates and lipids metabolism or from the transformation of essential amino acids.

Nitrogen Balance

The ratio of:

$$\frac{\text{Intake of N}}{\text{Output of N}}$$

= 1, i.e., nitrogen equilibrium. Normal adults are in nitrogen equilibrium.

> 1, i.e., Positive Nitrogen Balance, e.g., pregnancy, convulsions and growth.

< 1, i.e., Negative Nitrogen Balance, e.g., malnutrition and certain wasting diseases where there is tissue breakdown.

Ionic properties of Amino Acids:

The amphoteric (property of behaviour either as an acid or a base) properties of amino acids account for their separation of electrophoresis on paper at pH 6.0 (Fig. 4.1).

The amphoteric nature of α - amino acids determines that, in the absence of other acids or bases, the carboxyl and amino groups are both

Aspartic acid	Alanine	Lysine
COO^-	CH_3	NH_3^+
|	|	|
CH_2	$CH.NH_3^+$	$(CH_2)_4$
|	|	|
$CH.NH_3^+$	COO^-	$CH.NH_3^+$
|		|
COO^-		COO^-

negatively charged ↓ isoionic ↓ positively charged ↓

\+ ● ● ● −

↑
point of application of the mixture

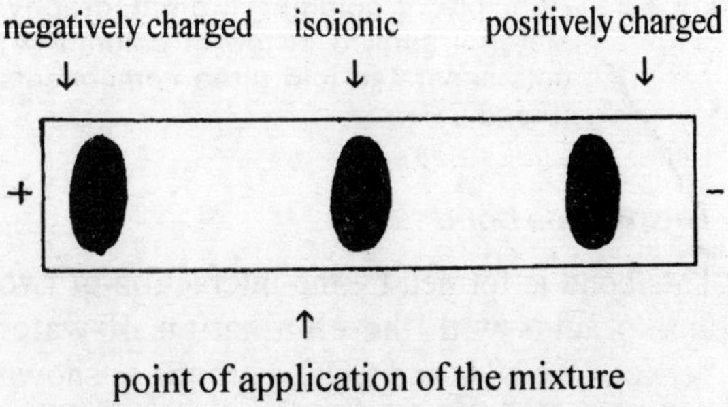

Fig. 4.1 : To show pattern of electrophoresis

ionized fully to give rise to the term zwitterion (German zwitter = hybrid or hermaphrodite). This kind of nature may be understood as follows:

Separation of Amino acids by Ion-Exchange Chromatography (Fig 4.2)

In addition to permitting the separation of amino acids by electrophoresis, their ionic properties also permit their separation by ion-exchange chromatography. Ion-exchange is performed using a resin to which positively charged groups (anion-exchange resin) or negatively charged groups (cation-exchange resin) are covalently bound and thus immobilized. Ions passed down a column of such a resin bind competitively to the charged groups. Principle of ion-exchange chromatography has been shown as in (Fig. 4.2):

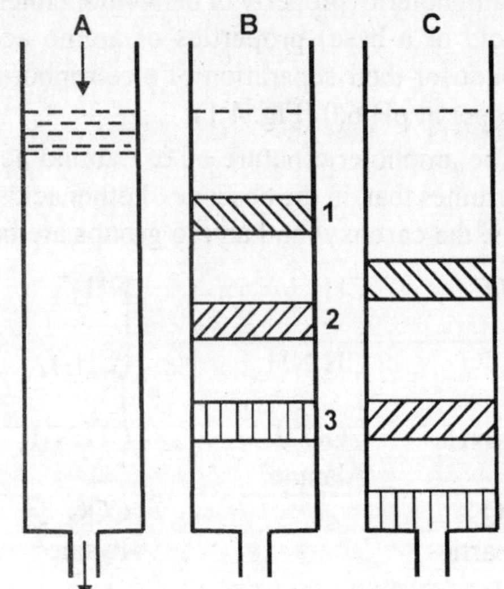

Fig. 4.2: Principle of column chromatography. Material applied at top of column (A) gets separated into three components (B and C)

The peptide bond

This bond is formed by the interaction of two amino acids with the elimination of water between the NH_2 and COOH groups as shown below.

$$\left(\begin{array}{cc} \text{O} & \text{H} \\ \| & | \\ -\text{C} - & \text{N} - \end{array} \right)$$

The Biuret Reaction

Biuret has the formula $NH_2CONHCONH_2$, and is a simple substance containing a peptide bond. **When *Biuret* is treated with $CuSO_4$ in alkaline solution, a purple colour is produced. This is known as the *Biuret Reaction*. All proteins give a positive reaction.**

Isoelectric point

The isoelctric point is that pH at which the protein carries a net charge of zero because at this pH the sum of positive charge is equal to the sum of negative charge. That is why proteins do not migrate in an electric field. At this pH, amino acids (constituents of a protein molecule) exist in the zwitterion form. According to the isoelectric point, proteins are described as basic, neutral or acidic depending or whether their overall charge at physiological pH is positive, approximately zero, or negative. Isoelectric points of some common proteins are as follows:

Protein	Isoelectric point
Serum albumin	4.7
α_1, - Globulin	2.0
γ_2, - Globulin	5.8
Fibrinogen	5.8
Hemoglobin	7.2
Pepsin	1.0
Insulin	5.4
Cytochrome	9.8
Lysozyme	11.1

High Performance Liquid Chromatography (HPLC)

This is the most latest kind of chromatography

in which an instrument named as Bio-Rad protein Chromatography system is used. **By this technique, separation of a variety of peptides may be done, for example:**

(i) Oxytocin
(ii) Met-Enkephalin
(iii) TRH
(iv) α - Endorphin
(v) α - MSH
(vi) β - Endorphin
(vii) Angiotensin II
(viii) Substance P
(ix) LHRH
(x) Neurotensin, etc.

The technique depends upon the use of microfine column matrixes to give high resolution rapidly.

α_1 Antitrypsin (AT) and its role in Emphysema

The predominant component of the α_1 - globulin band consists of a protein named as **α_1-antitrypsin (AT).** It has been wrongly named because it is active against elastase rather than trypsin and is a member of a group of **Serine Proteinase Inhibitors or, Serpins.**

In normal young, the destructive power of enzyme elastase released from the neutrophils in checked by AT. **Cigarette smoking increases the number and activity of lung neutrophils and consequently the amount of enzyme elastase.** Moreover, oxidation reduces the protection afforded by a given amount of circulating AT.

α_1- antitrypsin is less active after oxidation; elastase then causes tissue breakdown and loss of elasticity in the lungs vis-a-vis emphysema. **It means that smoking leads to a tendency of emphysema.**

Proteins

Proteins may be defined as extremely complex nitrogen containing organic compounds which are polymers of amino acids and possess high molecular weight. Amino acids present in the protein molecules remain linked to each other with the help of a special linkage known as a peptide linkage (– CO – NH –).In addition to carbon, hydrogen and oxygen, proteins invariably contain nitrogen and generally sulphur also.

Proteins have also been found to contain phosphorus, iron, copper, iodine, manganese, zinc and other elements.

Denaturation

A protein is said to be a native protein if its amino acid composition and stereochemical structures remain unchanged from the natural state. These properties control all the functions of a protein, whether solubility in dilute salt solutions, proteolytic activity, oxygen carrying capacity, or whatever it may be. These characteristics are altered and the process of denaturation is said to occur when a protein undergoes changes in structure or composition (Fig 4.3).

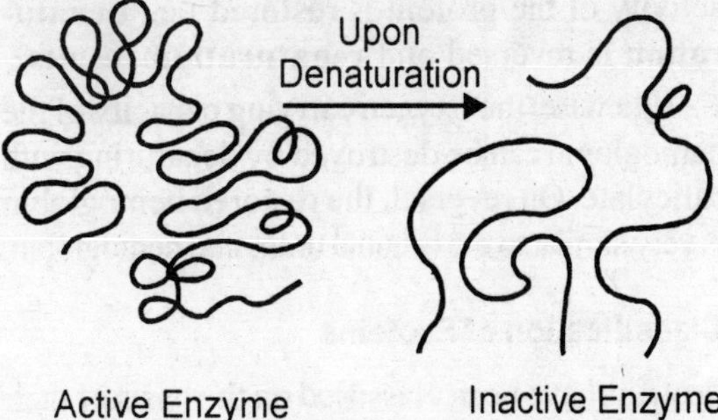

Fig. 4.3 : Representation of denaturation of protein

Chemical and physical agents that cause these changes are called denaturing agents. Their action involves the splitting of some or all the protein cross linkages with their possible reformation, in some cases, to cause a rearrangement of the peptide chains.

Denaturation may be caused by the following:

1. Heat
2. Mineral acids and alkalies
3. Shaking or stirring
4. Grinding
5. Ultraviolet radiations
6. Ultrasonic waves
7. Neutral Chemical agents, etc.

Renaturation

Denatured proteins may, however, under certain conditions, be restored to proteins with many of the properties of the original protein. This process is known as **'renaturation'**. It appears, however, that renaturation seldom results in the complete restoration of the denatured protein to its original state.

Pepsin can be denatured and so loses its proteolytic properties if it is warmed to the proper temperature.

When the solution is cooled, the proteolytic activity of the protein is restored i.e., **denaturation** is reversed and **renaturation results.**

Likewise, the oxygen carrying capacity of the hemoglobin can be destroyed by denaturing with salicylate. On reversal, the restored hemoglobin is very similar to the original untreated hemoglobin.

Classification of Proteins

Proteins have been classified on the basis of their composition as follows:

I Simple proteins

Simple proteins are made up of amino acids only and upon hydrolysis yield a mixture of amino acids only.

Examples

(A) **Fibrous (insoluble) proteins** : Also called as **scleroproteins.** They impart a supporting or protective function in the animal. These are insoluble in water.

(a) Collagens : Principal supporting proteins of skin, tendons and bones. They possess very large amount of hydroxyproline. They are **resistant to peptic and tryptic digestion.**

(b) Elastins : Found in elastic tissues like tendons and arteries. **Readily digested by trypsin and pepsin.** It contains smaller amount of hydroxyproline.

(c) Keratins : Found in animal skin, nails, horns, hoofs, hair, feathers, etc. They possess high cystine content.

(B) **Globular (soluble) proteins** : Are soluble proteins with definite molecular weights. Each molecule contains one or more peptide chains, held in a coiled configuration by disulfide bridges and other bonds.

(a) Albumins : Include ovalbumin from egg white, serum albumin from blood serum, and lactalbumin from milk. They are coagulable by heat and soluble in pure water. They are precipitated from solution by **full saturation of ammonium sulphate.**

(b) Globulins : Include serum globulins, lactoglobulin from milk, thyroglobulin from thyroid gland. Also found in many plant seeds, e.g. edestin from hempseed. Are soluble in dilute salt solutions and are precipitated from solution by **half saturation of ammonium sulphate.** Coagulated by heat.

(c) Plant proteins (glutenins, prolamins) : Cereal proteins such as glutelins of wheat, orygenin of rice and zein of maize. Soluble in very weak acids or alkalies but insoluble in all neutral solvents.

(d) Protamines : They are simpler polypeptides. Uncoagulable by heat and possess strong basic properties. Rich in arginine. **Example is salmine from salmon sperms.**

(e) Histones : Are soluble in water but insoluble in dilute ammonia. Rich in arginine and lysine and possess strong basic properties. Example scombrone from mackerel sperms.

(C) Denatured Proteins

When proteins are subjected to certain physical and chemical agents, they get denatured. In fact, they undergo intramolecular changes which cause changes in solubility and other properties. Soluble proteins for example albumins and globulins are converted by heat, ultraviolet light, mechanical agitation or long contact with alcohol, etc. into insoluble materials known as coagulated proteins. Such coagulated proteins are denatured one.

II Conjugated Proteins

Are those proteins which consist of protein combined with some non protein substance (the prosthetic group). They are classified according to the nature of the prosthetic group, as indicated below:

III Derived Proteins

Include those substances formed from simple and conjugated proteins. It is the least well defined of the protein groups. These are subdivided into primary derived proteins and secondary derived proteins.

1. Primary derived proteins : Slight change with little or no hydrolytic cleavage of peptide bonds.

(a) Proteans : Insoluble products, example fibrin from fibrinogen

(b) Metaproteins : Generally soluble in very dilute acids and alkalies but insoluble in neutral solvents. Examples are acid and alkali albuminates.

(c) Coagulated : Insoluble products formed by the action of heat or alcohol upon natural proteins. Examples are cooked egg albumin, cooked meat, etc.

2. Secondary derived proteins: These are formed in the progressive hydrolytic cleavage of the peptide unions of proteins. They represent very complex molecules of different size and amino acid composition. They are roughly grouped into following three categories :

(a) **Proteoses**

(b) **Peptones**

(c) **Peptides**

Structure of Proteins

Proteins exhibit four levels of organization

1. **Primary structure**
2. **Secondary structure**
3. **Tertiary structure**
4. **Quaternary structure**

Primary Structure: It refers to the sequence of individual amino acids in the polypeptide chain or chains that comprise the protein and the location of disulfide bonds, if any.

– Ala – Gly – Gly – His – Leu –

Secondary Structure: It refers to the conformation of polypeptide chains. The term *conformation* refers to the relative positions of each of the constituent atoms of a molecule in the space (Fig. 4.4).

Globular proteins (example insulin) indicate a coiled structure in which peptide bonds are folded in a regular manner. The foldings are the results of linking of the carboxyl and amino groups of the peptide chains by means of hydrogen bonds and disulfide bonds. Such foldings are referred to as the secondary structure of the protein (Fig. 4.4).

Conjugated Protein = Protein part + prosthetic group

		Prosthetic group	*Example*
1.	Nucleoproteins	= Nucleic acid	Virus proteins
2.	Glycoproteins and Mucoproteins	= Carbohydrate or a derivative of carbohydrate	Mucin of saliva
3.	Phosphoproteins	= Phosphoric acid	Casein of milk, ovovitellin of egg yolk
4.	Chromoproteins	= Metalloporphyrin or some similar substance which absorbs visible light	Haemoglobin
5.	Metalloproteins	= Metals(copper, Mn, Mg, Zn, Mo, etc.)	Tyrosinase, arginase,anhydrase, xanthine oxidase, etc.
6.	Lipoproteins	= Lipids (cholesterol, phospholipids triglycerides, etc.)	Serum lipoproteins, lipoproteins of egg yolk

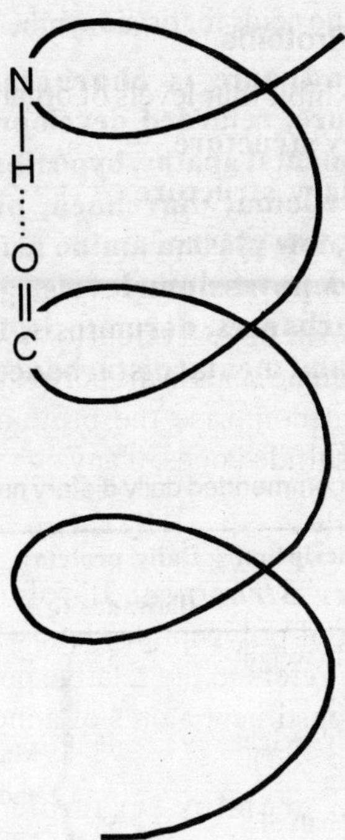

Fig. 4.4 : Secondary structure

Tertiary Structure: It refers to the coiling of several helical portions of single helix into a three dimensional structure (Fig. 4.5).

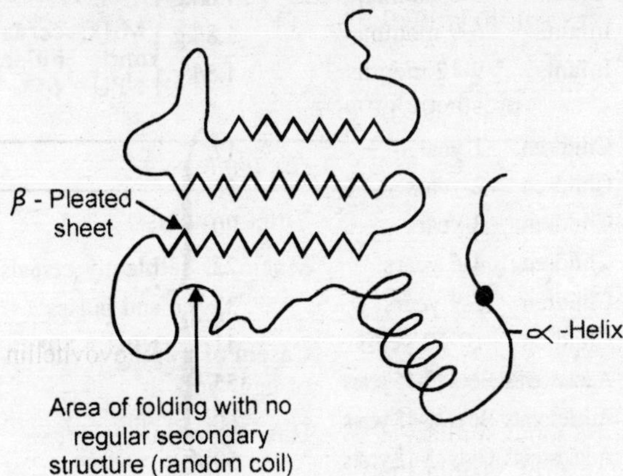

Fig 4.5 : Tertiary structure

The tertiary structure of proteins is stabilised and maintained by :

(a) Hydrogen bonding

(b) Disulfide bonding

(c) Ionic interactions

(d) Vander Waal's forces

(e) Hydrophobic interactions

(f) Ester bonding

Example of the tertiary structure of protein is the protein of tobacco mosaic virus (TMV) which resembles the kernel of the corn.

Quaternary Structure

Proteins containing more than one polypeptide chain display fourth level of structural organization called **quaternary structure**. In this type, the individual polypeptide chain is arranged in relation to each other so as to give a simple three dimensional structure on the overall protein molecule. Each polypeptide chain in such a protein is called a subunit. Depending upon the number of subunits present, such proteins are called as dimers, trimers, tetramers or polymers, etc. **Examples are haemoglobin, ferritin, etc.**

Biochemical functions/roles or biological importance of proteins

They play very important roles in the human body and are very essential substances. They play following important roles in the human body.

1. Proteins may be said as the essence of life processes.
2. All enzymes are made up of proteins.
3. Many of the hormones are proteinous in nature for example **insulin, glucagon, oxytocin, vasopressin, etc.**
4. They serve as building block units for subcellular, cellular and organic structures.
5. They act as defence against infections by way of protein antibodies.
6. They are involved in blood clotting through

thrombin, fibrinogen and other protein factors.

7. Cementing substances and the reticulum which bind the cells as tissues/organs are partly made up of proteins.
8. They perform hereditary transmission by way of nucleoproteins found in the cell nucleus.
9. They act as buffers.
10. They help in the transport of oxygen and CO_2 by way of haemoglobin and certain special enzymes which are found in red blood cells.

Dietary Requirement of Proteins

Requirement of proteins of an individual depends upon the age, sex and body weight. It is as mentioned in Table 4.2.

Now the chemists have reached the fact that the quantity of protein alone does not solve the entire purpose but the **quality** of a protein has got more significance hence one must give more emphasis on the quality of a protein. **By the quality of a protein, we mean that it must comprise of essential amino acids in it.**

Deficiency Diseases

Protein deficiency is generally encountered during infancy and childhood and is known as protein- energy malnutrition **(PEM)**. There are two severe forms of the disease known as **kwashiorkor** and **marasmus.**

Kwashiorkor is mainly a disease of rural areas, occurring in the second year of life. It occurs most commonly in the infants after weaning (breast feeding) when the diet which replaces mother's milk is markedly deficient in proteins but high in carbohydrate. This disease has its highest incidence **between the age group of 1 to 4 years** when the need for essential amino acids for tissue synthesis is more.

This syndrome is characterized by growth failure, retarded development, loss of appetite, mental apathy, hypoalbuminemia leading to edema, diarrhoea, pellagrous skin lesions, low plasma amino acids, lipids, glucose and potassium levels, gastrointestinal disturbances, dermatosis, fatty liver infiltration and mental disturbances are also frequent.

Table 4.2 : Recommended daily dietary protein intake

Category	Description	Daily protein allowance (g)	Nature of diet
Man	Body weight 55 kg	55	Mainly cereals and pulses NPU = 65*
Woman	Body weight 45 kg	45	
Woman	2nd half of pregnancy	55	
Woman	Lactation upto 1 year	65	
Infants	0-3 months	2.3 /kg	Entirely milk NPU=75-100*
Infants	3-6 months	1.8/kg	
Infants	6-9 months	1.8/kg	Milk, cereals and pulses, NPU = 65*
Infants	9-12 months	1.5/kg	
Children	1 year	17	Mostly cereals and pulses NPU = 50*
Children	2 years	18	
Children	3 years	20	
Children	4-6 years	22	
Children	7-9 years	33	
Children	10-12 years	41	
Adolescents: Boys 13-15 years		55	
Adolescents: Boys 16-18 years		60	
Adolescents: Girls 13-18 years		50	

** The essential amino acids requirement of adults is less exacting than those of infants and children, therefore, the same dietary has a higher NPU for adults than for children.*

Marasmus

Marasmus literally means "to waste". It results from a continued severe deficiency of both dietary proteins and the calories i.e. energy.

> Marasmus is predominantly due to the **deficiency of calories.** This is usually observed in children given watery gruels (of cereals) to supplement the mother's breast milk.

It generally occurs in the children below one year of age. The symptoms include growth retardation, muscle wasting, anaemia, weakness, and repeated infections. Attitude is irritable. Skin is shrunken, dry and atrophic.

A marasmic child does not show edema or decreased concentration of plasma albumin (usual level in them is 2 to 3 g/dl whereas in kwashiorkor cases it is always less than 2 g/dl) and the level of cortisol in serum gets increased in marasmic child whereas decreased in kwashiorkor ones.

Immunoglobulins

Immunoglobulins or *antibodies* are **synthesized in B lymphocytes or their derivatives, plasma cells** and with remarkable specificity bind to *antigenic sites* on their moelcules.

All immunoglobulins are composed of four polypeptide chains, two identical light (L) chains(MW 23,000) and 2 identical heavy (H) chains (MW 53,000-75,000) which are held together as a tetramer (L_2H_2) by disulfide bonds (Fig. 4.6). Each chain can be divided into specific regions that have structural and functional significance. The half of the *light* (L) *chain* towards the carboxyl terminus is referred to as the *constant region* (C_L), whereas the amino-terminal half is the *variable region* of the light chain (V_L). Nearly, one-quarter of the *heavy (H) chain* at the amino terminus is referred to as its variable region *(V_H)* and the remaining three quarters of the heavy chain are referred to as the constant regions (C_H1, C_H2, C_H3) of that H chain. The function of the immunoglobulin molecule that binds the specific antigen is formed by the amino-terminal portions (variable regions) of both the H and L chains i.e., the V_H and V_L regions.

As made clear in Fig. 4.6, digestion of an immunoglobulin by the enzyme papain produces 2 antigen binding fragments (Fab) and one crystallizable fragment (F_c). The area in which papain cleaves the immunoglobulin molecule i.e., the region between the C_H1 and C_H2 regions is referred to as the **hinge region.**

There are two general types of light chains i.e. *kappa* (k) and *lambda* (λ). A given immunoglobulin molecule always contains two *k* or two λ light chains, never a mixture of *k* and λ. In human the *k* chains are more common than λ chains in immunoglobulin molecules.

In human, 5 classes of H chains have been found which can be easily distinguished from

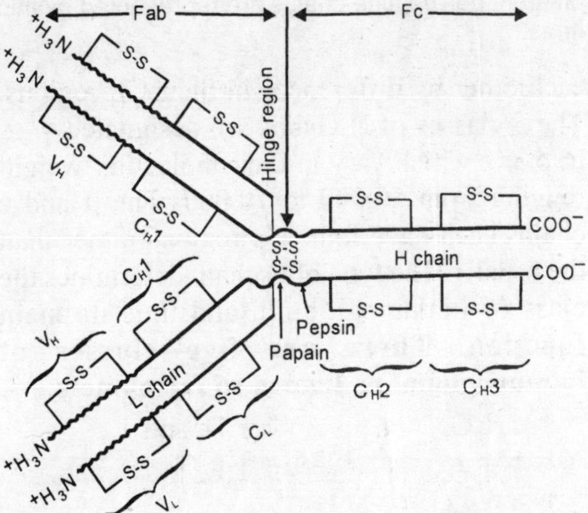

Fig 4.6 : A simplified model for an IgG human antibody molecule showing the 4-chain basic structure and different regions. V, indicates variable region; C, the constant region, and the vertical arrow, the hinge region. Thick lines represent H and L chains; thin lines represent disulfide bonds.

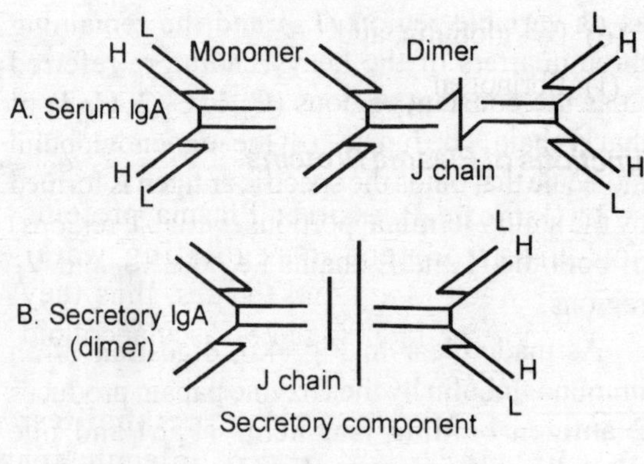

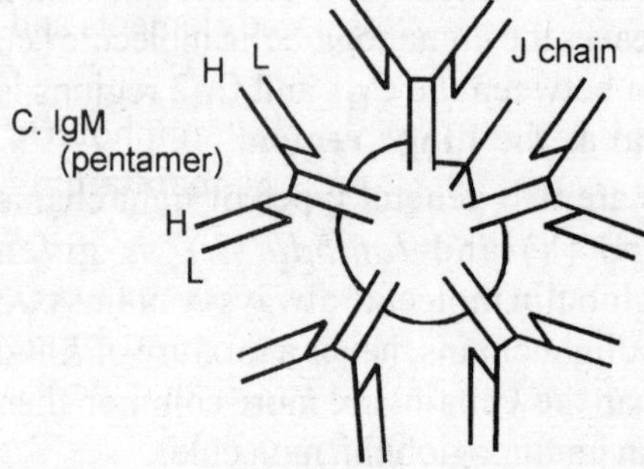

C. IgM (pentamer)

Fig. 4.7 : Highly schematic illustration of polymeric human immunoglobulins. Polypeptide chains are represented by thick lines; disulfide bonds linking different polypeptide chains are represented by thin lines.

each other by differences in their C_H regions. The 5 classes of H chains are designated γ, α, μ, δ & ε which vary in their molecular weight ranging from 50,000 to 70,000. The μ and ε chains each have four C_H regions rather than the usual 3. The type of H chain determines the class of immunoglobulin and thus its main function. **There are five classes of immunoglobulins known so far namely:**

1. I_gG,
2. I_gA,
3. I_gM,
4. I_gD, and
5. I_gE

Many of the H chain classes can be further divided, into subclasses on the basis of structural differences in the C_H regions.

Some immunoglobulins such as immune I_gG exist only in the basic tetrameric structure, while others such as I_gA and I_gM can exist as higher order polymers of 2, 3 (I_gA) or 5 (I_gM) tetrameric units (Fig. 4.7).

The L and H chains are synthesized as separate molecules and are subsequently assembled within the B cell or plasma cell into mature immunoglobulin molecules, **all of which are glycoproteins in nature.**

Schematic model of I_gG molecule is as shown below in Fig. 4.8.

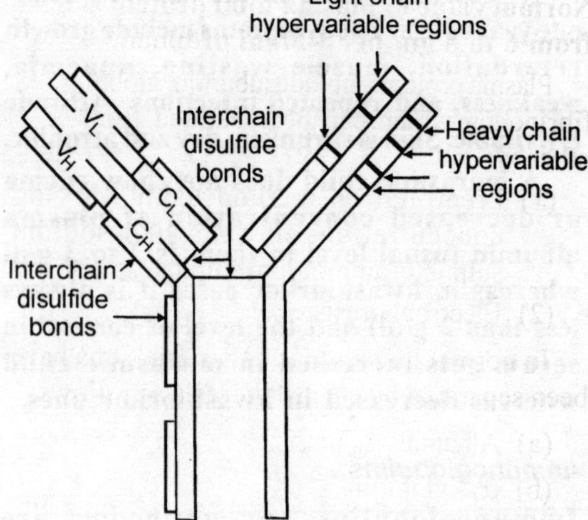

Fig. 4.8 : Schematic model of an I_gG molecule showing approximate positions of the hypervariable regions in heavy and light chains.

Each immunoglobulin light chain is the product of at least 3 separate structural genes i.e., a variable region (V_L) gene, a joining region (J) gene (bearing no relation to the J chain of I_gA or I_gM) and a constant region (C_L) gene. Each heavy chain is the product of at least 4 different genes i.e., a variable region (V_H) gene, a diversity region (D) gene, a joining region (J) gene and a constant region (C_H) gene. **In this way, the 'one gene, one protein' concept is no more valid.**

Each person is capable of generating antibodies directed against perhaps one million different antigens.

Various disorders of immunoglobulins include increased production of specific classes of immunoglobulins or even specific immunoglobulin molecules. **Hypogammaglobulinemia** may be restricted to a single class of immunoglobulin molecules (eg, I_gA or I_gG) or may involve underproduction of all classes of immunoglobulins (I_gA, I_gD, I_gE, I_gG and I_gM).

Plasma Proteins

Normal value of plasma total protein ranges from 6 to 8 gm per 100 ml of blood.

Plasma proteins include albumin, globulin and fibrinogen which can be separated from each other by:

(1) Precipitation method using varying concentrations of salts like sodium sulphate, ammonium sulphate, etc.

(2) Electrophoresis

In normal human plasma six fractions have been separated by electrophoresis as follows:

(a) Albumin

(b) α_1 - globulin

(c) α_2 - globulin

(d) β_1, - globulin

(e) β_2 - globulin, and

(f) fibrinogen

Functions of Plasma Proteins

1. **Osmotic Pressure:** Plasma proteins are important in regulating water between blood and tissues, thus they help in maintaining intravascular colloid osmotic pressure.
2. **As carrier of certain metabolites:** They act as a carrier molecule for bilirubin, fatty acids, trace elements and many drugs.
3. **As buffers:** Proteins are amphoteric in nature and thus help in maintaining the pH of blood.
4. The lipoproteins act as **carrier molecule** for different types of lipids and lipid-soluble molecules that are not soluble in the plasma water.
5. Some **metal-binding proteins** for e.g. trnasferrin have the properties of globulins and act as carriers for trace elements.
6. **As immunoglobulins:** The property of antibodies formation resides in the γ -globulin fraction of the proteins.

Proteins	*Biological role*
Collagen, keratins	Structural proteins
Pepsin, amylase, etc.	Enzymes
Insulin, prolactin	Hormones
Haemoglobin, ceruloplasmin	Transport proteins
Ferritin	Storage proteins
γ - globulins	Immune functions
Hormone receptors	Protein receptors

CHAPTER 5

NUCLEIC ACIDS

We are The carriers of genetic information from one offspring to another. We are very complex molecules. Scientists are pursuing us and shall continue to pursue us till the 'universe' is present as we are very complicated molecules. Many many thanks to the science- stalwarts like James Watson, Francis Crick, Morris Wilkins (forgotten man of DNA), Chargaff, etc., who dedicated their lives for us. Genome technology is only due to us.

If any group of compounds can be said to be **'controller'** in **biochemistry, it is the nucleic acids** which are found in every living cell and these may be defined as the nitrogen containing compounds of high molecular weight, **vis-a-vis polymers of nucleotides.** These are in fact macromolecules which remain present in most of the living cells, either in the free state or combined with proteins. The nucleic acid protein complexes are known as nucleoproteins, and these can be separated into the component proteins and nucleic acids by treatment with acid or high salt concentration. For the first time, they were reported by the scientist Miescher in 1871. Proteins associated with nucleic acids fall into two major classes as mentioned below:

Proteins
- protamines (e.g. salmine from salmon sperm)
- histones (are prepared from calf thymus and rat liver)

These proteins are basic in character, for example salmine which consists of 40 arginine

Nucleic acids may be defined as the macromolecules in which the nucleotides remain linked to each other by phosphodiester bonds between the 3' and 5' positions of the sugars.

A portion of a molecule of RNA, therefore, has the structure as given in Fig. 5.1 **where base can either be a purine or pyrimidine.**

Most nucleic acids are very large molecules, therefore, to show the complete formulae is rather very cumbersome. A useful form of shorthand for the structure is therefore employed which exhibits the bases present by using their first letter. The sequence of bases is extremely important so that a nucleic acid may be shown by the first letters of the bases only (Fig. 5.2).

residues out of a total of 120.

As the name suggests, nucleic acids are acidic in character at physiological pH and carry a high density of negative charge. Nucleic acids are mainly of the following two types:

Nucleic acids

Ribonucleic acid (RNA)	Deoxyribonucleic acid (DNA)

Hydrolysis of DNA and RNA under controlled conditions yields *nucleotides*, which can be regarded as the basic unit of nucleic acids just as amino acids are the basic unit of the proteins and monosaccharides of the polysaccharides. **Further hydrolysis of *nucleotides* yields *nucleosides*** and eventually phosphate, a sugar and number of purine and pyrimidine bases. Nomenclature and components of nucleic acids have been described in Table 5.1.

Our understanding regarding the nucleic acids has grown tremendously in the recent years. Several top scientists of the world's top laboratories are working day and night on 'nucleic acids', amongst whom good contributories are:

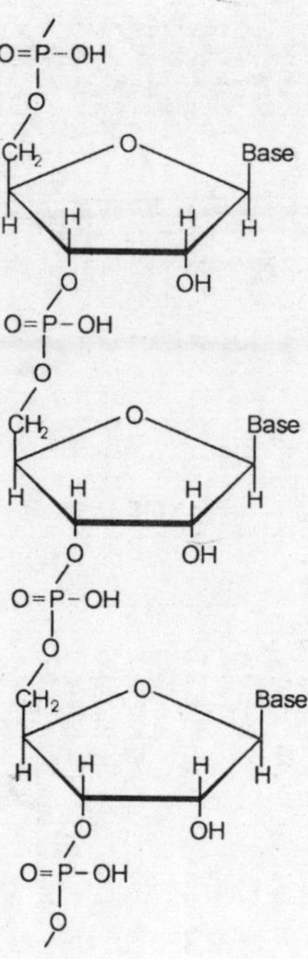

Fig. 5.1 : Part of the molecule of RNA

(i) Miescher,
(ii) A.R Todd,
(iii) **Har Gobind Khorana (Nobel Prize in 1968)***
(iv) Wilkins, (Nobel Prize in 1962)
(v) Watson, (Nobel Prize in 1962)
(vi) Crick, (Nobel Prize in 1962)

Table 5.1 : Nomenclature and Components of nucleic acids

RNA (cytoplasmic nucleic acid)	**DNA (nuclear nucleic acid)**
Polymer: (base-rib-phosphate)$_n$	(base-deoxyrib-phosphate)$_n$
Nucleotide : base-ribose— O—P(=O)—OH, with OH on P	base-deoxyrib — O — P(=O) — OH, with OH on P
Nucleoside: base-ribose-OH	base-deoxyrib-OH
Purine : adenine, guanine	adenine, guanine
Pyrimidines : cytosine, uracil and others	cytosine, thymine

* *He succeeded in synthesizing the first wholly artificial gene which contained in it 77 nucleotides. He was of Indian origin, later settled in U.S.*

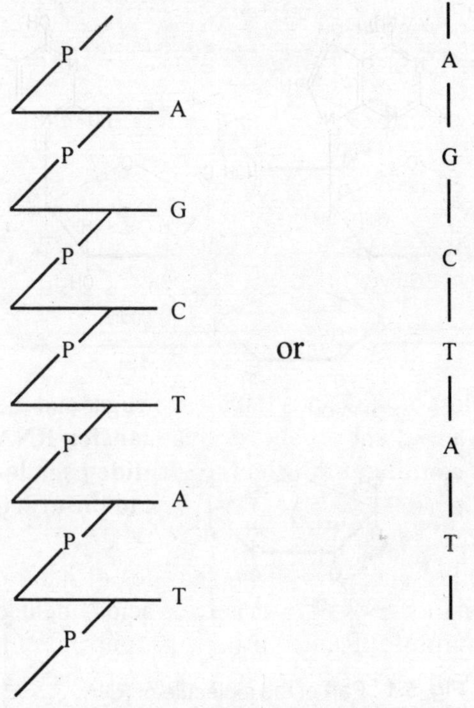

Fig. 5.2: Shorthand notation to exhibit the base sequence of a nucleic acid

(vii) Davidson,
(viii) Chargaff, etc.

Functions of the Nucleic Acids

(i) Nucleic acids are responsible for the direction of metabolism throughout the life of a cell.
(ii) They direct the synthesis of proteins.
(iii) They control the synthesis of enzymes.
(iv) They are responsible for the transfer of genetic information from one offspring to another.
(v) Nucleic acids, in fact, contribute the essential substance of the genes and the apparatus by which the genes act.
(vi) For the clinician, they are of major interest as they are undoubtedly involved in the causation of cancers **(malignancies).**

Chemical Composition

Nucleic acids fall into two principal classes according to the nature of the sugar they contain:

(i) the deoxyribonucleic acid, i.e., DNA which contains the sugar known as deoxyribose sugar, and
(ii) the ribonucleic acids i.e., RNAs which contain the sugar known as ribose.

RNA and DNA are polymers of nitrogenous bases, sugars, and phosphoric acid; thus

$$(\text{base-sugar-phosphate})_n$$

nucleic acid

where n is a large number.

The link between the polymer units is the phosphate diester bond as shown below:

$$-\text{sugar}-O-\overset{\overset{\displaystyle O}{\|}}{\underset{\underset{\displaystyle OH}{|}}{P}}-O-\text{sugar}-$$

phosphate diester bond

Nucleotides

When the phosphate diester bond gets hydrolyzed, the monomeric units of nucleic acids are separated which consist of a nitrogenous base, a sugar and a phosphate; such a unit is called as a nucleotide as shown below:

$$\text{base}-\text{sugar}-O-\overset{\overset{\displaystyle O}{\|}}{\underset{\underset{\displaystyle OH}{|}}{P}}-OH$$

nucleotide

Nucleotides and nucleosides are named after the bases contained in their structure, as below:

Base	Nucleoside	Nucleotide
Adenine	Adenosine	Adenylic acid
Guanine	Guanosine	Guanylic acid
Uracil	Uridine	Uridylic acid
Cytosine	Cytidine	Cytidylic acid
Thymine	Thymidine	Thymidylic acid

If the base is linked to deoxyribose, then the names are modified so that a nucleoside consisting of adenine and deoxyribose would be called deoxyadenosine. As well as the nucleotides indicated, a number of biologically important nucleotides such as adenosine di- and triphosphate (ADP and ATP), guanosine di- and triphosphate (GDP and GTP) and nicotinamide adenine dinucleotide (NAD) are known to occur in the free state.

Adenosine 5′-triphosphate (ATP)

Nucleosides

When the ester bond between the sugar and the phosphate group in a nucleotide is hydrolyzed, a fragment consisting of a nitrogenous base and a sugar moiety is obtained which is called as a *nucleoside,*

base – sugar – OH

nucleoside

The important examples of nucleosides include adenosine and uridine whose structures are as given below; others are guanosine, thymidine, cytidine, etc.

Adenosine

Uridine

Most of the bonds linking the sugar and the base are as shown above, **but transfer RNA does contain an unusual nucleotide pseudo-uridine in which ribose is linked to the uracil via the 5 position.**

Other examples of nucleosides of natural origin (not derived from nucleic acids) include the important antibiotics like puromycin, tubercidin, nebularine, cordycepin, etc., which are derived from moulds, fungi and also from a group of compounds isolated from sponges, among which the important examples are those of

Puromycin

Tubercidin

spongothymidine, spongouridine, and spongosine, etc.

Puromycin is an antibiotic which was discovered in **1952** in the culture filtrates of ***Streptomyces alboniger.*** It has got wide spectrum of activity but unfortunately is not being used in human beings because of its toxic nature to the mammalian cells.

The Pentose Sugars

Sugars found in the nucleic acids are either D-ribose as in RNA or D-2-deoxyribose as in DNA, structure of which are as given below. The 'type' of the presence of pentose sugars in nucleic acids is the basis of its classification, **if they contain 'ribose' sugar in its structure, then they are known as ribonucleic acids and if deoxyribose then deoxyribonucleic acid.**

The structures of these sugars are as given below:

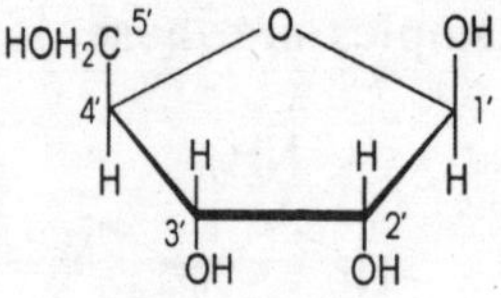

β-D-Ribofuranose

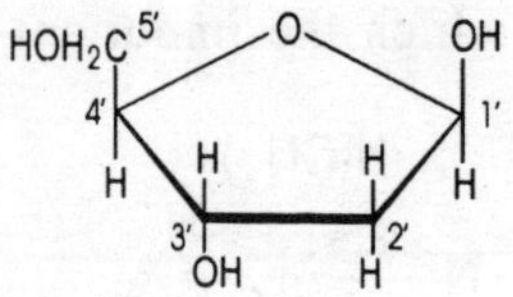

β-D-2- Deoxyribofuranose

The carbon atoms on the sugars are denoted as 1', 2', etc. in order to differentiate them from the atoms of the bases.

Nitrogenous Bases

The formulae of the main nitrogenous bases found in the nucleic acids are as shown below:

Purines

Adenine and guanine are substituted purines and remain present in all nucleic acids.

Small quantities of other bases have been detected in nucleic acids from some sources. It should be noted that both purine and pyrimidine bases can exist in the keto or enol form (Fig. 5.3).

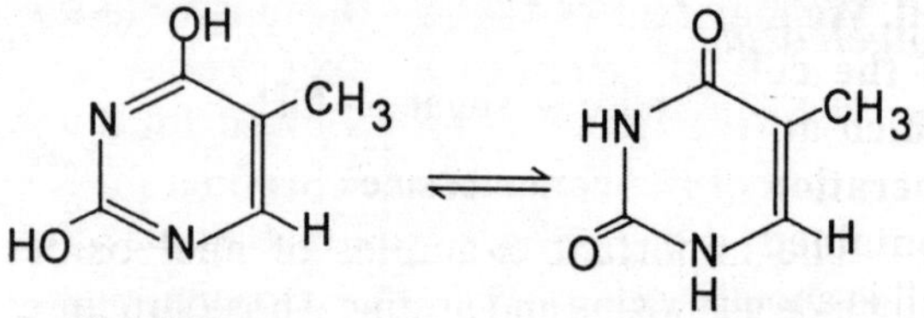

Purines

Purine

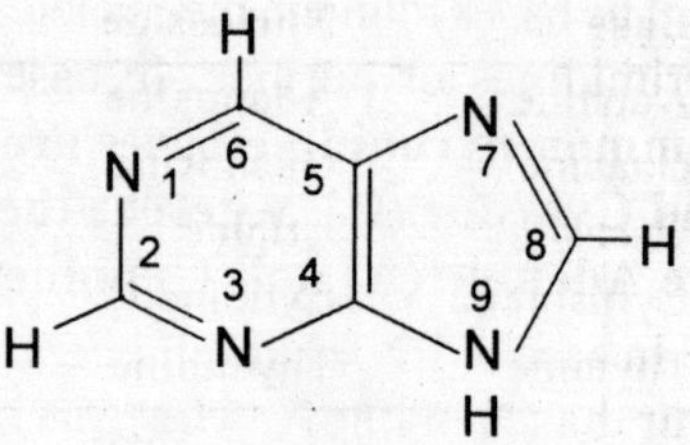

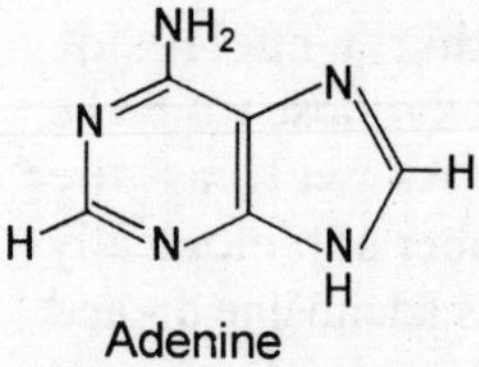

Adenine

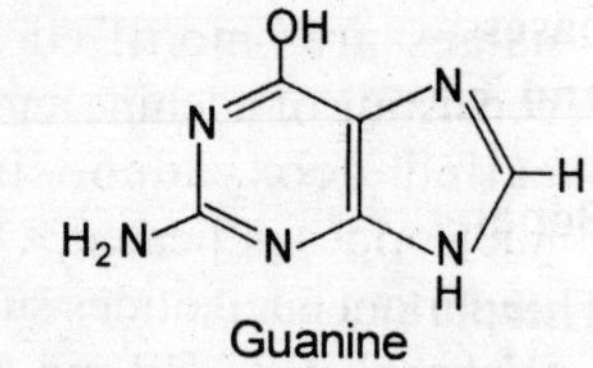

Guanine

Pyrimidines

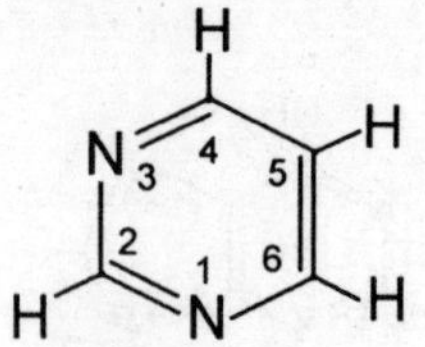

Pyrimidine

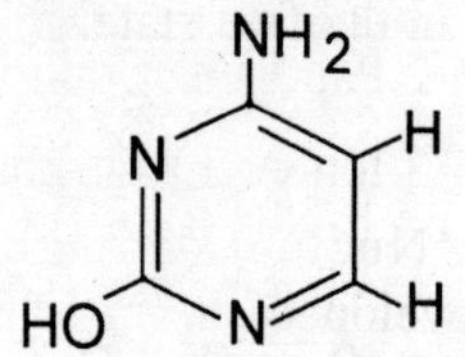

Cytosine

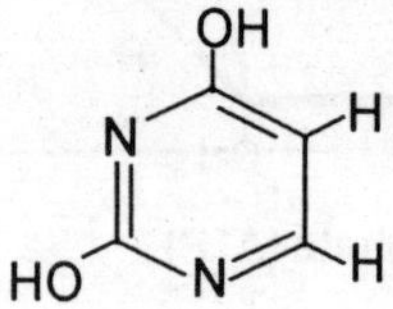

Uracil

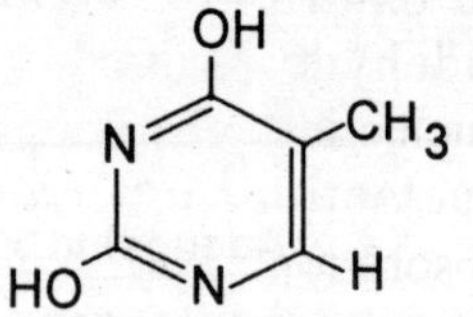

Thymine

Enol form

Keto form

Fig. 5.3 : The keto and enol forms of thymine

The bases found in the nucleic acids are either pyrimidines or purines. In case of DNA, **the common pyrimidine bases are Thymine (T) and Cytosine (C); whereas the purine bases are Adenine (A) and Guanine (G).**

In case of RNAs, they generally contain only four bases namely, **the purine bases are Adenine and Guanine and the pyrimidine bases are Uracil (not Thymine as in DNA), and Cytosine.**

Separation and Determination of Nucleotides

There are various methods by which nucleotides can be separated and determined, out of which the following three methods are generally used:

1. Paper chromatography,
2. Paper electrophoresis, and
3. Ion-exchange chromatography

Nucleotides can be identified on the developed chromatogram either by ultraviolet (UV) light absorption (dark spots) or fluorescence (light spots). Ribose derivatives can be oxidized by sodium iodate on paper by aldehyde reagents. The areas containing nucleotides can be cut out and the individual nucleotides determined quantitatively by absorption spectroscopy.

DEOXYRIBONUCLEIC ACID (DNA)

The genetic information of a cell is confined in its complement of deoxyribonucleic acid (DNA). This genetic information scientifically is known as the genome of the cell. We may regard DNA as the master tape of the cell, the computer programme in which all the information required for the operation of the cell and its reproduction is contained. It has been studied that an *E. coli* cell is about 1 μm long; its DNA is 1 mm long. **This DNA encodes for atleast 4,000 proteins and contains many regions that regulate the expression of these proteins.**

DNA is intimately associated with the genetic material of the cell. In some micro-organisms, a single strand of DNA seems to be the store for the genetic information; but, in higher organisms, the DNA is present as nucleoprotein in the chromosomes. The amount of DNA in the cell of a particular species is constant, whereas the germ cells with half the number of chromosomes contain half the DNA present in other cells. **The DNA occurs almost exclusively in the nucleus and in minute quantity in the mitochondria.** It plays following ***biological roles:***

Biological Roles of DNA

(i) The function of DNA is to act as a *store house of genetic information and to control the synthesis of proteins in the cell.*

(ii) *Cell replication:* Hereditary characteristics are passed on to daughter cells through replication of DNA; during cell division, the two strands of DNA get separated and free nucleotides are attached to each strand according to the *'base pairing'* rule. The nucleotides are then probably 'zipped' together by the action of a DNA polymerase to give two identical molecules of the original DNA (Fig. 5.4).

(iii) *Control of protein synthesis:* It is now clear from a number of experiments that the sequence of bases in the nuclear DNA determines the proteins synthesized in the cytoplasm of the cell. The ***'genetic code'*** is such that 3 non-overlapping bases known as a *'codon*" code for each amino acid. The code is 'degenerate' in that more than one triplet may code for a particular amino acid. The DNA therefore acts in the first instance as a *'template'* on which the messenger RNA (m-RNA) gets synthesized. The m-

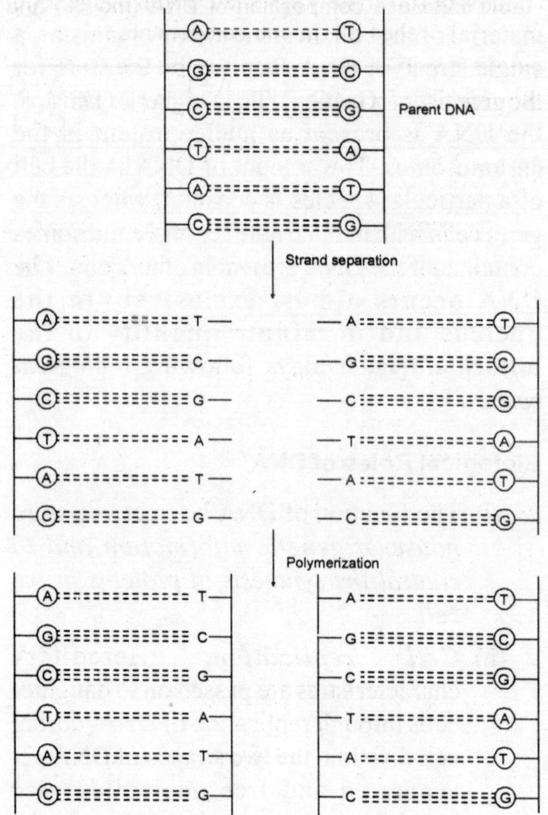

Fig. 5.4 : The replication of DNA (A, G, T and C represent the nucleotides on the newly synthesized strand of DNA).

RNA, with a complementary base sequence to the nuclear DNA, then carries the genetic message from the nucleus to the *protein synthesizing system on the ribosomes.*

Structure of DNA

For convenience, we may study the structure of DNA into three stages nan. ly:

(a) Primary structure,

(b) Secondary structure, and

(c) Tertiary structure

(a) Primary Structure

DNA is a linear polymer (double stranded in its native state) of 21-deoxynucleotide residues which remain linked to each other by phosphodiester bonds between 3' and 5' positions of the 2'-deoxyribosyl moieties (Fig. 5.5).

The most common bases in DNA are:

(a) Adenine

(b) Thymine

(c) Guanine, and

(d) Cytosine

The *primary structure* of DNA is referred to as the linear sequence of nucleotide residues comprising the polydeoxyribonucleotide chain.

The primary structure of DNA molecules from various sources range from a few thousand residues in some viruses to 10^6 residues in bacteria to 10^9 residues in a human chromosomal DNA. A single molecule of bacterial DNA is nearly 1 mm long; whereas the length of a DNA molecule of a human chromosome is estimated to be 8.2 cm. **Molecular weights and lengths of DNA from various sources vary widely.**

Base Composition of DNA

Base composition of DNA remained unidentified after its discovery for nearly a century because of the difficulty of separating the products of DNA hydrolysis from one another. Invention of paper chromatography provided a mean to overcome this difficulty and E. Chargaff was the first scientist to determine the base composition of many species in 1950. The base composition differs widely from one species to another. Each species has a characteristic base composition but every organ of higher organisms has the same base composition. Strikingly, for every organism the ratio of pyrimidines to purines, (A + G)/(C + T), is nearly unity as shown in Table 5.2.

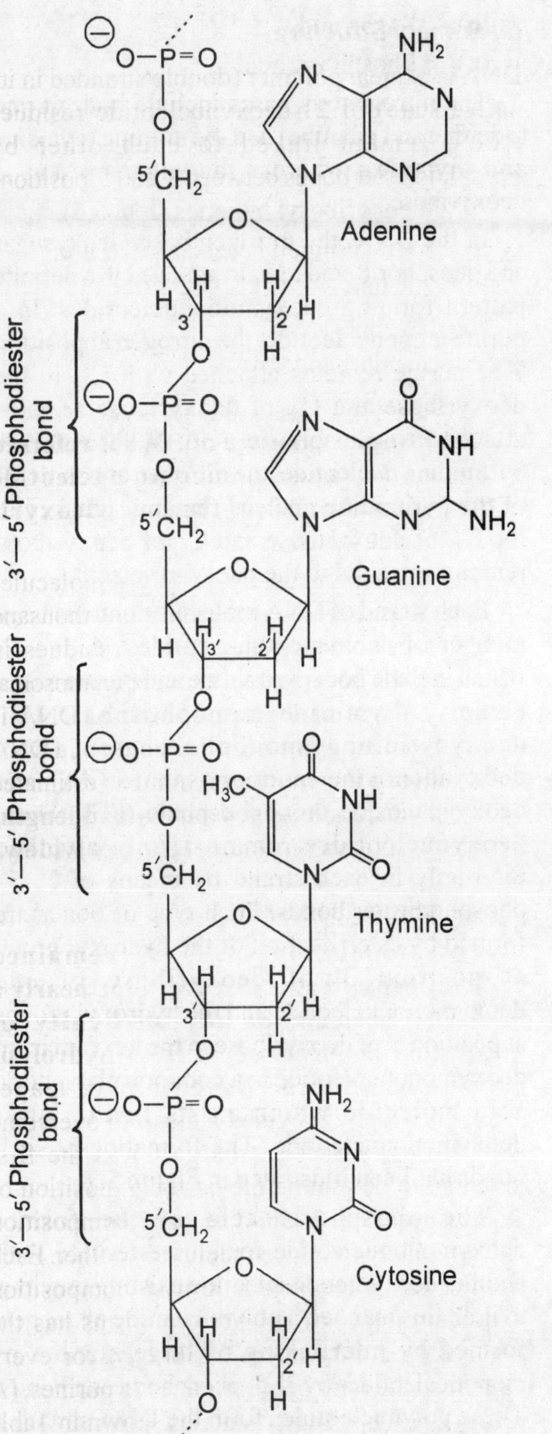

Fig. 5.5 : Covalent backbone of DNA

Table 5.2: Base composition of DNA (mol %) and ratios of various components

Source	A	G	C	T	$\frac{A+T}{G+C}$	A/T	G/C	$\frac{A+G}{C+T}$
Man	30.4	19.9	19.9	30.1	1.52	1.009	1.000	1.006
Ox	29.0	21.2	21.2	28.7	1.36	1.010	1.000	1.006

The mole percent ratio of guanine to cytosine (G/C) and adenine to thymine (A/T) are also nearly unity in each case as shown above. The (A + T)/(G + C) ratios, however vary widely.

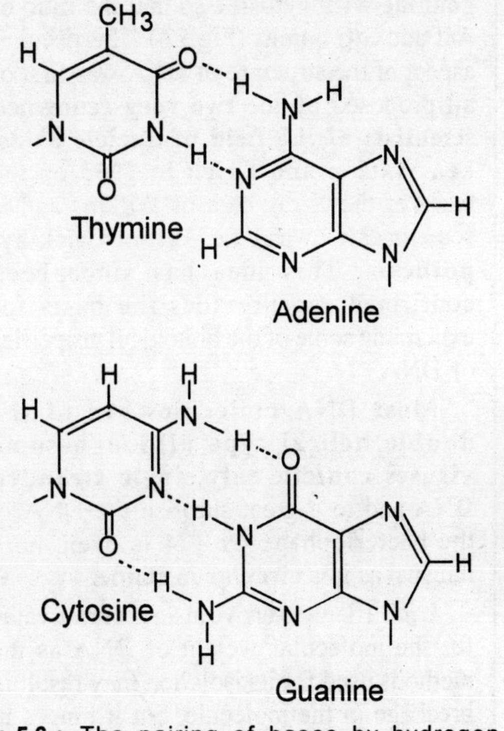

Fig. 5.6 : The pairing of bases by hydrogen bonding (- . - - - - -) as in DNA

(b) Secondary structure

Scientists Watson and Crick were responsible for deducing the structure of DNA in 1953; they were awarded Nobel prize in 1962 for this brilliant discovery. One key to the structure of DNA was Chargaff's observation that purines and pyrimidines are present in DNA in equimolar quantities.

DNA is a very complicated molecule which consists of two chains of polynucleotides which are interwoven in the form of a **spiral structure** which is stabilized by hydrogen bonding between particular base pairs. The stereochemistry of the bases is such that **adenine pairs with thymine and guanine with cytosine** so that the ratio of A/T and G/C is unity (Fig.5.6). This peculiar aspect of the structure of DNA was first of all proposed by the **two very renowned scientists of the field of nucleic acids, i.e., Watson and Crick in 1953** on the basis of the X-ray data of Wilkins and is sometimes known as the **Watson-Crick hypothesis.** This idea has since been confirmed and provides the basis for explaining some of the biological properties of DNA.

Most DNA molecules are of the double helical type although some viruses contain only single stranded DNA and to a great surprise the DNA in the bacteriophage **ϕx** 174 is even more unusual as it is **circular in shape.**

It is difficult to arrive at an accurate value for the molecular weight of DNA as the methods used for its isolation may result in breakage in the molecule, but it ranges in millions.

Deoxyribonucleic acids are very complex molecules which possess a molecular weight ranging from 6-100 millions. They are elongated in shape and consist mostly of two strands which remain coiled in a parallel helical manner.

Complete hydrolysis of DNA leads to the formation of the following:

(a) Various nitrogenous bases,

(b) Sugar, and

(c) Phosphoric acid

The nitrogenous bases include both purine (adenine and guanine) and pyrimidine (cytosine and thymine); whereas the sugar present is deoxyribose.

In the DNA, the nitrogen base, deoxysugar and phosphoric acid remain attached in a definite pattern forming deoxymononucleotides. In a purine mononucleotide, the nitrogen at position 9 of purine remains attached with C_1, in the deoxyribose and $C_{5'}$ of deoxyribose remains attached to phosphoric acid. Whereas, in a pyrimidine nucleotide, the nitrogen at position 1 of the pyrimidine nucleus remains attached to the C_1, of deoxyribose and $C_{5'}$ of deoxyribose remains attached to the phosphoric acid.

Each strand of DNA molecule contains large number of deoxymononucleotides (d- B-S-P) which include both pyrimidine and purine bases, namely, thymidine monophosphate (T), deoxycytidine monophosphate (dC), deoxyadenosine monophosphate (dA) and deoxyguanosine monophosphate (dG). These deoxynucleotides remain firmly attached internally in each strand by means of 3', 5'-phosphodiester bonds. Such type of bonds are formed by esterification of the hydroxyl group at position 3' of deoxyribose of one deoxymononucleotide and the hydroxyl groups at position 5' of deoxyribose in the next adjacent deoxymononucleotide to a common phosphoric acid molecule which exists in the latter deoxymononucleotide. The formation of such bonds has been illustrated in Figure 5.7.

The phosphoric acid of the former deoxymononucleotide remains esterified with another deoxymononucleotide existing previous to it. In this manner, a polynucleotide chain gets formed by interlinking of large number of mononucleotides by 3', 5'-phosphodiester bonds. These polynucleotides form the DNA strand.

In different DNAs, the sequence of

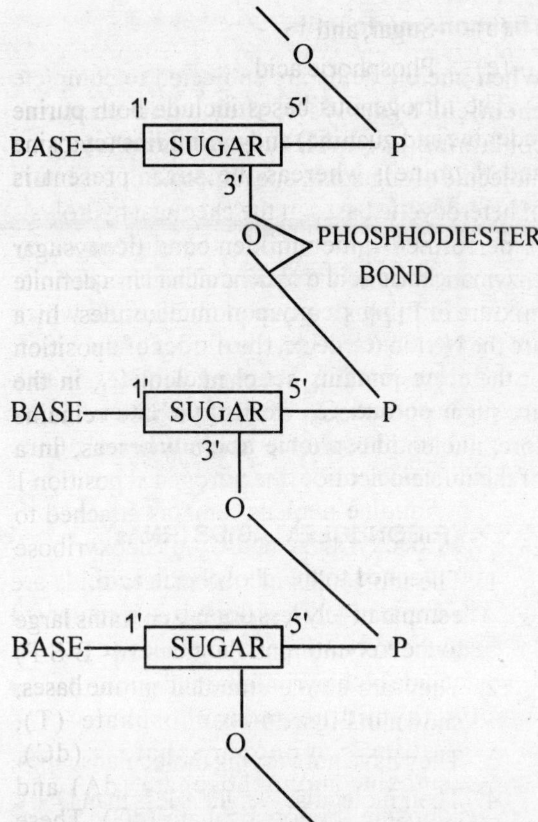

Fig. 5.7: Formation of 3', 5'-phosphodiester linkages between mononucleotides

deoxymononucleotides is found to vary. The specific properties exhibited by the DNA - molecules are governed by this sequence. The two strands of DNA molecule are complementary to each other. Their base sequence is interdependent which follows the base pairing rule.

In a double-helix, formed by parallel coiling of the two strands along a longitudinal axis, the placing of the bases is such that **adenine is placed in the plane of thymine and guanine is placed in the plane of cytosine or vice versa, the so called base-pairing rule.**

(c) *Tertiary structure*

The two strands are kept in position and the structure is stabilized by means of hydrogen bonds, each amino group being joined to a keto group, i.e., adenine to thymine, guanine to cytosine, etc. Formation of two hydrogen bonds between adenine and thymine; and three hydrogen bonds between guanine and cytosine is maximally possible. The formation of the H-bonds between such bases has been shown in Figure 5.8.

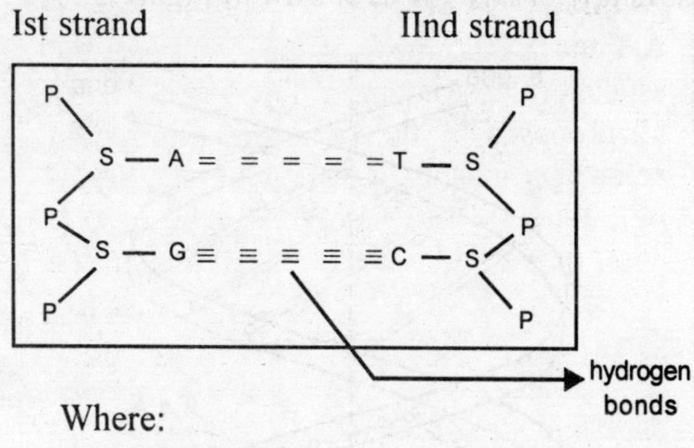

Where:

A = Adenine, G = Guanine, T = Thymine, C = Cytosine, S = 2-deoxyribose, and P = Phosphoric acid

Fig. 5.8: To show formation of H-bonds between purine and pyrimidine bases

The molar content of adenine equals the molar content of thymine; and the molar content of guanine equals that of cytosine in DNA The ratio of adenine plus thymine to guanine plus cytosine however is not equal and varies from DNA to DNA obtained from different sources.

DNA (Fig. 5.9) helix consists of several million turns. The two strands of a DNA helix run parallel but in opposite directions. **The double helical structure is although quite stable but may be denatured by heat treatment or extremes of pH.** Denaturation of DNA results in uncoiling of the two strands as a result of which two separate chains are formed; the molecular weight also gets halved and absorbance at 260mμ (characteristic of nucleic acids) also gets increased.

DNAs are mainly present in the nucleus of the cells and are the carriers of hereditary characters. DNA can reproduce itself by the phenomenon of replication. **Genes are composed of the DNA proteins which are believed to be associated with the mechanism of retention of memory in the brain.** Viruses which infect the bacterial cells are also purely DNA-proteins. Double helical structure of DNA is as shown in Figure 5.9.

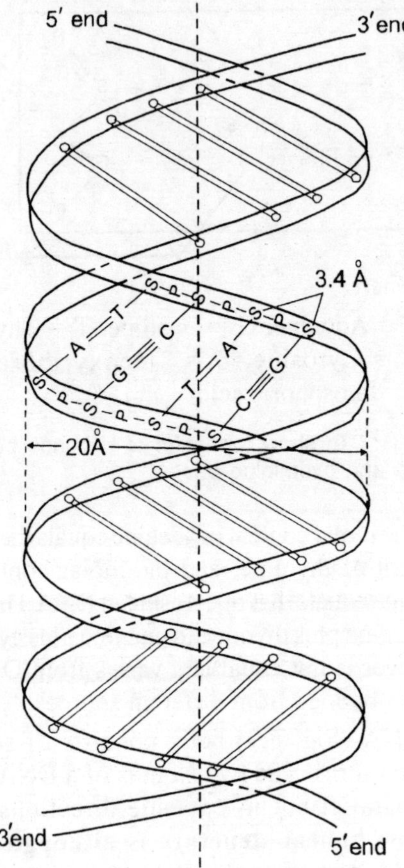

Where: (i) P means phosphate diester

(ii) S means deoxyribose sugar

(iii) A = T is the adenine thymine pairing

(iv) G ≡ C is the guanine cytosine pairing

Fig. 5.9 : Double helical structure of DNA

The monomeric units

When nucleic acids are subjected to complete chemical hydrolysis; they yield mixtures containing one molecule of phosphate, one molecule of sugar and one molecule of a mixture of heterocyclic bases. If the chemical hydrolysis is performed under milder conditions or by enzymatic means, one obtains either an equimolar mixture of Pi plus a group of nucleosides which are the N-ribo (or deoxyribo) sides of the bases, or the corresponding set of nucleotides, which are sugar phosphate esters of the latter. Therefore, nucleotides are the true monomeric units of the nucleic acids.

RIBONUCLEIC ACIDS (RNAs)

1. The molecules of ribonucleic acids are comparatively less organized if compared to their counterpart molecules i.e., DNA.
2. They are single stranded molecules as shown in Figure 5.10.
3. They have got varying molecular shapes.
4. Their molecular weight is less than DNA.
5. They have been shown to possess 60-6,000 mononucleotides in their molecules.
6. Complete hydrolysis of ribonucleic acids yields a mixture of purines, pyrimidines, sugar and phosphoric acid. The purines found in the hydrolysates are generally adenine and guanine whereas the pyrimidines are cytosine and uracil.
7. Certain purines and pyrimidines are also sometimes found in some RNAs which include:
   (i) 5-methylcytosine,
   (ii) 5-hydroxymethylcytosine
   (iii) 1-methylguanine,
   (iv) 2-methylamino-6-hydroxypurine,
   (v) 6-methylaminopurine, and
   (vi) 6-dimethylaminopurine.

RNA molecule consists of a single strand of nucleic acid in the form of a random coil with only limited regions of base pairing, therefore, the simple relationship of A/U = G/C = 1 does not hold true for most forms of RNA. The molecular weight of transfer RNA is nearly 25,000, whereas other forms of RNA have a high molecular weight of a million or near about.

RNA is distributed throughout the cell, most of which remains present in cytoplasm as soluble and ribosomal RNA,but about 10% is found in the nucleus with minute quantities being also present in the mitochondria. There are three types of RNA present in the cells of higher organisms, viz :

(i) messenger RNA (m-RNA),
(ii) ribosomal RNA (r-RNA),
(iii) transfer RNA or soluble RNA (t-RNA or s-RNA).

All the above RNAs remain actively involved in the synthesis of protein.

8. The sugar in all types of RNAs has been identified to be a pentose sugar named as D- ribose.
9. Different mononucleotides existing ordinarily in the RNAs are:
   (i) adenylic acid (A),
   (ii) uridylic acid (U),
   (iii) guanylic acid (G), and
   (iv) cytidylic acid (C)

The sequence of these mononucleotides varies from RNA to RNA. **Different mononucleotides in a RNA strand are interlinked by the 3',5'phosphodiester bonds which are formed in a similar manner as in DNA molecules.**

Types of RNAs

At present, following four types of RNAs are known to exist:

(a) m-RNA (messenger RNA),
(b) t-RNA (transfer RNA) or S-RNA (soluble RNA),
(c) r-RNA (ribosomal RNA), and
(d) viral RNA

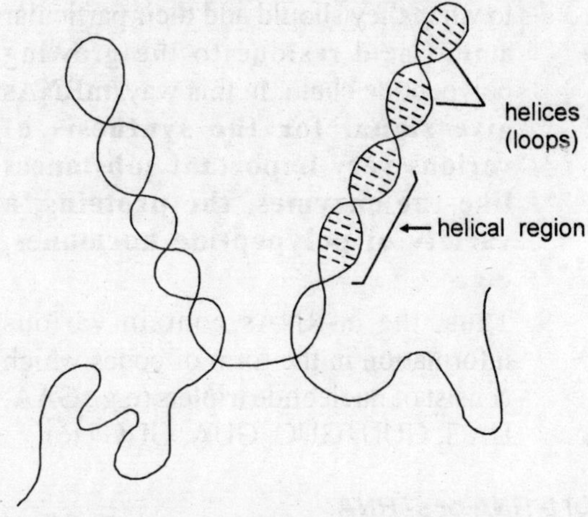

Fig 5.10 : Single stranded helical structure of a RNA molecule. The helical regions are stabilized and maintained in their shapes by A to U & G to C interactions; such interactions (bindings)are maintained by H-bonds.

(a) m-RNA

1. These nucleic acids exhibit highest molecular weight amongst all RNA.
2. Their M.W. ranges from 2-5 lacs.
3. They are highly elongated molecules.
4. They possess varying molecular shapes.
5. They are very short lived.
6. They are synthesized as a result of transcription of the DNA molecules within the nucleus and their base sequence strongly resembles to one of the corresponding DNA strand; the difference occurs only in a pyrimidine base. **In place of thymine, m-RNA**

contains uracil.

7. These have been shown to contain 60-6,000 mononucleotides in their molecules.
8. **They are known as "informational molecules" which carry message from nuclear DNA to the site of protein synthesis i.e. ribosomes,** informing various aminoacyl-t RNAs as to when they should add their particular amino acid residue to the growing polypeptide chain. In this way, **mRNAs give signal for the synthesis of various very important substances like the enzymes, the proteins, a variety of polypeptide hormones, etc.**
9. Thus, the m-RNAs contain various information in the form of codes which consist of nucleotide triplets (e.g., GAA, UAG, GUU, GUC, GUA, GUG etc).

(b) t- RNA or s- RNA

This is also known as soluble RNA (s-RNA); it constitutes nearly 10-20 per cent of total RNAs of the cell. Its M.W. ranges from 20,000 to 40,000 and it bears 70 to 80 mononucleotides in its molecule.

They are found in the soluble fraction of tissue homogenates after centrifugation at high speed i.e. 100,000 x g. There is evidence of the existence of atleast 21 transfer RNAs, each being specific for each naturally existing amino acid. It has been further studied that many amino-acids have more than one different t-RNA. Their main function is just to get attached with the activated amino acid and to carry it to the site of protein synthesis i.e. ribosomes so that it be added to the growing polypeptide chain.

Besides the presence of regular bases i.e. adenine, guanine, uracil and cytosine, t-RNAs have been found to contain some very unusual bases like ribothymidine, dihydrouracil, inosine, dihydrouridine, pseudouridine etc., which possess an unusual linkage between the sugar ribose and the base.

Messenger RNA

The first step in the synthesis of protein is the transfer of genetic message of the DNA to messenger RNA, the process is known as **'transcription'.**

The messenger RNA migrates into the cytoplasm and it is here, in association with ribosome and transfer RNA, **that the 4 letter code is converted to the 20 letter code of proteins. This stage is known as 'translation'.** Part of the DNA strand is only transcribed, so that m-RNA is smaller than the nuclear DNA. The actual molecular weight of a particular m-RNA is determined by the number of amino acid residues in the protein being synthesized, but is often of the order of a million or so. The mRNA, unlike the other forms, is metabolically unstable.

Transfer RNA

Each amino acid has a specific t-RNA which transfers the activated amino acid to the site of protein synthesis. Unlike the other forms of RNA, transfer ribonucleic acids have low molecular weights and are made up of relatively few nucleotides. The complete sequence of nucleotides has been determined for some t-RNAs and speculations made about the **'recognition sites'** on the molecule. There are two of these sites on each t-RNA molecule, one that identifies a particular amino acid and the other which recognizes and binds to the triplet base on the codon. This triplet of bases on the t-RNA is known as an **anti-codon.** All t-RNAs have the same terminal group of bases CCA and it is the adenine that reacts with the activated amino acid.

The molecule of alanine-t-RNA has been fully studied which is a single stranded molecule. Its structure resembles to that of clover-leaf (clover is a kind of grass) and is as shown below. This has been confirmed by x-ray diffraction techniques.

All transfer RNAs have been found to possess a terminal adenosine which bears a free hydroxyl group at 2' or 3' position of ribose and cytidylic acid at second and third positions. (Fig. 5.11).

Studies have also revealed that t-RNA molecules have a complex structure with extensive internal base-pairing (Figure 5.11). The following points are common to all known t-RNA structures:

1. Guanosine at the 5′-terminal, and the sequence of CCA at the 3'-terminal. The amino acid becomes attached through its carboxyl group, by an ester link to a ribose hydroxyl group of the 3'-terminal adenosine.
2. A 'DHU' loop of 8-12 unpaired bases, which always contains an unusual base called as dihydrouracil.
3. A loop of 7 unpaired bases, containing the sequence Ψ CG, where Ψ is pseudouridine.
4. A loop of seven unpaired bases containing the anticodon which always has uridine base at its 5'-side, and a purine, often methylated on its 3'-side.
5. A smaller loop of variable size is found between the T ψ CG loop and the anticodon loop as shown in the Fig. 5.11).

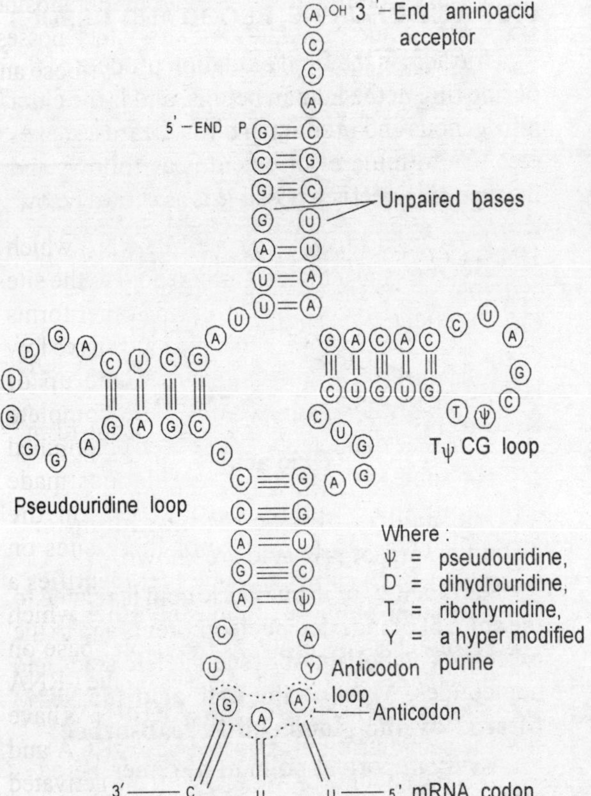

Fig. 5.11 : A possible structure of alanine-t-RNA

(c) r-RNA

These RNAs constitute nearly 50 to 60 per cent of the total ribonucleic acid of the cells and are single stranded molecules which are highly elongated. The r-RNA strands are found to be helical at certain portions. The helical portion exhibits hydrogen bonding as per base-pairing rule.

Most of the r-RNA is found to be combined with proteins in macro molecular aggregates called as ribosomes which are found in the cytoplasm and on the cytoplasmic surface of granular endoplasmic reticulum. They are also often called *cytoribosomes.* On the granular endoplasmic reticulum, 5-8 ribosomes are linked by a m-RNA strand to form a linear cluster called **polyribosome** or **polysome** (Fig. 5.12).

Ribosomes may be characterized by their sedimentation constant. Ribosomes possess a sedimentation constant of 80 S and mass of 4.4×10^6 daltons. The 80 S ribosome is made up of two subunits namely a large subunit of 60 S and a small subunit of 40 S.

Primary structure of r-RNA referred to

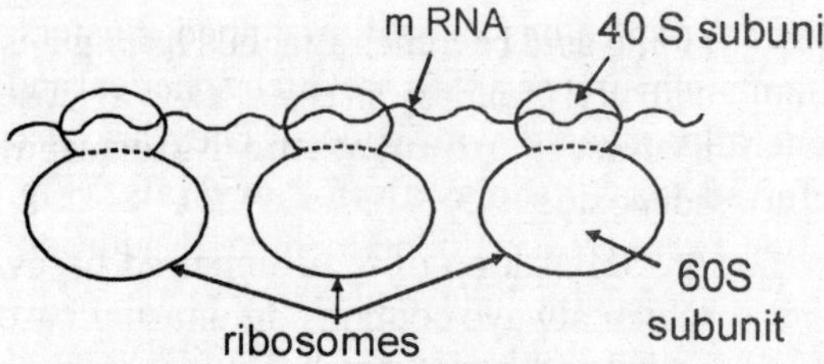

Fig. 5.12 : Polyribosome

the number and sequence of nucleotide (i.e., their bases). For instance, mammalian 5 S, 5.8 S, 18 S and 28 S rRNAs consist of about 120, 160, 1900 and 4,700 bases respectively

> **Ribosomal RNA**
>
> Ribosomes are microscopic particles in the cell which are visible only under the electron microscope with a fairly uniform composition of about 60% protein and 40% RNA. These are made up of two parts which can be separated in vitro. In animal cells, the 80 S ribosomes consist of 60 S and 40 S subunits of different chemical composition. Several ribosomes may be attached to a particular strand of m-RNA to form a **'polysome'**, rather like beads on a string.

which include mainly adenine, guanine, cytosine and uracil and a few pseudouridines. Besides the major bases, some minor nitrogenous bases may also be found.

Secondary structure of r-RNA consists of many short double-helical stems interconnected by single stranded loops. Each double-helical stem is formed by hydrogen bonds.

(d) Viral-RNA

Viruses which infect the animal and plant cells are mostly ribonucleoproteins. The percentage of RNA in such viruses ranges from 1 to 44. So far, the most studied viral-RNA is that of tobacco mosaic virus (TMV). **TMV is rod like in shape,** approximately 3,000 Å in length and 170 Å in diameter.

Viral-RNAs are single stranded helical molecules which generally possess molecular weight of nearly 2.2×10^6. However, the M.W. of different types of viral-RNAs may range from 1.2×10^6 to 32×10^6. They have been found to have 6,400 mononucleotides in their molecules. Each helix has a radius of 40 Å and has been found to contain some 49 nucleotides per turn. Adenylic acid remains present at the terminal nucleotide at each end. The fact that the RNA molecule remains covered by the protein molecule has been established. Careful separation of the protein part of viral nucleoproteins by the sophisticated latest techniques has revealed that it is the nucleic acid portion which is infective and not the protein portion.

URIC ACID OF URINE, BLOOD AND TISSUES

Uric acid is the final oxidation product of the purine ring in the human beings, and is the chief nitrogenous end product in birds, lizards, snakes etc. The formula of uric acid is as follows and the type of isomerism possible is as shown below:

```
HN – CO                      N═C.OH
 |    |                      |    |
OC   C–NH              HO–C    C–NH
 |    ||    >CO ⇌          ||    ||     >C.OH
HN–C–NH                      N – C–N  ═
Keto-form                              Enol-form
```

Uric acid

Uric acid is dibasic. Monosodium and disodium salts of uric acid are known.

The quantity of urinary uric acid is related to the amount of ingested nucleoproteins and to the extent of catabolism of tissue nucleic acids and nucleotides. **Most of the uric acid (85-90%) filtered by the glomeruli is reabsorbed.**

A very important point to be remembered is that in leukemia where the destruction of leukocytes takes place rapidly, output of uric acid gets tremendously increased. This is also true in the diseases of the liver and organs rich in nucleoproteins. There is always found disturbed metabolism of uric acid in the disease **'gout'**, the biochemistry of which is not yet very clear. It is seen that prior to an attack of gout, the urinary output of uric acid gets somewhat decreased and after the attack, it gets increased and remains increased for several days. Uric acid forms salts with sodium, calcium, magnesium, ammonium and potassium to give corresponding urates. Uric acid crystals may be easily distinguished in a sediment of urine sample under microscope (Figs. 5.13 and 5.14).

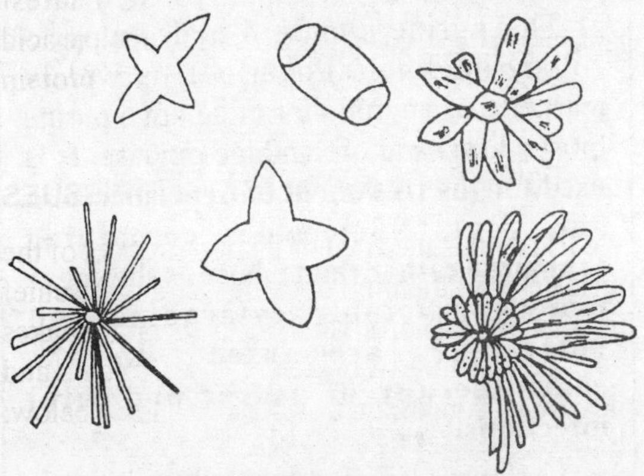

Fig. 5.13 : Uric acid crystals

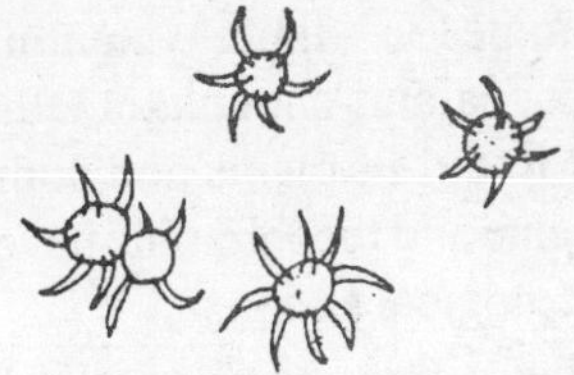

Fig. 5.14 : Ammonium urate crystals

Uric acid crystals when aggregate to form clusters, give rise to troublesome stones either in the kidneys or the bladder. The largest contribution in the formation of stones in the kidneys is that of calcium oxalate crystals; then phosphate crystals and then the least contribution is of uric acid crystals. The acid sodium urate may form clusters of needles or stellar-shaped clusters. Ammonium urate crystals are often spherical and generally covered with spikes. They are also referred to as **"thorn apple" crystals.** (Fig. 5.14). These are usually pigmented. In addition, they may exhibit many ***'bizarre'*** shapes. **The range of uric acid in normal human plasma is from 2 to 6 mg per cent, averaging 4 mg%. Values for females is a little on lower side averaging to about 3.5 mg% than their counterparts i.e. males who have an average value of about 4.5 mg%.** Red blood cells appear to contain about half as much uric acid as in plasma. Uric acid appears to be very irregularly distributed in tissues.

Following are the four types of "Gout'

1. ***Primary metabolic gout:*** This is caused due to an overproduction of uric acid, **due to genetic defects which promote the *de novo* purine synthesis. It is characterized by high levels of blood and urinary urates, rise in the miscible uric acid pool, accumulation of uric acid and urates in cartilages and joints, urate calculi in kidneys and renal damage.** These urate deposits are referred to as ***tophi.*** Such deposits in the joints provoke a painful inflammatory condition; for some reason it has been observed that the joints at the base of the big toe get especially susceptible; such a condition is known as **acute gouty arthritis.** The chronic inflammatory changes induced by the depositions of sodium urate tophi can generate **chronic gouty arthritis,** eventually resulting in the destruction of joints. The exact mechanism for the deposition of such urates is not yet clear.
2. ***Secondary metabolic gout:*** **It results from a secondary increase**

in the catabolism of purines in various states like prolonged fasting, leukaemia and polycythaemia etc. In this type, more breakdown of tissues takes place as a result of which system gets loaded with unusually high amount of nucleotides.

3. **Primary renal gout: This is caused due to the failure of urate excretion by the renal tubules which is due to the genetic deficiency of the urate transport system in renal tubules.** This type of gout does not involve any over production of uric acid.
4. **Secondary renal gout: This results from a failure of urate elimination in the glomerular filtrate** which is due to a generalized renal failure in the kidney disorder called **glomerulonephritis.**

Effect of Diet

Excretion of uric acid continues at a rather constant rate during starvation and purine-free diet due to the so-called endogenous (tissue) purine metabolism. **The ingestion of foods high in nucleoproteins, such as glandular organs, produce a marked increase; whereas a diet of milk, eggs, and cheese (very low in purine content), causes practically no elevation in uric acid excretion.**

Treatment of Gout

The classic treatment for gout is the administration of **colchicine, a drug which has got the tendency to interrupt the mitosis of leucocytes** and thus prevents development of inflammation. It is believed that the inflammation is a consequence of phagocytosis of urate crystals by the leucocytes that invade the

---

Cancers are made up of cells that continue to divide indefinitely. Since cell division requires a net synthesis of nucleic acids, there has been considerable effect made to find compounds that will selectively inhibit the formation of nucleic acids and check the uncontrolled growth of cancer.

Synthetic analogs of nucleobases, nucleosides and nucleotides are widely used in medical sciences and clinical medicine. One of the most important components of the oncologist's pharmacopeia is the group of synthetic analogs of purine and pyrimidine nucleobases and nucleosides.

The purine analog 4-hydroxypyrazolopyrimidine (allopurinol) is widely marketed as an inhibitor of de novo purine biosynthesis and of xanthine oxidase. **It is used for the treatment of hyperuricemia and gout. Nucieosides containing arabinose rather than ribose as the sugar moieties, notably cytarabine and vidarabine are used in the chemotherapy of cancer and viral infections.**

Caffeine (1,3,7 - trimethylxanthine) is found in coffee, tea and other plants; theobromine (3,7-dimethylxanthine) occurs in tea, cocoa and chocolate. Other purines are also found in plants and some of these like caffeine and theobromine have important pharmacological actions.

Nuclease may catalyze the hydrolysis specifically of DNA and RNA or they may attack both kinds of polynucleotide. These enzymes are generally of two types:

(i) **Exonucleases:** Which require a terminus at which to initiate hydrolysis, and

(ii) **Endonucleases:** Which do not require a terminus and which may attack at one or many sites within a polynucleotide.

---

affected area. Various compounds which promote the excretion of urate by the kidneys have been introduced as a means of controlling gout.

More recently, **a competitive inhibitor of xanthine oxidase has been developed to control gout by preventing the formation of urate** so that excess purines are excreted as hypoxanthine and xanthine; **this compound is known as allopurinol** and differs from hypoxanthine in the distribution of ring nitrogens. The rationale for its use is that hypoxanthine and xanthine will not precipitate in the joints. Hypoxanthine is more soluble than urate, although xanthine is not. Allopurinol also is not a completely safe drug.

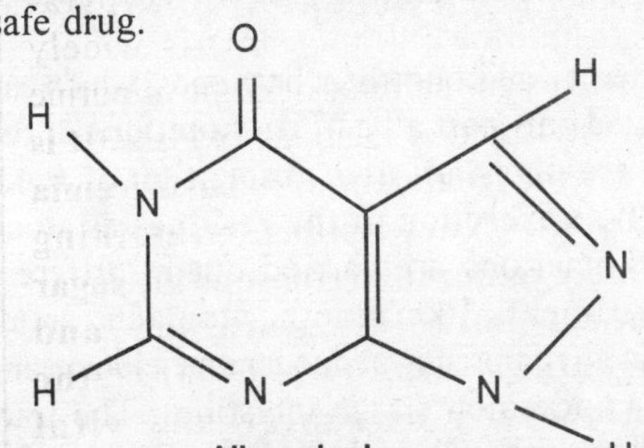

O
H H
N
N
H N N
H

Allopurinol

LESCH-NYHAN SYNDROME

Rare patients afflicted with a condition named as **Lesch-Nyhan Syndrome** may be met with once in a while; **this disease is caused by a hereditary deficiency of GMP pyrophosphorylase. This x-linked recessive disease is peculiarly horrifying because children suffering from it mutilate (damage their own organs/body parts) themselves.** Characteristically, they will bite off the tips of their own fingers or bite their lips if their hands are protected i.e. tied upon with some string/ rope etc. The aggressive attacks may be of serious nature like biting of others or as age advances, may use obscene abusive language. The pathos of the affliction is accentuated by the tendency of the children to be very likeable and open, quick to laugh and capable of warm affection. The climax is that such children get sometime terrified of their own aggression; they may even scream under the cover of fear and may bite their fingers seriously. Patients suffering from this disease have a tendency to excrete large quantities of uric acid - more per unit of body mass than is seen in any other condition. Their synthesis of purines is extraordinarily rapid (of course, they also become gouty as an additional distress).

The missing enzyme i.e. GMP pyrophosphorylase is responsible for the salvage (protection from loss) of free guanine and hypoxanthine by converting them to the corresponding nucleoside monophosphates. This enzyme is found to be more active in brain, which has over 10-fold more enzyme than does the liver.

Genetic Tracing of Fatherhood

DNA finger printing technology now available in our country in various upgraded well equipped laboratories is a very good mean in establishing **paternity.**

This technology is responsible in establishing fatherhood while dealing with cases where a husband has abandoned his wife. Previously there did not exist any specific law to take action against culprits who abandoned their wives and children taking advantage of absence of any legally admissible evidence of their marriage to these women. **This technology is a 'full proof' method in establishing paternity scientifically.**

CHAPTER 6

DIGESTION AND ABSORPTION

Introduction

The alimentary tract extends from the mouth to the anus (Fig. 6.1) which remains in contact to the external environment at both ends, which can be sealed only partially. **Main functions of the tract are digestion and absorption of food, as well as excretion of the residues as stool.** These functions are carried out in different compartments like mouth, stomach, small intestines (comprising of duodenum, jejunum and ileum) and colon (large intestine). The tract terminates in the sigmoid and the rectum.

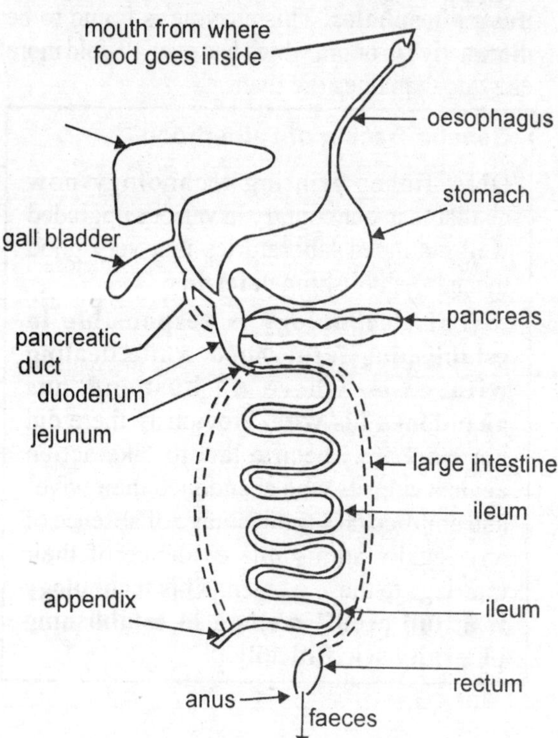

Fig. 6.1: Diagrammatic presentation of the alimentary tract

All movements and secretions are controlled by nerve impulses. An involuntary wave like contraction of muscles lining the walls of the tract (peristaltic movement) facilitates the passage of the food. The mucus present in the mucosal lining of the epithelial cells acts as a lubricant, and also protects these cells from being digested by the enzymes of the secretions from different glands. It further prevents the entry of infectious viruses and microbes into the body through these cells. The mucosal cells are regenerated very rapidly to compensate the physical and chemical damage during their function.

Only a small portion of the food we eat is in the proper form for absorption into the blood or the lymph system of the body. Such things as water, uncombined mineral salts, and uncombined vitamins may not need digestive action prior to absorption. Side by side, the bulk

A number of factors assist the digestive processes. Cooking of food produces several changes. It softens certain tissues, breaks the cellulose covering around starch granules allowing better access to digestive enzymes, partially hydrolyzes some food components, brings about coagulation of liquid proteins of eggs and other foods and also improves the flavour of some, which may result in increased flow of saliva and gastric juice.

Mastication greatly increases the surface area of food for better contact with the digestive juices. The most important factor in digestion, is of course, the action of the enzymes and other specific components of the digestive juices.

The enzymes and other compounds important in digestion are secreted by various glands of the body. The control of these secretions is nervous, hormonal or both.

of our food undergoes many chemical changes before the resulting molecules can be absorbed. The proteins and protein split products must be hydrolyzed to amino acids; the polysaccharides and the oligosaccharides to hexose sugars and the lipids to fatty acids and glycerol, in part at least. Other lipids are also hydrolyzed to smaller product molecules.

Digestion of Carbohydrates

Carbohydrates being used most by human beings in food consist of polysaccharides i.e. starch (vegetables, grains, cereals, pulses etc.) and glycogen (animal sources like liver, muscles etc.). To a lesser extent are the disaccharides i.e., lactose of milk and sucrose of molasses and the ordinary sugar. Other related compounds less commonly present are lactic acid, alcohol, pectins etc.

The digestive process involves the enzymatic hydrolysis of the poly and disaccharides to the simplest constituent units i.e., monosaccharides, consisting mainly of glucose with small amount of fructose and galactose. First of all ptyalin (an (α- amylase) secreted from the parotid glands in the mouth, hydrolyzes starch to maltose mainly with few other smaller polymers of glucose containing 3-9 units (e.g., maltotriose, dextrin). The action of ptyalin continues in the fundus of the stomach till the food is mixed with the gastric secretion producing a low pH at which ptyalin gets inactivated. However, this appears to cause at the most 30% digestion of starch. When the food passes into the duodenum and the upper jejunum, the pH gets raised by the bicarbonate in the pancreatic secretion. **Virtually, whole of the starch gets hydrolysed to maltose and other polymers in about 30 minutes by the action of pancreatic amylase which remains present in the pancreatic secretion. At this site, glycogen is also hydrolysed to smaller fragments due to the splitting of (α -1→ 4 linkages for which this amylase is specific.**

$$\text{Lactose} \xrightarrow{\text{(lactase)}} \text{glucose + galactose}$$

$$\text{Maltose} \xrightarrow{\text{(maltase)}} \text{glucose + glucose}$$

$$\text{Sucrose} \xrightarrow{\text{(sucrase)}} \text{glucose + fructose}$$

$$\text{Dextrin} \xrightarrow{\text{(dextrinase)}} \text{glucose (several molecules)}$$

Further digestion of maltose and other disaccharides as well as of small polymers of glucose takes place in the epithelial cells lining the intestinal lumen.Enzymes i.e., lactase, maltase, sucrase and dextrinase are found to be located in the membrane of the microvilli brush border and the sugars are hydrolysed as soon as they come in contact with these membranes.

In this way, the final product of the digestion of carbohydrates is almost wholly glucose with little fructose and galactose and are absorbed immediately after formation.

Another polysaccharide i.e., cellulose remains abundantly present in the vegetable food; but the enzyme necessary for its breakdown remains absent in humans, therefore, it's excreted as such in stool. Cellulose is a polymer of β - glucose; herbivorous animals i.e., cattles do possess the corresponding enzyme i.e., cellulase, therefore, they can digest it.

Absorption of Carbohydrates

Be it known that glucose is the most abundant monosaccharide available after digestion of carbohydrates; however, there may be found small amounts of other monosaccharides viz., fructose, galactose and perhaps mannose also. Some amount of the disaccharides, i.e., sucrose and maltose may also remain unhydrolysed. All these are absorbed easily through the intestinal mucosa. Glucose and galactose are also absorbed by the same process. The latest theory is that these carbohydrates are not absorbed by simple diffusion, but by the sodium ion dependant transport mechanism requiring special carrier protein. This is well established in case of glucose and galactose, whereas, other carbohydrates may have a facilitated diffusion mechanism with special carrier proteins. The disaccharides are hydrolysed into the monosaccharides by specific enzymes inside the epithelial cells and it is only the monosaccharides that are passed into the portal blood.

Fructose is absorbed much more slowly than glucose and galactose. It does not require any extra energy and more Na^+ ions. Some of it may be converted to glucose during absorption. Mannose and pentoses are absorbed even more slowly than fructose.

Digestion of Lipids

The most abundant fat in the human diet is triglycerides or neutral fats with smaller proportion of some phospholipids and cholesterol (mainly in the form of esters).

Fats are digested due to hydrolysis by the action of enzyme lipase into fatty acids plus glycerol; **in case of cholesterol ester, it is fatty acid + steroid.**

Gastric lipase digests small amount of fat in the stomach which is mostly tributyrin (butter fat). Most of the fat is digested in the intestines by pancreatic lipase which remains present in bulk in the pancreatic secretion. There is some enteric lipase also secreted in the intestine, the role of which is not important.

The enzyme lipase is soluble in water but its substrates, the lipids are water-insoluble. So lipase can attack on a lipid only at the water-oil interface. This is facilitated by emulsification of lipids by bile supplied from the liver, it is present in the aqueous medium of the intestinal lumen. Bile contains bile salts and phospholipids (mostly lecithin). These are in ionised form with negatively charged organic part and positively charged sodium ions. The organic ion behaves as an amphipathic lipid and its polar part is soluble in water. The nonpolar part is soluble in fat and is dissolved in the surface layer of the dietary fat globule, while the polar part remains outward dissolved in the aqueous medium (Fig. 6.2) which lowers the surface tension, and the fat globule becomes liable to easy fragmentation by the mechanical agitation of the peristaltic

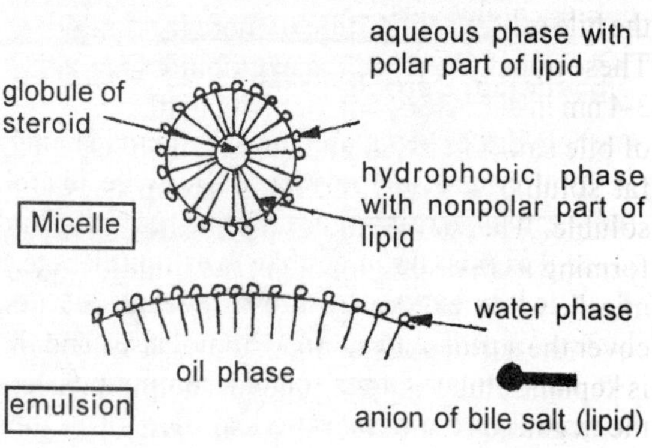

Fig. 6.2: Emulsification and micelle formation by bile acids

movement of the intestine. **As a result, an emulsion is formed by the dispersion of the minute fat globules in the aqueous medium, thus increasing the surface area of the fat by nearly 1000 fold.**

The attack of lipase, therefore gets immediately increased though it is not in a common solvent with its substrate. The action of pancreatic co-lipase and phospholipase A_2 (both are released from their precursor by the action of enzyme trypsin) in the presence of Ca^{2+} ions facilitates the firm binding of the enzyme pancreatic lipase to the substrate at the water-oil interface. In this way, by the action of pancreatic lipase ester bonds in the α - positions of a neutral fat i.e., a triglyceride are rapidly hydrolysed by firstly forming one molecule each of α–β- diglyceride and a fatty acid and finally one molecule each of β- monoglyceride and a fatty acid as shown below in Fig. 6.3. Now by the action of yet another enzyme known as intestinal isomerase β - monoglyceride is converted to α - monoglyceride which in turn by the action of enzyme intestinal lipase in the presence of water molecule in finally broken down to yield one molecule each of glycerol and a fatty acid (Fig. 6.3).

Products so formed are capable of blocking the digestion of more fat globules but as they are removed quickly in the micelles formed by the bile salts, the digestion of more fat continues. These micelles are spherical globules (Fig. 6.2), 3-4 nm in diameter, composed of 20-40 molecules of bile salt. The sterol nucleus of the bile salt is fat soluble whereas the polar group is water soluble. The sterol nuclei aggregate together, forming a small fat globule in the middle of the micelle while the polar groups projecting outward cover the surface of the micelle, whole of which is kept in solution in the aqueous medium due to the negative charge on the polar part.

Bile salt micelles do also have a tendency to transport the monoglycerides and fatty acids engulfed in them to the brush borders of the

α $CH_2 - O - CO - R$
|
β $CH_2 - O - CO - R$
|
α $CH_2 - O - CO - R$
Triglyceride

$+H_2O$ (Rapid) ↓ pancreatic lipase

$CH_2 - OH$
|
β $CH - O - COR + R.COOH$ (fatty acid)
|
α $CH_2 - O - COR$
α - β - diglyceride

$+H_2O$ (Rapid) ↓ pancreatic lipase

$CH_2 - OH$
|
β $CH - O - COR + R.COOH$ (fatty acid)
|
CH_2OH
β - monoglyceride

↓ intestinal isomerase (slow action)

α $CH_2 - O - COR$
|
$CH - OH$
|
CH_2OH
α - monoglyceride

$+H_2O$ ↓ intestinal lipase

CH_2OH
|
$CHOH + R.COOH$ (fatty acid)
|
CH_2OH
glycerol

Fig. 6.3 : Hydrolysis of triglycerides

epithelial cells and then the bile salts return to the chyme to be reused. The lipase present in the epithelial cells slowly hydrolyses the monoglyceride but not completely. Free fatty acids and unhydrolysed monoglycerides are absorbed. Fig. 6.3 represents the scheme of hydrolysis.

Phospholipase A_2 has got a tendency to hydrolyse ester bond of phospholipids at β - position forming free fatty acid and a lysophospholipid. Cholesterol esterase enzyme which is found in pancreas hydrolyses cholesterol esters yielding free fatty acid and free cholesterol. These digested products are also 'ferried' to the brush border by the bile salt micelle.

Absorption of Lipids

Lipids are mostly absorbed in the duodenum and the jejunum. Lipids are hydrolysed yielding a mixture of glycerol, diglycerides, monoglycerides and free fatty acids. Dietary lipids are never digested completely in the alimentary canal. Hydrolysis of the trigycerides to diglycerides and β - monoglycerides occurs easily but hydrolysis of the β - monoglycerides is relatively very difficult. The mixture of these intermediary hydrolytic products promotes the process of emulsification of the unhydrolysed dietary fats.

Glycerol is fairly water- soluble and hence no difficulty is faced in its absorption. As soon as glycerol is formed, it is quickly absorbed. Most of the glycerol is absorbed through the blood capillaries.

Generally, fatty acids up to the chain length of 10 carbon atoms are primarily absorbed through the blood capillaries but fatty acids of higher chain length are primarily absorbed through the lymphatic route. The low molecular weight fatty acids are absorbed without much difficulty but the complexity goes on increasing as the molecular weight of the fatty acids goes on increasing. This is due to the fact that low M.W. fatty acids are relatively hydrophilic whereas the high M. W. fatty acids are hydrophobic. The hydrophobic fatty acids can not be absorbed till these are brought into some soluble form. This is brought about by the formation of fatty acid-bile salt complexes which are more soluble and can be absorbed without much difficulty. Fatty acids can also be absorbed in combination of the steroids by forming more soluble esters. The fatty acid present in the β monoglycerides is hydrolysed within the mucosal cells by a distinct lipase which is found in these cells.

The short chain fatty acids (upto 10 carbon atoms) are transported directly into the blood stream in the free form and get bound to the plasma albumin. These fatty acids comprise nonesterified fatty acid (NEFA) fraction. The fate of the longer chain fatty acids is different. These are converted into triglycerides by intermediate formation of the phosphatidic acids and then carried away by the lymphatic system to the venous blood. The triglyceride thus synthesized in the mucosal cells are transported into the lymphatic circulation in two forms, namely, chylomicrons and invisible fatty particulates. **An enzyme lipoprotein lipase present in the blood stream is responsible for splitting of the complexes of chylomicrons and thus removes milky appearance of blood. Previously, the name clearing factor was given to this enzyme.**

The undigested fat is finely emulsified by the intestinal movement in the presence of bile salts, monoglycerides and diglycerides to give fine particles of the dimensions of 0.1 to 0.5 μ. These particles have been named as micelles. These micelles can be easily absorbed as such without undergoing any further hydrolysis. The micelles thus absorbed get accumulated in the space of the endoplasmic reticulum of the mucosal cells and are subsequently discharged into the intercellular space and corium of the villus. The diglycerides and monoglycerides absorbed in this manner are resynthesized into triglycerides.

These triglycerides are then transported by the lymphatic circulation. Thus, about 95% of the total ingested lipids may be absorbed by both the mechanisms.

Cholesterol has been shown to be absorbed mostly in the free state and not as esters as was being previously believed. However, absorption of cholesterol is followed by its re-esterification in the lymphatic circulation. Absorption of cholesterol has been reported to be facilitated by the presence of unsaturated fatty acids in the intestine. Bile salts are necessary for the absorption of cholesterol. Plant sterols are not absorbed. Out of the different sterols, cholesterol is absorbed most easily.

Absorption of different types of lipids gets markedly lowered in states like biliary-obstruction and liver dysfunction. **In some cases, an abnormal link gets established between lymphatic system and the urinary tract which results in the formation of milky urine and loss of the absorbed fats through urine. Such a condition is known as chyluria.**

Similarly, a connection might sometimes be established between lymphatic system and the pleural space as a result of which fats may pass into the pleural fluid giving it a milky appearance. Such a condition is clinically known as chylothorax.

Digestion of Proteins

Proteins are large polypeptide molecules coiled by weaker bonds in their tertiary structure. The Digestion of proteins involves gradual breakdown of this polypeptide by enzymatic hydrolysis into the constituent units i.e. amino acid molecules which are absorbed in the blood stream. The breaking of a peptide bond by a specific enzyme is shown below:

$$-NH-CO- \xrightarrow[+H_2O]{\text{enzyme}} -NH_2 + HOOC-$$

Presence of HCl in the stomach denatures proteins by breaking the weaker bonds of the tertiary protein structure and the enzyme pepsin converts this denatured protein into polypeptides like peptones and proteoses. **These along with other polypeptide fragments, reach the duodenum and jejunum where several enzymes secreted by pancreas for example trypsin, chymotrypsin, carboxypeptidase and elastase attack these protein fragments producing dipeptides, tripeptides and small polypeptides.** Carboxypeptidase is an exopeptidase, whereas the others are endopeptidases. These enzymes are nonspecific to the nature of the protein, but specific to the peptide bond. Trypsin attacks the peptide bonds with basic amino acids; chymotrypsin with uncharged amino acids, and elastase with small amino acids of wide range. Carboxypeptidase attacks individual amino acid at the carboxyl end. However, only a small portion of the protein gets converted to the single amino acids at this stage- the products being mostly dipeptides, tripeptides and some small polypeptides. Further digestion is carried out in the epithelial cells where the brush border with its microvilli possesses other peptidases protruding into the exterior. These are mainly amino-peptidases and some dipeptidases. Specific nucleases are believed to hydrolyse RNA and DNA at this stage. The action of these enzymes produces dipeptides and tripeptides along with some individual amino acids which are passed into the interior of the epithelial cells where other specific peptidases convert almost all of them to single amino acids that are transported to the blood stream by the opposite side of the cell membrane.

Absorption of Proteins

Proteins are rarely absorbed in the intact form except in the cases of foetal and new-borns. These are absorbed in the form of amino acids through the blood route. Almost negligible amount may also be absorbed through the lymphatic route. Amino acids obtained during the process of digestion do not accumulate in the intestine indicating that these are absorbed very rapidly. **L-amino acids are absorbed more rapidly as compared to the corresponding D- forms.** The D-amino acids are absorbed passively but the L- forms are abosrbed actively. **Absorption of the L-amino acids, therefore requires energy. Hypoxic conditions or addition of respiratory uncouplers such as cyanide, azide or dinitrophenol, therefore, lower the rate of absorption of the L-amino acids. Vitamin B_6 is involved in the active transport of the L-amino acids.**

In a mixture of the amino-acids, specially in cases of the neutral amino acids, the absorption of one amino acid is inhibited by the other which is suggestive of a competition amongst neutral amino acids probably for a common carrier. The possibility of a different mechanism for the absorption of arginine, ornithine and lysine is indicated by the observation that the neutral amino acids do not compete with these amino acids for getting absorbed and their rate of absorption remains unaffected by the presence of arginine, ornithine or lysine. The absorption of neutral amino acids is only partially affected by the presence of proline and hydroxyproline which indicates the possibility of a third type of mechanism for the absorption of proline and hydroxyproline.

Small amounts of proteins may remain undigested which are absorbed by pinocytosis. Although, their amounts may be insignificant from nutritional point of view, such proteins may act as antigen to form antibody. **However an excess may lead to allergy.** In the new borns, the proteins may not be digested completely; the immunoglobulin, IgA from mothers's milk is absorbed as such which contributes to the immunity in the child.

Disorders of the Alimentary tract

Derangement in the function of the organs concerned with the alimentary system is associated with various disease conditions as mentioned below:

(A) Stomach disorders

The alteration in the normal secretion of the gastric juice is reflected primarily in the concentration of HCl in the stomach. There may be hyperchlorhydria (increased concentration of HCl) or hypochlorhydria (decreased concentration of HCl). **In hyperchlorhydria, the acid together with pepsin released from pepsinogen, may attack the very cells of their origin exposing the wall of stomach. Contact of acid with this may produce ulcer, accompanied with pain and other discomforts.**

The final result of continued hyperchlorhydria is the development of peptic ulcer, that may further be aggravated by the reduced secretion of alkaline fluid from the pancreas and/or inability of the layer of mucus to protect the wall of that part of the duodenum from the action of gastric acid in the chyme. **Peptic ulcer is a common ailment especially amongst malnourished and undernourished people.**

Hypochlorhydria evidently leads to digestive insufficiency. **There may even be achlorhydria (absence of HCl) and *achyla* when associated with the absence of enzymes and the intrinsic factor secreted in the stomach. Pericious anemia presents the latter condition. Carcinoma of stomach has hypochlorhydria or even achlorhydria.**

(B) Pancreatic disorders

Disorder in the external secretion of the pancreas may cause a wide range of digestive disorders since the enzymes necessary for the hydrolysis of carbohydrates, lipids and proteins are all originated from the pancreas. The reduction in the acidity of the chyme from the stomach is also due to the bicarbonate secreted by the pancreas. **The important internal secretions of the pancreas are insulin and glucagon.** In pancreatitis, benign or malignant, there may be found excessive secretion of enzymes amylase and lipase and also elevated levels of the same in blood. One may also find elevated urinary levels of these enzymes.

(C) Bile disorders

Liver is the site of formation of bile which excretes bile acids, bilirubin, cholesterol, etc., besides being the most important factor in the emulsification of fats in the small intestine. Any disorder in the liver affecting the bile formation will certainly disturb the above functions. Cholesterol is insoluble in water, but is solubilized in bile due to the presence of phospholipids and bile acids, water content also having an important role. Alteration in the proportion of these substances in bile may reduce the solubility of cholesterol. This, as well as too much concentration of bile in the gall bladder by excessive absorption of ions and water through the mucosa and too much secretion of cholesterol in the liver, will cause a supersaturated condition for the dissolved cholesterol. **Any seeding agent, say an infection, will then initiate the formation of cholesterol crystals, accumulation of which will lead to gallstones. This is a common pathology in the middle aged or older perosns. Obstruction to the passage of bile due to gallstones or pancreatitis produces jaundice.**

(D) Disorders in the small intestine

A large number of clinical conditions are related to the digestion and absorption in the small intestine. Deficiency of enzyme lactase (inherited or otherwise) leads to the accumulation of lactose (milk intolerance) with abdominal cramps and diarrhoea. Similar condition may also take place from the deficiency of enzymes sucrase and maltase. Hereditary defect in the carrier protein may cause reduced absorption of glucose and galactose. Under certain conditions, a few proteins or small polypeptides (for instance wheat gluten or its fraction) get absorbed and produce their antibodies in the system which may produce coeliac disease in children and a similar one in adults (non-tropical sprue). Anemia results from reduced absorption of iron, folic acid, and vitamin B_{12}. Protein deficiency syndrome is the result of malabsorption of amino-acids; tetany may take place with the malabsorption of Ca^{2+}, Mg^{2+} and vitamin D. Steatorrhea (excess fat in the faeces) is mostly the result of unabsorbed fat and fat soluble vitamins. Deficiency of vitamin K (lack of production and/or absorption) contributes to bleeding diseases/disorders.

CHAPTER 7

ENZYMES AND ISOENZYMES

ENZYMES

Enzymes are biological catalysts (biocatalysts) which bring about chemical reactions in living cells. They accelerate the rate of the reaction and are usually present in very small amount in various cells. They can also exhibit their activity when they have been extracted from the source. They are organic compounds and a number of them have been obtained in crystalline form. **Today, more than 840 enzymes are known.**

General properties of the enzymes:

1. They are proteinous in nature.
2. They accelerate the rate of the reaction by:
   (a) not altering the reaction equilibrium.
   (b) being required in minute quantity.
   (c) being not consumed in the overall reaction.
3. They act as catalysts, deficiency of which may diminish the rate of a particular reaction; whereas complete absence of it may completely block a particular reaction.
4. They are very specific for their substrates.
5. They possess active sites at which interaction with substrate occurs.
6. They are responsible for lowering the activation energy.
7. **Some enzymes are regulatory in function.**

Enzyme Cofactors, Coenzymes, Prosthetic Groups

In addition to the protein component, many enzymes require nonprotein constituents for their proper functioning. In some cases these components, broadly described as cofactors, may be metal ions and, in other cases, organic molecules of relatively low molecular weight. When the small organic molecules are tightly bound either by covalent or coordinate bonds, they are called as **prosthetic groups. The heme group of the cytochromes is an example of a prosthetic group.**

Pyridoxal phosphate, a slightly modified form of vitamin B_6 (pyridoxine), is an essential cofactor or coenzyme, for an important group of enzymes known collectively as *transaminases.* As the name implies, these enzymes transfer α-amino group from an amino acid to a α -keto acid.

Coenzymes

Coenzymes are organic molecules, often derived from the B vitamins, that participate directly in enzymatic reactions. Some coenzymes are attached to their companion enzymes as tightly bound prosthetic groups, whereas others can be easily removed by dialysis. The complete functional complex of enzyme and cofactors is called a ***holoenzyme;*** the protein part, free of the cofactors, is called an ***apoenzyme.***

Characteristics of coenzymes:

1. They are stable towards heat.
2. Generally derived from vitamins.
3. Function as co-substrates.
4. They participate in:
   (a) Electron transfer reactions, e.g. NAD^+, NADH, FMN, FAD, etc.
   (b) Group transfer reactions e.g., CoA,TPP, pyridoxal phosphate, tetrahydrofolic acid, etc.

Coenzymes	Functions performed
1. NAD^+	Hydrogen transfer
2. $NADP^+$	Hydrogen transfer
3. FAD	Hydrogen transfer
4. FMN	Hydrogen transfer
5. TPP(Thiamine pyrophosphate)	Acetyl group transfer
6. PP (Pyridoxal phosphate)	Amino group transfer
7. Biotin	Carboxyl group transfer
8. Coenzyme A	Acyl group transfer

Nicotinamide nucleotides

NAD^+, $NADP^+$ and their reduced forms are involved in a great variety of dehydrogenase reactions in the mitochondria, cytosol and endoplasmic reticulum of the cell. They are water soluble, and are usually free to diffuse away from the enzyme after conversion to the oxidized or reduced form, to take part in another dehydrogenase reaction catalysed by another enzyme.

NH_2 adenine Ribose Nicotinamide

*$NADP^+$ has PO_4 here

Nicotinamide adenine dinucleotide (NAD); NADP is nicotinamide adenine dinucleotide phosphate.
* $NADP^+$ has got PO_4 in place of OH

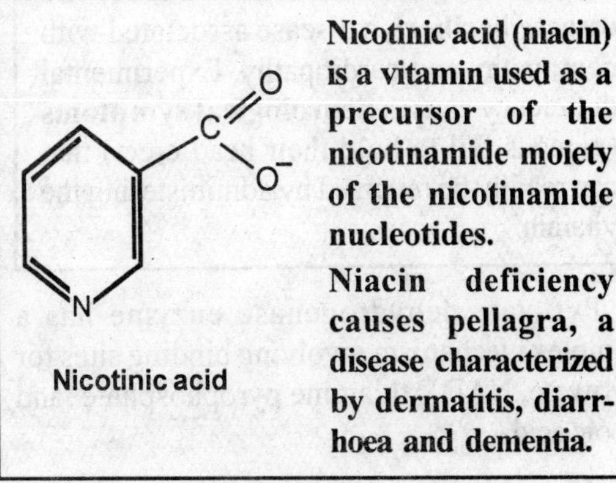

Nicotinic acid (niacin) is a vitamin used as a precursor of the nicotinamide moiety of the nicotinamide nucleotides.

Niacin deficiency causes pellagra, a disease characterized by dermatitis, diarrhoea and dementia.

Flavin nucleotide coenzymes:

FAD is the coenzyme of a class of dehydrogenases known as flavoproteins. The flavin moiety of the molecule is derived from riboflavin (vitamin B_2).

Flavin mononucleotide (FMN) is an important coenzyme in some flavoproteins, including NADH coenzyme Q reductase, etc.

FMN consists of riboflavin phosphate (i.e., FAD without the adenosine monophosphate moiety).

Flavin coenzymes remain tightly bound to the enzyme protein throughout the reaction, in contrast to the nicotinamide coenzymes that bind reversibly to the enzyme.

A number of mitochondrial dehydrogenases are flavoproteins; for example, NADH dehydrogenase, succinate dehydrogenase and fatty acyl CoA dehydrogenase.

Thiamine pyrophosphate

Thiamine (Vitamin B_1) is the precursor of thiamine pyrophosphate, the coenzyme for some important oxidative decarboxylation reactions (pyruvate dehydrogenase, oxoglutarate dehydrogenase).

In oxidative decarboxylation, loss of CO_2 is accompanied by oxidation of an aldehyde to an acid.

Deficiency of thiamine causes the disease beriberi, a disease associated with neuropathy and cardiopathy. Experimental deficiency causes **neurological symptoms** (pigeons fail to hold their head erect) that can readily be reversed by administering the vitamin.

Pyruvate dehydrogenase enzyme has a complex mechanism involving binding sites for pyruvate, NAD^+, thiamine pyrophosphate and lipoic acid.

Pyridoxal phosphate

Pyridoxal phosphate (derivative of vitamin B_6) acts as a coenzyme in transamination and decarboxylation reactions. In a transamination reaction the aldehyde group of pyridoxal phosphate first forms a Schiff's base with the amino group of the amino acid, which is then converted to keto acid. Pyridoxal phosphate is thereby converted to pyridoxamine phosphate which transfers the amino group to another keto acid to form an amino acid.

Pyridoxal phosphate also acts as a coenzyme in decarboxylation reactions of amino acids such as :

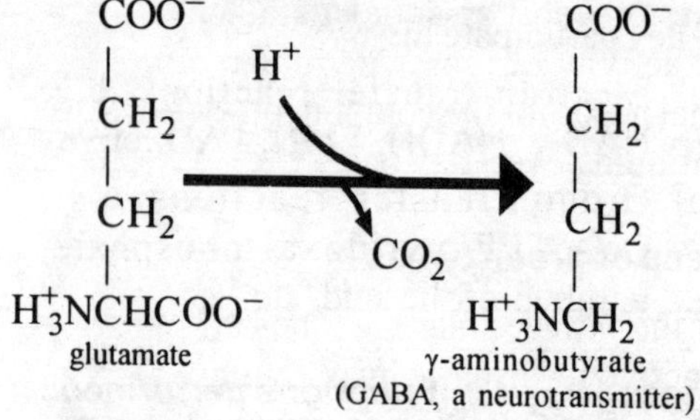

Vitamin B_6 deficiency is rare in man, because the vitamin is widely distributed in common foodstuffs and in addition is synthesized in appreciable quantities by intestinal flora. The main abnormality seen in B_6 deficiency is dermatitis which is readily cured by the administration of the vitamin.

Biotin

It is an essential food factor and is a coenzyme for carboxylation reactions (e.g. pyruvate carboxylase). These reactions involve ATP, which is necessary in the first step of the reaction; this is the conversion of biotin to carboxybiotin by the addition of CO_2 to C-1 of biotin.

Pantothenic acid is an essential food factor which forms part of coenzyme A.

Coenzyme A

It is a complex molecule which contains a free sulfhydryl (-SH) group. This group can react with a carboxyl group to form a thioester. Such thiolesters are involved in many reactions involving acyl groups, including acetyl and fatty acyl groups.

Enzyme and cofactor turnover

Like all biologic materials, enzymes have a finite half-life; that is, they are subject to turnover and replacement. Therefore, a diet must include sufficient essential amino acids, metals and vitamins to provide enzyme replacement, among other needs. Human beings have only a limited ability to store most essential metal ions and the biologic activity of most vitamins requires the nutritional needs for the components of enzymes on a continuing everyday basis.

Zymogens or proenzymes

Most of the intracellular enzymes are secreted in their active forms known as **Zymase** form of the enzyme but side by side few enzymes are secreted in their inactive forms known as **proenzymes** or **zymogens.**These enzymes (proenzymes/zymogens) have a tendency to undergo prior change in structure after coming into contact with certain activating agents.Activating agent may be H^+, another enzyme on the active form of the zymogen itself. For instance gastric juice contains pepsin which is secreted by pepsinogen (a zymogen). **Pepsinogen (Fig 7.1) is changed into its active form pepsin** by H^+ of the gastric juice.

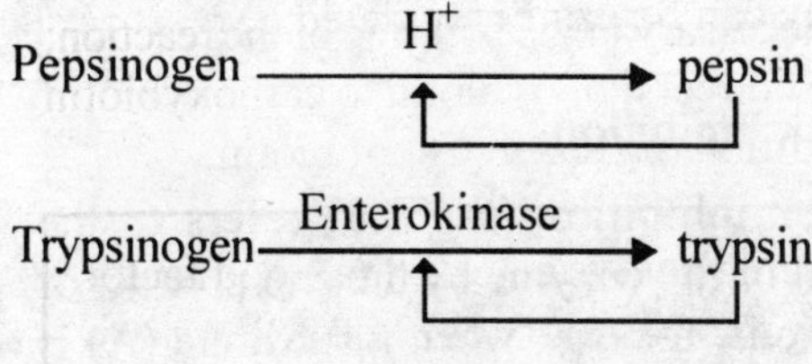

Fig. 7.1 : Activation of a zymogen

Once formed pepsin itself acts on pepsinogen and catalyses its own conversion into pepsin;such a process is called as **autocatalysis** (Fig 7.1)

Thus, **zymogens** are inactive precursors of enzymes that are primarily concerned with proteolytic activity. The important examples of this category are the enzymes found in the gastrointestinal tract that act on dietary proteins. This unique process is probably involved with the protection of tissues from digestion by their own proteolytic enzymes.

Important examples of the enzymes that occur as zymogens are as follows:

Zymogem	*activator*	*active enzyme*
Pepsinogen	H^+, pepsin	pepsin
Trypsinogen	trypsin, enterokinase	trypsin
Chymotrypsinogen	trypsin	chymotrypsin
Procarboxy-peptidase	trypsin	carboxy-peptidase
Proelastase	trypsin	elastase
Prorennin	H^+, rennin	rennin

Pepsin is the major proteolytic enzyme found in the stomach. Pepsinogen has a M.W. of 42,500 and is converted by acid or pepsin itself to active pepsin with a M.W. of 34,500. The conversion is accompanied by the removal of one-fifth of the peptide chain(in the form of six peptides).

Allosteric Enzymes

Some of the enzymes possess additional sites known as allosteric sites (Greek:allo-other) besides the active site. Such enzymes are known as allosteric or regulatory enzymes. The allosteric sites are the unique places on the enzyme molecule.

These enzymes are regulated by certain substances called allosteric modulators (effectors) which reversibly bind to the enzyme at the allosteric site. An interaction with the effector molecule brings about conformational changes in the catalytic site of the enzyme. The binding of the effector molecule may inhibit the enzymatic reaction (called as allosteric inhibition); such an effector molecule is called as a negative effector (allosteric inhibitor). Contrarily, an effector may also activate the enzymatic reaction (called as allosteric activation) and is called a positive effector (allosteric activator).

Examples of this category are (i) HMG CoA reductase is a regulatory enzyme of cholesterol biosynthesis, where as aspartate transcarbamoylase is the regulatory enzyme for pyrimidine synthesis.

If the effector substance is the substrate itself then it is called as **homotropic effect;** contrarily, if the effector molecule is a substance other than the substrate then it is called as the **hetrotropic effect.** Removal of inhibition can be brought about by increasing the amount of the inhibitor. Mechanism of action of allosteric enzymes can be very well understood by the following Figure 7.2.

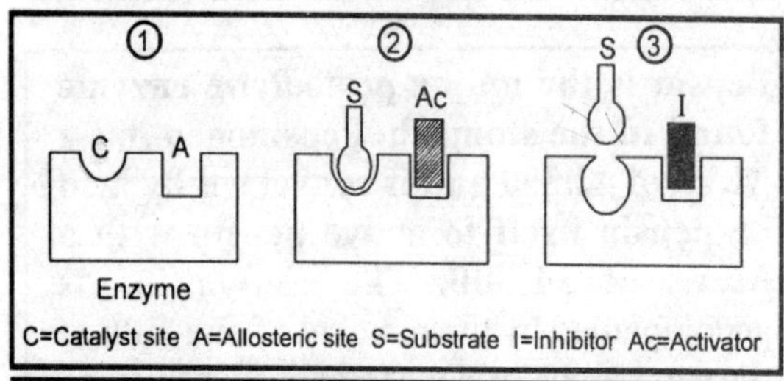

Fig. 7.2 : Action of allosteric enzymes: (1) The enzyme has separate catalytic (C) and allosteric (A) sites (2) When activator (Ac) is fixed, the catalytic site assumes correct three dimensional structure, so that substrate(S) can combine, (3) When inhibitor (I) is attached, catalytic site is altered, so that substrate is not engaged.

A few examples of allosteric enzymes are as follows:

(a) succinylCoA+glycine $\xrightarrow{\text{ALA synthase}}$ δ-amino-levulinic acid (ALA)

This is the first step in the synthesis of heme. Here the end product i.e., heme will allosterically inhibit the enzyme ALA synthase which is the key enzyme of heme synthesis.

(b) Carbamoyl phosphate + asparate

$\downarrow$ Asparate transcarbamoylase

carbamoyl asparate

This is the first step in the biosynthesis of cytidine triphosphate(CTP).Here ,the end product i.e.,CTP will allosterically inhibit the enzyme asparate transcarbamoylase.

(c) Inhibition of enzyme HMG CoA reductase by cholesterol (the end product of cholesterol biosynthesis) is another example of allosteric inhibition.

(d) **Phosphofructokinase (PFK) which catalyzes the phosphorylation of fructose-6-phosphate to fructose- 1, 6 -diphosphate is the rate limiting enzyme of glycolysis. This enzyme is allosterically inhibited by ATP and citrate but allosterically activated by AMP and fructose-6-phosphate.**

Allosteric enzymes are utilized by the body for regulating various metabolic pathways. Such a regulatory enzyme in a particular pathway is called as a **key enzyme or rate limiting enzyme.** The flow of the whole pathway is constrained as if there is a bottle-neck at the level of the key enzyme. The allosteric inhibitor is most effective when substrate concentration is low. This is metabolically very significant. When more substrate molecules are available, automatically there is less necessity for stringent regulation. In this way, the whole pathway can be easily regulated.

Feedback inhibition

Feed back inhibition (Fig 7.3) refers to the inhibition of the enzyme by the end product of the reactions, for e.g., when a substrate (A) is converted to a product (P) through various intermediates (B, C,D, E, etc), the end product of the reaction inhibits the first enzyme of the pathway (Fig 7.3). In this type of inhibition, the accumulation of the end product slows down the whole reaction sequence and since the end product continues to be consumed, its synthesis continues. Since it is partially competitive, both V_{max} and K_m are altered.

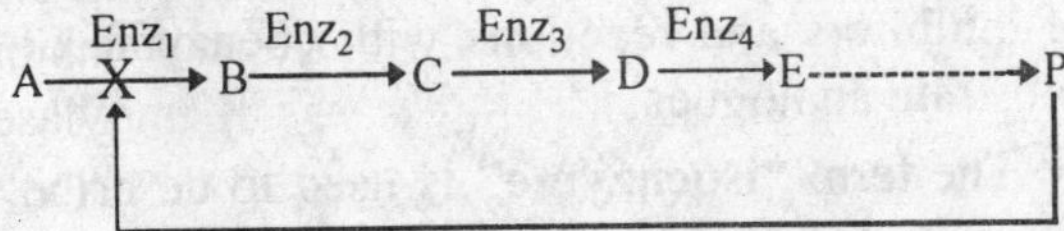

Fig. 7.3 : Feedback Inhibition

As it is a mixed type of inhibition, the inhibitor binds to the enzyme at a site other than the active site called as **allosteric site** which is encountered in **allosteric enzymes.**

Feedback inhibition is a type of regulatory mechanism which has been identified in many instances and is especially interesting since it is a self- regulatory device allowing a cell to adjust the rate of synthesis of a metabolic intermediate to its everchanging needs. One important classical example of it involves the synthesis of CTP in **Escherichia coli.** Early in this reaction sequence, carbamoyl phosphate is converted to carbamoyl aspartate by the enzyme **aspartate transcarbamoylase.** This reaction is crucial, since its inhibition affects the subsequent reactions leading to CTP. This enzyme is sensitive to inhibition by CTP. As the reaction sequence produces CTP, and when the CTP is not used rapidly enough in subsequent reactions (e.g., incorporation into nucleic acids), a critical concentration of CTP is reached, which inhibits aspartate transcarbamoylase. The result is a decrease in the synthesis of CTP until its concentration is lowered below the level at which the enzyme is inhibited.

Classification of Enzymes

As per international classification, **the enzymes have been classified into six major classes,** each with several subclasses; within each subclass, formal names have been assigned to the known enzymes to describe the reactions they catalyze. Trivial names for many enzymes, for example, pepsin, trypsin, urease, etc. are still very common and easy to remember as well. Many enzymes are still easier to recognize them by their trivial names. The newer nomenclature has been less widely adopted due to its own complications.

No.	Major classes	Examples
1.	Oxidoreductases	Alcohol dehydrogenase, xanthine oxidase.
2.	Transferases	Hexokinase, etc.
3.	Hydrolases	Glucose-6-phosphatase, pepsin, carboxypeptidase
4.	Lyases	Aldolase, pyruvate decarboxylase
5.	Isomerases	Phosphotriose isomerase, phosphoglucomutase
6.	Ligases	Glutamine synthetase, glutathione synthetase

Six major classes are:

1. ***Oxidoreductases:*** They catalyze a wide variety of oxidation-reduction reactions and frequently employ coenzymes such as NAD^+, $NADP^+$, FAD, or lipoate as the hydrogen acceptor. Other acceptors include coenzyme Q or molecular oxygen. **Common trivial names include dehydrogenase, oxidase, peroxides, and reductase.**
2. ***Transferases:*** They catalyze various kinds of group transfers. Many important steps in metabolism require transfer from one molecule to another of amino, carboxyl, carbonyl, methyl, acyl, glycosyl, or phosphoryl groups. **Common trivial names include amino transferase (transaminase), acyl carnitine transferase and transcarboxylase.**
3. ***Hydrolases:*** They catalyze cleavage of

bonds between a carbon and some other atom by addition of water. **Some common trivial names include esterase, peptidase, amylase, urease, phosphatase, pepsin, trypsin and chymotrypsin.**

4. ***Lyases:*** They catalyze breakage of carbon-carbon, carbon-sulphur and certain carbon-nitrogen (excluding peptide bonds. **Common trivial names include decarboxylase, aldolase, citrate lyase and dehydratase.**
5. ***Isomerases:*** They catalyze racemization of optical or geometric isomers and certain intramolecular oxidation-reduction reactions. **Trivial names include epimerase, racemase, and mutase.**
6. ***Ligases:*** These catalyze the formation of bonds between carbon and oxygen, sulphur, nitrogen and other atoms. The energy required for bond formation is frequently derived from the hydrolysis of ATP. **Some trivial names include synthetase and carboxylase.**

Isomeric enzymes or isoenzymes or isozymes (Multiple molecular forms of enzymes)

A particular enzyme obtained from different times often has certain physicochemical properties which are characteristic of the tissue of origin, although the same chemical reaction is catalyzed in each case. Electrophoresis and chromatography in particular are the two techniques which are most frequently used to separate and 'finger print' these multiple molecular forms. Different physicochemical properties of the enzymes frequently affect their catalytic activity, so that they often differ in such properties as their Km, sensitivity to heat, effect of inhibitors and reactions with coenzyme or substrate analogues.

Examples of Isoenzymes are:

1. Lactate dehydrogenase **(LDH)**
2. Creatine phosphokinase **(CPK or CK)**
3. Alkaline phosphatase **(ALP)**
4. Malate dehydrogenase
5. Carbonic anhydrase
6. Hexokinase
7. Phosphorylase
8. Glucose-6-phosphate dehydrogenase, etc.

The term **"isoenzyme"** is used to describe the multiple form of an enzyme which are distinct proteins, such as those of lactate dehydrogenase, creatine phosphokinase, alkaline phosphatase etc. A single tissue may contain more than one form of an enzyme, for instance, kidney contains isoenzymes of alkaline phosphatase which may be separated from each other with the help of column chromatography on diethylaminoethyl-cellulose (DEAE-Cellulose).

Lactate dehydrogenase which has thoroughly been studied is composed of four subunits. There are two different subunits that can be combined into tetramers in five ways. The possible combinations can be separated by electrophoresis as shown in Figures 7.4 and 7.5. If one subunit type is identified as "M" (the major form found in muscle or liver) and the second as "H" (the major form found in heart), then the tetramers could have the compositions M_4, M_3H, M_2H_2, MH_3, or H_4. These can be separated from each other by electrophoresis.

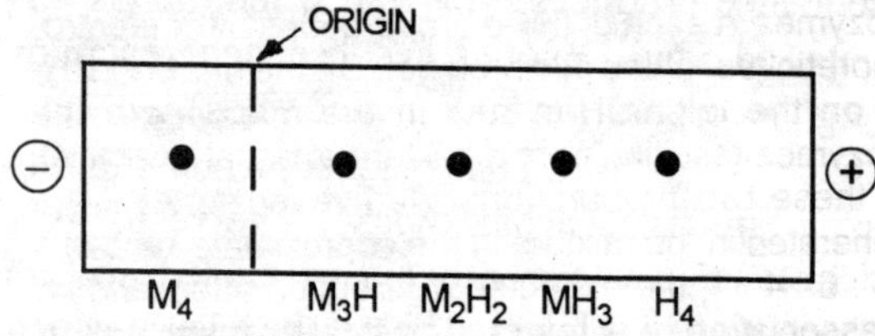

Fig. 7.4: Electrophoresis of lactate dehydrogenase isoenzymes at pH 8.6

In man, the content of several isoenzymes differs in heart and liver. Although the reason for this is not known, use is made of the fact in diagnostic differentiation of diseases of the liver and myocardium. In both types of disease states, lactate dehydrogenase leaks out of the damaged cells and increases the concentration of the enzyme in blood serum. Differentiation can be based in part on the pattern that appears on electrophoresis and in part on the fact that some of the isoenzymes from the myocardium are more resistant to heat denaturation than the corresponding hepatic isozymes. In the simpler differential test situation, a serum sample may be analyzed twice, once before and once after heat denaturation under carefully controlled conditions.

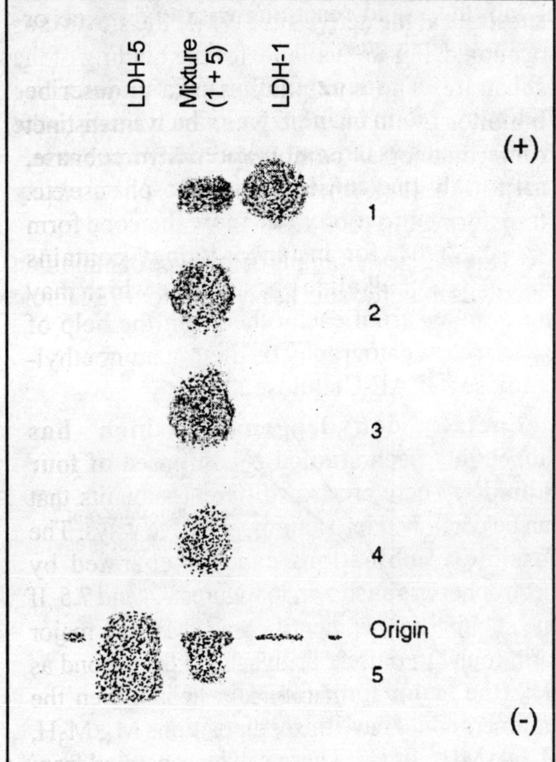

Fig. 7.5: This photograph shows the LDH isozymes in each of three preparations after electrophoretic resolution in starch gel. On the right is LDH-1, on the left LDH-5, and in the middle are the isozymes resulting from a mixture of equal quantities of these two preparations. All five isozymes were generated in the mixture in the approximate ratio of 1 : 4 : 6 : 4 : 1, the expected distribution after random reassociation of subunits. The total enzyme activity in the mixture was the sum of the activities of the single isozyme preparations. All three preparations were placed in 1 M NaCl and frozen overnight before electrohoretic resolution.

Clinically Important Enzyme Inhibitors

Enzymes may also be inactivated or denatured by a variety of chemical means, several of which have clinical importance. Many enzymes depend on essential sulfhydryl groups, which form tight covalent bonds with various heavy metals. For this reason mercury, lead, silver, etc are extremely toxic. **Even iron and copper, although they are classed as essential minerals, can produce intoxication when ingested in excess.**

Another class of inhibitors affects enzymes by introducing foreign alkyl groups into the structure. Most of these substances were initially developed as chemical warfare agents and are highly toxic in nature. Two best known are:

(a) diisopropylfluorophosphate (DFP), and
(b) the so called nitrogen mustards, for example, methachloramine and 2, 2'-dichloro-N-methyldiethylamine.

These, so called, nitrogen mustards are now employed clinically as enzyme inhibitors in the treatment of certain types of neoplastic diseases.

Enzyme inhibitors are:

1. Mercury
2. Lead
3. Silver
4. DFP
5. Various insecticides used in agriculture
6. Nitrogen mustards

The organic phosphates, of which DFP is only one example, are particularly good inhibitors of acetylcholinesterase, which breaks down the neurotransmitter substance known as acetylcholine. **Inactivation of acetylcholinesterase produces violent spasms of the pulmonary system and interferes with normal neuromuscular and cardiac functions.** Similar agents employed as insecticides in agriculture may be severely or fatally toxic.

Enzyme Inhibition

The rate of an enzyme-catalyzed reaction can be decreased by specific inhibitors, i.e., compounds that combine with the enzyme and prevent normal enzyme substrate interactions in the active site, thus diminishing the rate of the reaction. Certain enzymic inhibitors are poisonous for living organisms, including cyanide, hydrogen sulfide and carbon monoxide. Many drugs are also inhibitors of metabolic reactions and molecular pharmacology is largely dependent on the knowledge of inhibition of enzymes.

Application of enzyme inhibition

1. Studies on enzyme inhibition have led to the development of hundreds of new drugs for use in medicine and veterinary science.
2. Enzyme inhibition studies have been directed specifically toward increasing our understanding of specific reactions or metabolic pathways in animals and plants.
3. Enzyme inhibition studies have also led to the development of nerve gases, insecticides and herbicides (weed killers).

Types of Inhibition

Many substances inhibit enzymes and reduce the initial velocity (increase 1/v). The Lineweaver-Burk plots reveal the mechanism of the inhibition. **Following four types of inhibitions are known:**

1. **Competitive inhibition,**
2. **Non-competitive inhibition,**
3. **Partially competitive inhibition, and**
4. **Uncompetitive inhibition.**

1. Competitive Inhibition

In this type of inhibition (Fig. 7.6), competitive inhibitors can combine reversibly with the active site of the enzyme and compete with the substrate at the active site. While the site is thus occupied, it is unavailable for the binding of the substrate. The combination of a competitive inhibitor I with enzyme E can be written in the same manner as combination with substrate, although the inhibitor is not chemically transformed to products.

One classical example of this type of inhibition involves malonic acid as an inhibitor of succinic

$$E + I \rightleftharpoons EI$$

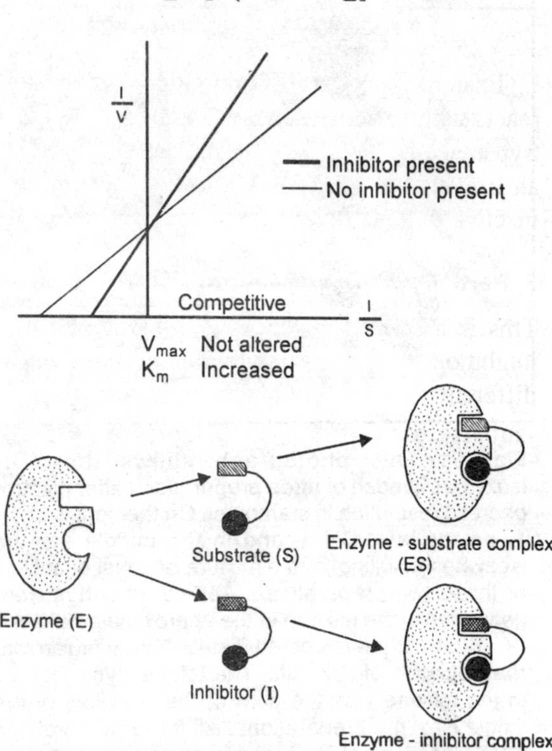

Fig. 7.6 : Showing Competitive Inhibition of an enzyme

dehydrogenase. This enzyme forms complexes and with the proper concentrations of reactants, succinate is not dehydrogenated (oxidized) to fumaric acid. On the other hand, with sufficient succinate present, the inhibition by malonate can be completely overcome.

2. Noncompetitive Inhibition

In this type, inhibition occurs when the inhibitor binds to a site on the enzyme other than the active site or binds irreversibly to the active site.

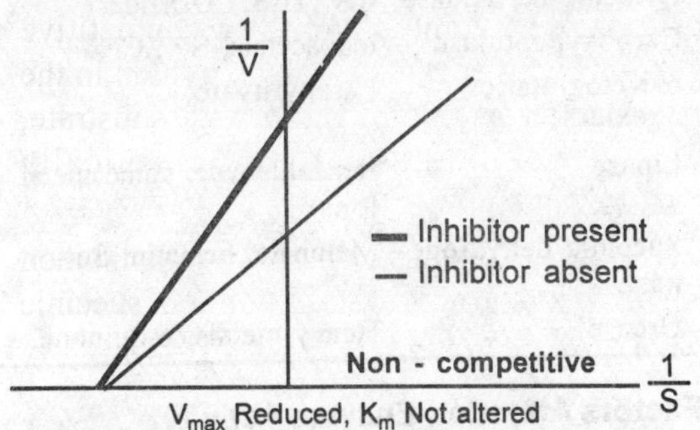

Examples include diisopropylfluorophosphate reacts with various esterases including chymotrypsin which has some esterase activity. This is an irreversible reaction. Urease is irreversibly inactivated by ultraviolet light.

3. Partially Competitive Inhibition

This is a special instance of non-competitive inhibition, where the inhibitor binding constant is different for the free enzyme and the enzyme -substrate complex. Two alternatives are

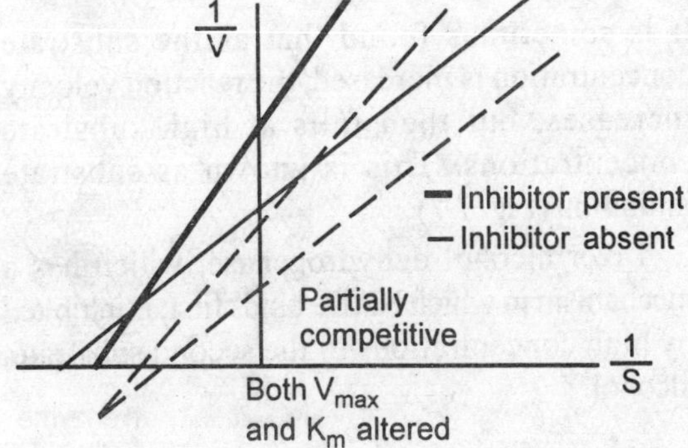

indicated by the solid and broken lines.

4. Uncompetitive Inhibition

It occurs when the inhibitor binds after the substrate has bound to the enzyme, and then stops the reaction from occurring; eventually no product is formed. This type of inhibition is not reversed by increasing substrate concentration. This type of inhibition is most frequently found in enzymic reactions with two or more substrates.

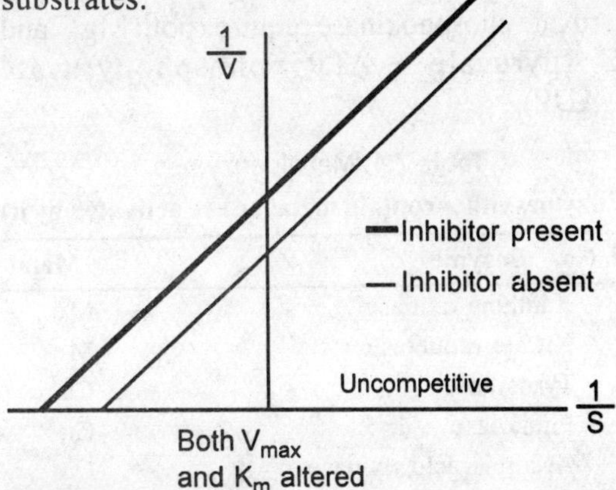

Enzyme Activators

Many ions and molecules have the capacity to activate some enzymes. Metal ions are activators of a number of enzymes. Following Table 25.1 shows this relationship. **Pepsin (as proenzyme pepsinogen) is activated by H^+ to form the active enzyme.** Many reducing agents (cysteine, glutathione) act as enzyme activators of-SH enzymes. Enzymes themselves activate other enzymes or proenzymes; i.e., enterokinase activates trypsinogen to form active trypsin.

Enzyme activators are :

1. Mg^{++}	2. Mn^{++}
3. Cobalt	4 Molybdenum
5. Calcium	6. Copper
7. Iron	8. Zn^{++}
9. Cysteine	10. Glutathione

Many enzymes require a metal ion (Table 7.1) for activity. In some cases, the requirement is specific for a particular metal. Carbonic anhydrase shows no activity upon removal of zinc, and no other metal is known to replace zinc in this enzyme. In other cases, more than one metal is able to bring about activation; for example, Mg^{++}, Mn^{++}, or Zn^{++} activate enolase (2-phosphoglycerate→phosphoenolpyruvate + H_2O). In a few cases it appears that two metal ions may be required by the enzyme; for example, pyruvate phosphokinase requires both Mg^{++} and K^+ (pyruvate + ATP→ phosphopyruvate + ADP).

Table 7.1: Metalloenzymes

(Enzymes either contain metal or are activated by it)

Sl. No.	Enzyme	Metal
1.	Xanthine oxidase	Mo
2.	Nitrate reductase	Mo
3.	Tyrosinase	Cu
4.	Phenolase	Cu
5.	Ascorbic acid oxidase	Cu
6.	Cytochrome enzymes	Fe
7.	Catalase	Fe
8.	Peroxidases	Fe
9.	Tryptophan oxidase	Fe
10.	Homogentisicase	Fe
11.	Lecithinases A and C	Ca
12.	Lipases	Ca
13.	Carbonic anhydrase	Zn
14.	Lactic dehydrogenase	Zn
15.	Carboxypeptidase	Zn
16.	Peptidases	Mg
17.	Phosphatases	Mg
18.	ATP-enzymes, such as hexokinases	Mg
19.	Arginase	Mn
20.	Phosphoglucomutase	Mn
21.	Dipeptidases	Mn
22.	Peptidases	Co

Enzyme inhibitors are those which have a tendency to inhibit/ retard or stop the activity of an enzyme.

Some important examples of enzyme inhibitors are as given in Table 7.2:

Table 7.2 : Enzymes and their inhibitors

Enzyme	Inhibitors
Arginase	Ornithine, lysine, L- amino acids
Alkaline phosphatase	Chelating compounds, arsenate, F^-
Carboxylase	HCHO, CH_3CHO, C_6H_5CHO
Cholinesterase	Physostigmine, neostigmine
Carbonic anhydrase	CO, sulfanilamide
Cytochrome oxidase	CN^-, H_2S, CO, azide
Carboxypeptidase	Iodoacetate, S^{--}, CN^-
α-Ketoglutaric oxidase	Parapyruvate
Lipase	Benzaldehyde, some metal ions
Succinic dehydrogenase	Malonate, hematin, Se
Urease	Heavy metals, o-quinone

Factors Affecting Enzyme Activity

Major factors responsible to affect the enzymic activity are the following:

1. Concentration of substrate
2. Concentration of enzyme
3. Concentration of reaction products
4. Effect of pH
5. Effect of temperature and
6. Effect of time

Substrate concentration

It is sometimes found that as the substrate concentration is increased, the reaction velocity increases, but then falls at high substrate concentrations. This is known as substrate inhibition (Fig. 7.7).

Liver alcohol dehydrogenase, which has a mechanism in which NAD^+ binds first, is inhibited by high concentrations of the second substrate, alcohol.

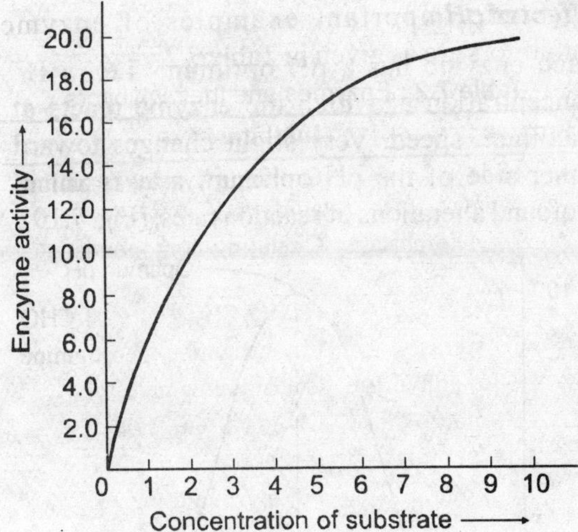

Fig.7.7 : Effect of substrate concentration on enzyme activity

The Michaelis-Menten Equation

The Michaelis constant (K_m) corresponds to the substrate concentration that produces half-maximal velocity. K_m is independent of enzyme concentration (Fig. 7.8).

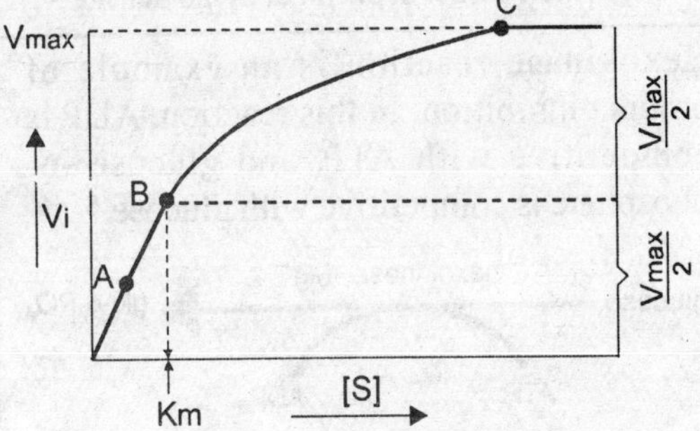

Fig. 7.8 : Determination of Km and V max

Derivation of the Michaelis-Menten equation

A mathematical analysis of the kinetics of an enzyme-catalysed reaction was proposed by Michaelis and Menten, whose names are always associated with the equation derived below. The derivation is based on a model of enzyme action in which the enzyme (E) binds to a single substrate (S) to form an enzyme-substrate complex (ES), which breaks down to form products (P) and to liberate free enzyme (E):

$$E + S \underset{k_{-1}}{\overset{k_1}{\rightleftharpoons}} ES \xrightarrow{k_2} E + P$$

k_1, k_{-1} and k_2 are rate constants for the various reactions as indicated above.

It is assumed that the reaction is in the steady state, with the concentration of ES constant, and the analysis applies only to the start of the reaction, at which point negligible amounts of products have been formed, so that the reverse reaction E+P→ES is also negligible. Then

$$\frac{d[ES]}{dt} = k_1([E_1] - [ES])\,[S] - k_{-1}[ES] - k_2[ES]$$

$$k_1[E_1]\,[S] - k_1\,[ES]\,[S] - k_{-1}\,[ES] - k_2\,[ES] = 0$$

$$k_1\,[E_1]\,[S] = [ES]\,(k_1[S] + k_{-1} + k_2)$$

$$\frac{k_1[E_1]\,[S]}{k_1[S] + k_{-1} + k_2} = [ES]$$

Divided by k_1

$$ES = \frac{[E_1]\,[S]}{[S] + \dfrac{k_{-1} + k_2}{k_1}}$$

Then initial rate (V) of formation of product $= k_2\,[ES]$

and when the enzyme is saturated with substrate maximum rate

$$(V_{max}) = k_2\,[E_1]$$

and the Michaelis constant

$$K_m = \frac{k_{-1} + k_2}{k_1}$$

Therefore,

$$\upsilon = k_2\,[ES] = \frac{k_2\,[E_1]\,[S]}{[S] + K_m}$$

$$\upsilon = \frac{V_{max}\,[S]}{[S] + K_m}$$

Strictly, this derivation is restricted to a single substrate reaction.

Concentration of enzyme

Within fairly wide limits the speed of an enzymatic reaction is proportional to the enzyme concentration. This can be shown to hold for many enzyme systems, provided interfering conditions do not develop and the substrate concentration is maintained constant (Fig. 7.9).

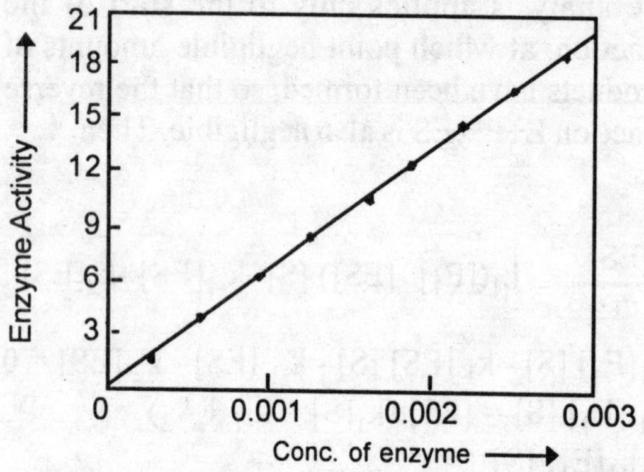

Fig 7.9: Effect of enzyme concentration on enzyme activity

Concentration of reaction products

An enzyme-product complex is part of the reaction sequence of enzyme-catalysed reactions. In the presence of large concentrations of product, this complex is dominant and product inhibition is observed. This is one of the reasons why the velocity of the reaction falls as the equilibrium is approached and it is of physiological importance in controlling pathways by negative feedback. In single-product enzymes as shown below in equation, addition of the product causes reversal of the reaction, but if there are two or more products, both are needed for reversal to occur, so inhibition of the forward reaction by each can be studied separately.

$$E + S \underset{k_2}{\overset{k_1}{\rightleftharpoons}} ES \xrightarrow{k_3} E + P$$

Usually each product is competitive with the substrate from which it is derived, e.g. see 'box'.

Effect of pH

Each enzyme has a pH optimum- i.e., a H^+ concentration at which the enzyme reacts at maximum speed. Very slight changes toward either side of the pH optimum may result in profound alterations of reaction rates, (Fig. 7.10).

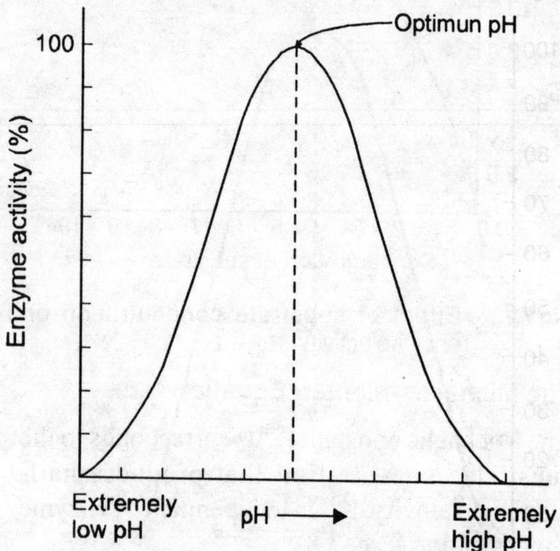

Fig. 7.10 : Effect of pH on enzyme activity

Hexokinase reaction is an example of product inhibition. In this reaction, ADP is competitive with ATP, and glucose -6-phosphate is competitive with glucose.

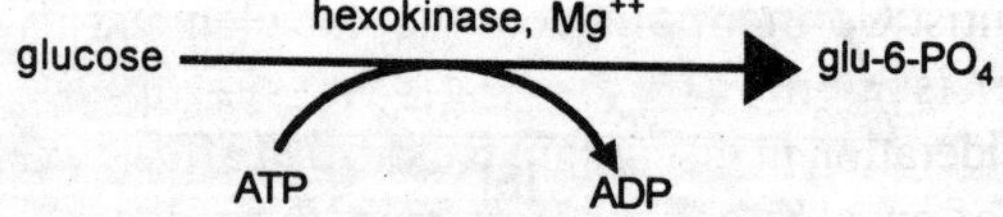

G-6-P may also act as a product inhibitor if it is not removed rapidly.

Effect of temperature

Chemical reactions, both catalyzed and noncatalyzed proceed at a faster rate as the reaction temperature is increased. This is true of enzymatically catalysed reactions in general only up to about 50°C. Above this temperature, heat inactivation of enzymes becomes a more important factor than the increased reaction rate and in all but a few exceptional cases, the speed of reaction slows and ceases around 70^0 to 80°C.

The optimum temperature of an enzyme is that temperature at which the greatest amount of substrate is changed in unit time. (Fig. 7.11).

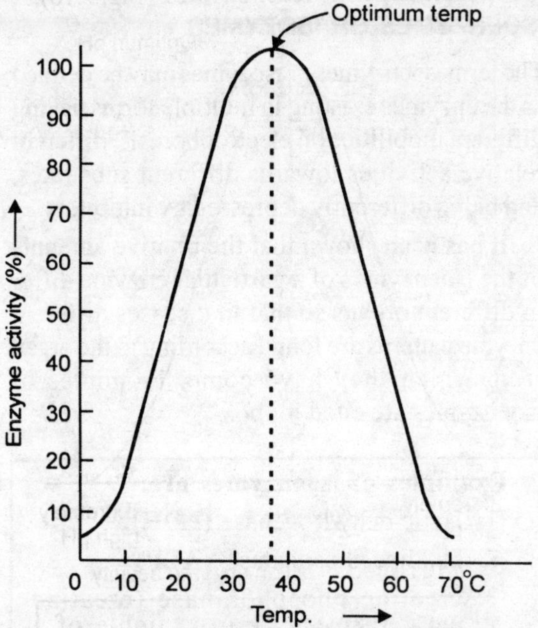

Fig 7.11: Effect of temp. on enzyme activity

Effect of time

Scientist Gortner points out that the element of time is generally not given sufficient consideration in discussing factors that affect the rate of enzyme action. He states, there cannot be an optimum hydrogen ion concentration or an optimum temperature independent of time. He indicates further that the optimum temperature of many enzymes from warm blooded animals is approximately 37°C only if time is measured in hours. It has been established that the time element is important in defining other conditions which regulate the rate of enzyme action.

Feedback Inhibition or Feedback Control

A significant control mechanism operating in living cells is known as feedback inhibition or control of enzymes. Specifically, this refers to the inhibition of the activity of an enzyme in a biosynthetic pathway by an end product of that pathway. A general representation of this kind of control is shown below:

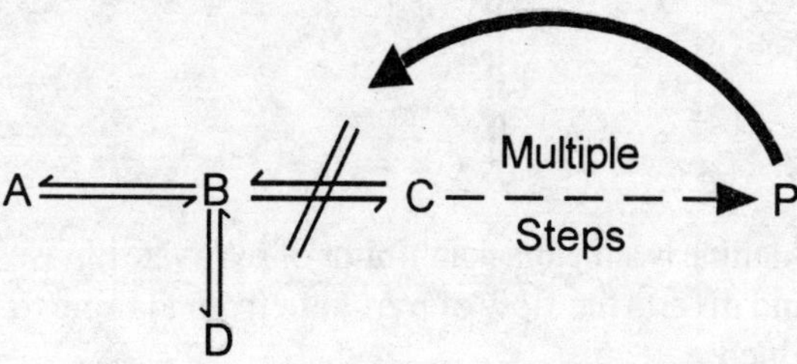

As seen in the diagram, the product (P) acts to inhibit some early step in the pathway, but not necessarily the first (product exerts a negative effect either on the first reaction or on a very early reaction). Frequently, substance B can be converted to more than one product; in this case the intermediate products are C and D. By feedback control it is possible not only to inhibit the production of P, but also to divert the flow of B from one pathway to another.

Several examples of this type have been studied in some detail. One of these systems involves the synthesis of pyrimidines. In this case, cytidine triphosphate (CTP) is an end product in a series of reactions and CTP markedly inhibits the enzyme concerned with the first specific step in this biosynthesis, namely, aspartate transcarbamoylase, which catalyzes the reaction between aspartate and carbamoyl phosphate to form ureidosuccinate. A series of further reactions leads to the synthesis of cytidine triphosphate.

Cholesterol synthesis is also regulated by feedback inhibition.

Yet another example of this phenomenon is the scheme involving pyruvate kinase, which converts phosphoenolpyruvate (PEP) to pyruvate. Major isoenzymes of this enzyme are found in muscle (M) and liver (L). The L-isozyme is subject to negative feedback, as shown below:

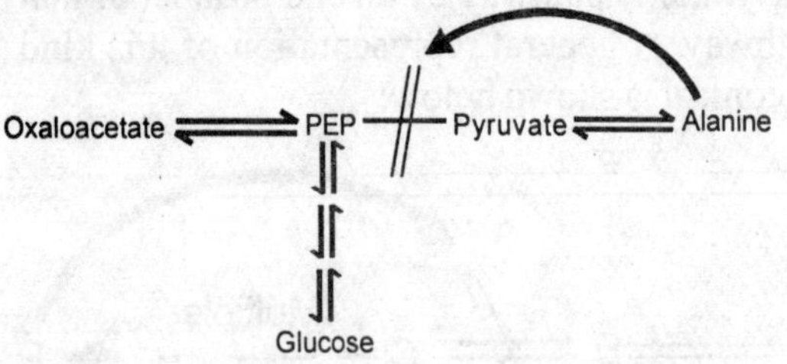

Alanine is a feedback inhibitor of pyruvate kinase and diverts the flow of pyruvate from alanine to glucose.

Enzyme Induction

Cellular enzymes can be divided into two primary classes:

(a) Constitutive Enzymes,

(b) Inducible Enzymes.

Constitutive enzymes

Enzymes of this class are present at virtually a constant concentration during the life of the cell. Presumably this is caused by a more or less constant relationship between the processes of enzyme synthesis and those of enzyme degradation.

Inducible enzymes:

Enzymes of this class are variable in the cell and as the need for the particular enzyme increases, the rate of synthesis gets increased or induced with respect to the rate of enzyme degradation. Thus, some of the enzymes responsible for glucose metabolism may be induced by increasing the load of glucose that an animal is required to metabolize. **Similarly, some of the enzymes involved in amino acid metabolism are inducible either by loading doses of the amino acid itself or by certain hormones.** During the wasting process, it is possible to measure increased serum concentrations of creatine phosphokinase, aldolase and other enzymes not regarded as inductive in the normal sense of the term.

ISOENZYMES OR ISOZYMES

The term isoenzymes or isozymes may be defined as the enzymes existing in multiple forms having different mobilities on electrophoresis, different relative activities towards different substrates, and being differently depressed by inhibitors.

It has been shown that the relative amounts of the isoenzymes of a particular enzyme differ in different organs so that in diseases different enzyme patterns are found according to the organ from which they have come. Examples of isoenzymes are cited in 'box'.

Examples of isoenzymes are:

1. lactic dehydrogenase **(LDH),**
2. alkaline phosphatase **(ALP)**
3. creatine phosphokinase (creatine kinase), **CPK or CK**
4. acid phosphatase, **(ACP)**
5. amylase
6. malate dehydrogenase,
7. cholinesterase,
8. hexokinase,
9. phosphoglucomutase,
10. pyruvate kinase, etc.

In clinical biochemistry till date most of the work has been done on the following isoenzymes:

(a) lactic dehydrogenase (LDH),

(b) alkaline phosphatase (ALP) and

(c) creatine kinase i.e. creatine phosphokinase (CK or CPK)

Today, nearly 100 enzymes have been detected to exist as 'isoenzymes'. Starch gel gives a clear electrophoretic separation than any other media. The vertical form is recommended. Other media include cellulose acetate, agar gel, etc.

Clinical significance of enzymes

The relative abundance of certain enzymes or their isoenzymes in serum has found application in the diagnosis of several diseases as mentioned below:

Alkaline Phosphatase

Measurement of the activity of alkaline phosphatase in serum in the investigation of bone diseases constituted one of the earliest applications of enzyme tests in diagnosis and has remained one of the most useful. The value of serum alkaline phosphatase assays in various disorders of bone has been confirmed by more than 50 years' experience, while isoenzyme studies have demonstrated that bone is indeed the source of the raised serum enzyme activity in these conditions. In contrast, no other enzyme test has emerged of comparable value in bone diseases, inspite of the systematic attention which has been devoted to the development of diagnostic enzymology in recent years.

Raised serum alkaline phosphatase was shown to accompany rickets of various aetiologies, **Paget's disease,** and **hyperparathyroidism with skeletal involvement.**

γ-glutamyl transferase is probably the most sensitive enzymic test of liver function yet described.

The normal range of serum alkaline phosphatase activity in adults is usually taken as **3-13 King-Armstrong units/100 ml.**

The serum alkaline phosphatase activity of the new-born infant is rather above the normal adult level, and it rises rapidly to as much as two and a half to three times the adult upper limit of normal during the first year of life. The activity falls somewhat by the end of the second year to values which are of the order of one and a half to two and a half times of 20-30 King-Armstrong units/100ml. These elevated values are maintained approximately constant throughout childhood and early adolescence with perhaps some upturn at the onset of puberty, typically declining to adult levels during the later teenage years.

When hepatobiliary disease is suspected, it is advisable to resort to an alternative enzyme test. The activities of several enzymes in serum reflect impaired biliary function in ways similar to (but not completely identical with) the behaviour of alkaline phosphatase in this situation. These enzymes typically show normal activities in osteoblastic bone disease. **Two such enzymes, i.e., 5'-nucleotidase and γ-glutamyltransferase,** have been shown to exhibit serum activities within the adult normal range in children and their use has therefore been recommended as a liver function test in young patients.

The highest serum alkaline phosphatase levels are generally encountered in Paget's disease of bone (Osteitis deformans) and the raised enzyme activity is often the only abnormality in the composition of the serum seen in this condition. The activity in serum may reach levels of 100-200 King-Armstrong units/100 ml or more, **the higher values being associated with cases in which a greater proportion of the skeleton is involved.**

While, determination of serum alkaline phosphatase activity is of great value in the detection of osteomalacia and rickets, the same is not true of hyperparathyroidism, in which an increased serum alkaline phosphatase is only seen in those cases in which bone changes are present.

Successful treatment of hyperparathyroidism (e.g. by the removal of a parathyroid adenoma) is followed by a fall in serum alkaline phosphatase activity which may, however be preceded by an initial rise due to healing of the bony lesions: this contrasts with the immediate fall in serum calcium.

Infiltration of the bones by malignant disease is accompanied by a rise in serum alkaline phosphatase activity whenever the process stimulates osteoblastic activity.

ISOENZYMES OF ALKALINE PHOSPHATASE (ALP)

On careful electrophoresis of plasma, four isoenzyme bands of ALP can be distinguished (liver, placenta, intestine, bone), but unfortunately there is a major difficulty in distinguishing the bone enzyme from the liver enzyme, as they migrate very close together in the support systems used. With these difficulties ALP isoenzyme detection has so far had to remain as a semi research procedure.

Acid Phosphatase

Acid phosphatase is an important enzyme and is found to be in abundance in adult prostate and seminal fluid, while significant amounts are found in several other tissues such as red cells, liver, kidney, bone, spleen and pancreas.

Normal Range

1 to 3.5 K.AU./100 ml or

1.8 to 6.5 I.U./litre

Most of the activity in normal serum is nonprostatic in origin and is found in both sexes at all stages. Less than 0.8 K.A. units is tartarate labile and so represents prostatic fraction.

Elevation

Clinical significance of acid phosphatase is chiefly in metastatic cancer of prostate, both in detection and following the progress of disease. **Raised values mostly between 5 to 50 K.A.U. are seen in over 75% cases of metastasizing prostatic carcinoma. Some times, values over 100 and very rarely even over 1,000 may be found.** Most of the increased enzyme activity is tartarate labile. Very high levels may be found in some cases of malignant prostate with secondaries (most often in bones).

A small increase has also been found in acute retention and following prostate massage, but values soon return to normal. Similar increases are noticed in Paget's disease and carcinoma of breast but in such cases the determination is not of much clinical significance.

If the increase in tartarate labile fraction is not significant and the total level is found raised, the increase may be due to red cells or other sources of acid phosphatase.

Isoenzymes of Acid Phosphatase

By polyacrylamide gel electrophoresis, various isoenzymes designated arbitrarily as 0, 1, 2, 3, 3b, 4 and 5 have been identified from different sources in normal and disease conditions. Zero represents the slowest moving and 5 the fastest moving fraction. Most of these isoenzymes are labile even at the room temperature and become inactivated. Therefore, in the serum only stable isoenzyme is found. The isoenzyme pattern in the leukocytes found is as follows:

Isoenzymes	*Sources*
1,2,4	in neutrophils
1,4	in monocytes
3	in lymphocytes and platelets
3b	in primitive blasts
5	in reticulum cells of leukaemic reticuloendothelosis

ISOENZYMES OF ACID PHOSPHATASE (ACP)

At the most, there do exist 14 isoenzymes on electrophoresis. One finds clear cut 14 bands on electrophoretogram. **The only isoenzyme of clinical importance is prostatic acid phosphatase.**

Normal plasma contains a tartarate resistant isoenzyme 5.

In variety of diseases, other isoenzymes may appear in plasma.

In metastatic prostatic cancer — changes in plasma enzyme activity are due to the presence of isoenzyme 2, which is tartarate labile.

Many acid phosphatase isoenzymes are cell specific i.e. derived from a specific type of cell.

Aminotransferases (Transaminases)

The enzymes which are involved in the transfer of an amino group (CH_2-NH_2) from an alpha amino acid to a alpha keto acid are called as transaminases and the process is called as transamination. Transamination reaction is an important step in the metabolism of amino acids.

Two enzymes occur in human tissues which catalyze reaction of this type:

(a) Aspartate aminotransferase, popularly known as **GOT (glutamic-oxaloacetic transaminase)** and

(b) Alanine aminotransferase, **popularly known as GPT (glutamic-pyruvic transaminase).**

Both transaminases are widely distributed in human tissues, GOT activity almost always being greater than GPT activity.

Serum GOT and GPT catalyse the following reactions of transaminations respectively:

$$\alpha\text{ KG} + \text{Aspartic acid} \underset{}{\overset{\text{GOT}}{\rightleftharpoons}} \text{Glutamic acid} + \text{Oxaloacetic acid}$$

$$\alpha\text{ KG} + \text{Alanine} \underset{}{\overset{\text{GPT}}{\rightleftharpoons}} \text{Glutamic acid} + \text{Pyruvic acid}$$

Interpretation

The normal range for serum GOT is 4-17 IU/l or 8-40 units/ml and for GPT 3-15 IU/l or 5-35 units/ml.

According to Wroblewski, in the newborn, values upto 120 units for GOT and 90 units for GPT must be considered normal.

Determination of GOT is particularly useful in myocardial infarction (M.I.) when ECG findings are not very clear. GOT rises rapidly after myocardial infarction; peak values which may be 2-20 times of normal, are reached within 24-48 hours and return to normal levels typically within 3-5 days.

Elevated level of GOT has been observed in almost 97% clinically proved cases of M.I.

Normal values have been reported in heart conditions without infarction, such as angina and pericarditis, in patients with pulmonary embolism and also in patients with acute abdominal attacks.

Foulk and Fleisher found an increase in over 50% patients with acute pancreatitis.

SGPT is not usually elevated in M.I. unless the lesion is a large one or there is associated liver damage.

Both the enzymes exhibit raised levels in hepatocellular damage e.g. due to hepatotoxic drugs, infective hepatitis and primary or secondary liver cancer. Raised levels are also seen in **Lannec's cirrhosis,** biliary cirrhosis and obstructive jaundice. In infective hepatitis, the increase is particularly marked and highest values are obtained. In early stage GOT is more increased than GPT, but SGPT exceeds SGOT in advanced stage. In infective hepatitis, estimation of serum transaminases is the most sensitive diagnostic index.

Very high values are obtained in toxic hepatitis due to carbontetrachloride poisoning.

Serum transaminases particularly SGOT gets elevated in certain muscular disorders, e.g. progressive muscular dystrophy, dermatomyositis and also following extensive muscle trauma, but is usually normal in progressive muscular atrophy, myasthenia gravis and rheumatoid arthritis.

Recommendations on the Use of Serum Enzyme Assays in the Diagnosis of Acute Myocardial Infarction

1. A single set of cardiac enzyme values in the emergency room is not sufficiently sensitive to exclude myocardial infarction. **Although a single, markedly positive CK-MB value will greatly increase the probability of acute infarction,** data are insufficient to support or reject a policy whereby low-risk patients, who otherwise would be sent home, would be observed until one or more CK-MB values are obtained.
2. If a myocardial infarction is inspected, then samples of total CK andCK-MB levels should be measured on admission and about 12 and 24 hours later, although condensed versions of this strategy may ultimately prove to be equally efficacious and more cost effective. If MI may have occurred more than 24 hours before admission, and if CK and CK-MB levels are not diagnostic, a total LDH level should be ordered. If the total LDH level is elevated, an assay of LDH isoenzymes should be obtained. If the first LDH1/LDH2 ratio is only slightly less than 1.0, a second assay is probably indicated.
3. If chest pain occurs after admission, CK and CK-MB assays should be done at 0, 12 and 24 hours.
4. **Routine use of enzyme assays other than those for CK, CK-MB, and LDH isoenzymes is not recommended.**
5. If more than 2 hours may pass before CK isoenzymes will be assayed, the serum sample should be preserved on ice.

Other Laboratory Measurements

Blood sugar

Hyperglycemia occurs frequently following AMI (acute myocardial infarction), not only in diabetic patients, in whom ketoacidosis may be precipitated, but also (with a lower frequency) in nondiabetics, in whom several weeks may elapse before carbohydrate tolerance returns to normal.

Serum lipids

These are often determined in patients with AMI. However, the results may be misleading, since numerous factors that can alter the values are operating at the time of the patient's admission to the hospital; for example, **stress increases serum cholesterol, whereas recumbency (the state of taking rest by lying down) decreases it.** Serum triglycerides are affected by calorie intake, intravenous and recumbency.

During the first 24-48 hours after admission, total cholesterol and HDL cholesterol remain at or near baseline values but generally fall precipitously after that. The fall in HDL cholesterol after AMI is greater than the fall in total cholesterol, thus the ratio of total cholesterol to HDL cholesterol is no longer useful for risk assessment early after MI. Therefore, unless values are obtained very early in patients admitted for AMI, it is the best to defer determinations of serum lipid levels until at least 8 weeks after the infarction has occurred.

Serum Amylase

Amylase is a starch splitting enzyme which hydrolyses starch and other high molecular dextrins to maltose at an optimum pH of 7.1. It is present in the pancreas and parotid gland. The major activity of this enzyme, called amylopsin, is in pancreatic juice, some is also found in saliva.

Interpretation

Normal range of serum amylase is given as 80-180 Somogyi units/100 ml. **The clinical significance of this enzyme chiefly lies in the diagnosis of acute pancreatitis in which values frequently exceed 2000 units.** Usually activities over 550 units strongly suggest a diagnosis of acute pancreatitis. The rise is rapid and transient, reaching a peak within the first 12-24 hours after the onset and returning to normal usually in 2 to 3 days.

In chronic disease of the pancreas, whether due to neoplasm or due to chronic pancreatitis, such high values are not seen (rarely exceeds 200 units/ 100 ml). In these conditions either duct obstruction is more gradual or progressive destruction of secreting tissues largely counteracts its effect.

High activities may also occasionally occur in variety of conditions in which pancreatic damage is secondary to other abdominal disturbance such as perforated gastric ulcers, peritonitis, intestinal obstruction. In these conditions values over 500 units may be found. These usually develop 5 to 10 days after the onset of symptoms and appear to be due to increased pressure on pancreatic duct.

ISOENZYMES OF AMYLASE

Although techniques are becoming available for the separate estimation of amylase isoenzymes (pancreatic, salivary), the measurement of isoenzymes is unlikely to resolve the major diagnostic problem of differentiating acute pancreatitis from non-pancreatic abdominal emergencies (perforated peptic ulcer, gut obstruction, etc.). This is because in the later situation, the pancreatic amylase that is normally present in the gut lumen leaks through the intestinal wall into the peritoneal cavity and from there it is absorbed into the blood stream.

Drugs such as morphine which cause contraction of sphincter of oddi increase serum amylase.

Creatine Kinase (CK or CPK)

CPK is a dimer consisting of one subunit which is found in the brain (designated as B) and another in muscle (designated as M). It exists in the following three isozymic forms namely:

1. **MM (found in skeletal and heart muscle)**
2. **MB (found in cardiac muscle, also found in striated muscle)**
3. **BB (found in brain and a variety of other tissues)**

About 15% of the heart CK is in the form of MB isoenzyme, the remaining 85% being MM. It should be noted that skeletal muscle also contains some MB isoenzyme (<0.4%). The amount of MB isoenzyme increases in the plasma after a myocardial infarct, and therefore

MB isoenzyme of CK increases in plasma after a myocardial infarction.

in theory provides a fairly specific test.

The most useful application of estimating plasma MB activity is in the investigation of those patients suspected of having an infarct.

Heart and skeletal muscles are the richest sources of serum creatine phosphokinase, an enzyme which reversibly catalyzes the phosphorylation of creatine with ATP to form adenosine diphosphate and creatine phosphate.

$$\text{Creatine Phosphate + ADP} \xrightleftharpoons{\text{CPK}} \text{Creatine + ATP}$$

This enzyme is also found in cerebral tissue. Consequently, damage or disease (e.g. myocardial infarction, acute cerebrovascular disease, muscular dystrophy or injury) of these tissues will result in elevated serum CK levels.

High levels of CPK are also found after

In the wake of myocardial infarction, CK activity begins to rise within 4 to 6 hours; reaches to peak between 18 to 30 hours and returns to normal by the third day. Marginally increased levels may be found due to severe exercise and by large multiple intramuscular injections. **Besides the diagnostic importance in M.I, it's also of diagnostic importance in progressive muscular dystrophy of Duchenne type, polymyositis and in other muscular dystrophies.**

severe exercise, in hypothyroidism, acute cerebrovascular accidents and strokes and motor neuron disorders.

Normal levels in men and women differ with the methods employed. Normal values in men and women according to the method of Hughes (modified) are as given below:

Men	:	20 - 50 IU/litre
Women	:	10 - 37 IU/litre

The magnitude of elevation of CK in M.I. is found to be greater than those of SGOT and LDH elevations. CPK may be a more sensitive indicator of myocardial ischaemia than the other enzymes and may be potentially more useful in subendocardial infarctions. No increase in activity is noted in heart failure cases.

CPK activity is not elevated in liver disease, blood dyscrasia, chronic pulmonary diseases and chronic renal diseases. Minimal elevation has been infrequently noted in isolated cases of pulmonary infarction. Rarely, positive reactions have been reported associated with gangrene of the gallbladder, carcinoma of the pancreas, and diabetic acidosis. CPK activity levels may be altered by the presence of thyroid disease. Extremely high enzyme values are found more frequently in severe myxoedema than in the milder forms. When the disease is controlled with thyroid hormone, the enzymic activity returns to the normal range.

In contrast to SGOT and LDH, CPK is not elevated in patients with primary hepatic disease or with hepatic congestion from heart failure. In rare instances of pulmonary embolism or pulmonary infarction, one may find abnormal serum CPK activity, but the elevation in CPK is slight and may be due to local irritation of skeletal muscle by phlebitis.

Lactic Dehydrogenase (LDH or LD)

Lactic dehydrogenase is an enzyme which catalyzes the reversible conversion of lactic acid to pyruvic acid (Fig. 7.12).

$$\underset{\text{Lactic acid}}{\begin{matrix} CH_3 \\ | \\ HC-OH \\ | \\ COOH \end{matrix}} + DPN \underset{\text{dehydrogenase}}{\overset{\text{lactic}}{\rightleftharpoons}} \underset{\text{Pyruvic acid}}{\begin{matrix} CH_3 \\ | \\ C=O \\ | \\ COOH \end{matrix}} + DPNH$$

Fig. 7.12 : Biochemistry of lactic dehydrogenase

This enzyme is found in varying concentration in all the tissues of the body, namely in decreasing order-liver, skeletal muscle, kidney, heart muscle, lung, serum etc.

LDH rise is usually noted within the first 12 to 24 hours after myocardial infarction, peak is reached in two to four days and gradual return to normal is seen from the eighth to the fourteenth day. The peak elevations in LDH are roughly proportional to the extent of injury to the myocardial tissue. **In myocardial infarction, LDH elevations above 3,000 units suggest a grave prognosis.**

LDH levels get increased in megaloblastic anaemia, carcinomatosis, acute leukaemia, granulocytic leukaemia, heart failure, pulmonary infarction, renal necrosis, muscle disease and sickle cell anaemia. Less pronounced LDH increases are seen in inflammatory hepatic disease.

The disadvantage of LDH determinations is that this enzyme is also relatively non-specific for myocardial tissue. It is so widespread in body cells that coexistent disease processes in other organ systems can cause elevations.

Isoenzymes of Lactic Dehydrogenase (LD)

Mammalian lactic (lactate) dchydrogenases are tetramers composed of two types of subunits, designated as M (the major form found in muscle or liver) and H (the major form found in heart). Five combinations of subunits are possible i.e.,

HHHH (H_4)
HHHM (H_3M)
HHMM (H_2M_2)
HMMM (HM_3)
MMMM (M_4)

The possible combinations can be separated by electrophoresis as shown in Fig. 7.13.

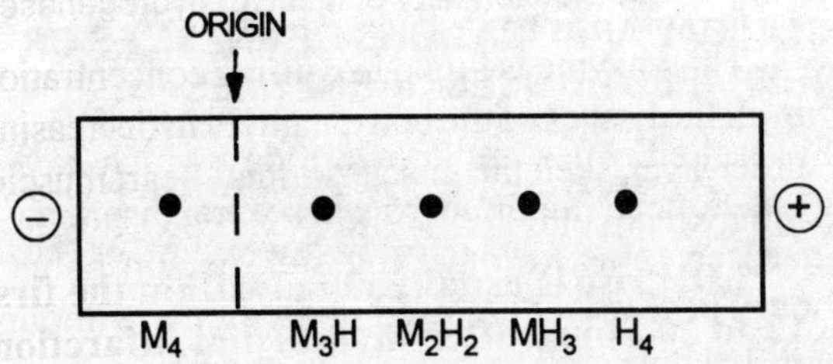

Fig. 7.13: Electrophoresis of lactate dehydrogenase isoenzymes at pH 8.6

It is clear from the Fig 7.13 that the net charge on the isozyme differs, those with an increasing content of the H subunit have an increasingly larger negative charge, while M_4 isozyme has a slightly positive net charge. These five forms of lactate dehydrogenase are isozymes that catalyze the same reactions, but they are found to different extents in different tissues. In man, the context of the several isozymes differs in heart and liver. Although the reason for this is not yet known, use is made of the fact in diagnostic differentiation of various diseases of liver and myocardium (heart). In both types of disease states, LD leaks out of the damaged cell and increases the concentration of the enzyme in blood serum.

In liver and heart muscle the predominant isozyme has subunit composition H_4 whereas in skeletal muscle, the predominant isozyme is M_4. The H_4 and M_4 isozymes have different K_m values for pyruvate. **Raised levels of LD_1 and LD_2 are characteristic of myocardial infarction; whereas LD_4 and LD_5 get elevated in liver disorders.**

Five isoenzymes of LD are known to exist:

LD_1 LD_2, LD_3, LD_4 and LD_5 (based on electrophoretic mobility)

1. Heart-LD_1 and LD_2
2. Liver-LD_5
3. Skeletal muscle-variable

Plasma LD may be elevated in:

(a) Myocardial disease
(b) Liver disease
(c) Skeletal muscle disease
(d) Miscellaneous

LDH of serum and various tissues consists of five different components which are separable by electrophoresis. These fractions are known as isoenzymes because they catalyze the same chemical reaction, i.e; the reduction of pyruvate to lactate.

Cellular damage to tissues such as myocardium and liver results in characteristic abnormalities in the relative proportions of various isoenzymes, demonstrable by electrophoresis. The plasma of normal adults contains five plasma isoenzymes, i.e. LDH_1, LDH_2, LDH_3, LDH_4 and LDH_5. These isoenzymes may be differentiated by physical (thermal stability), chemical (mobility on starch gel) and immunological characteristics.

LDH_1 and LDH_2 fractions of lactic

dehydrogenase become predominated in cases of myocardial infarction during electrophoresis. These isoenzyme changes occur earlier in the course of infarction and persist longer than the total plasma LDH enzyme activity.

Haemolyzed specimens cannot be used and the amount of serum subjected to electrophoresis must contain an adequate amount of enzyme activity.

Normal range

It differs with the method employed. For the spectrophotometric method, Wroblewski has given the normal range as 200-650 units (85-300 I.U. per litre), Elliot and Wilkinson as 150-500 units (72 to 240 I.U. per litre) whereas King, using his own method as 70-240 I.U. per litre.

> **There is a marked increase in the proportion of LD_1 in serum in myocardial infarction and LD_5 in liver disease.**
>
> **An increase in the level of lactate dehydrogenase activity in cerebrospinal fluid has been reported in cases of tumours of the Central Nervous System.** The normal range has been given as 10-25 I.U./l by King and as 3-20 by Wroblewski.

Antienzymes

Antienzymes may be referred to as the enzymes possessing antagonistic property to the proteolytic enzymes of the human system. Such enzymes are synthesized within our body. **Because of the availability of such enzymes, the wall of the alimentary canal is not digested itself by its own proteolytic enzymes.** Likewise, intestinal parasites (which are very common especially amongst children for example round-worms, hook-worms, pinworms, etc.) are also not digested by the proteolytic enzymes present in the alimentary canal. **Reports are also available regarding production of antienzymes in the serum when certain enzyme preparations are given parenterally.** The mucous membrane is also believed to contain anti-proteolytic enzymes. **Ascaris has been shown to contain anti-trypsin and anti-pepsin activity.**

> **Some well known antienzymes are:**
>
> 1. Anti-trypsin
> 2. Anti-pepsin
> 3. Anti-rennin
> 4. Anti-urease etc.

> **Radioimmunoassay can also be used to measure serum trypsin activity in suspected cases of cystic fibrosis.**

CLINICAL APPLICATIONS OF ENZYMES OR THERAPEUTIC USES OF ENZYMES

Several enzymes are known today which have got beneficial important role in several disorders/ diseases so as to make the sick person better one. These are being used in medicine without any hesitation. Their use in medicine is on increase day by day. More and more researches are going on in this direction. Since, the enzymes are inactivated in gastrointestinal tract, hence these are administered parenterally. Some of the important examples of such enzymes are as follows:

Trypsin

This has proved to be of value in the treatment of several clinical conditions. The purified enzyme has been administered parenterally, orally and intramuscularly. **In the treatment of acute thrombophlebitis (a blood clot and inflammation in a vein), small recurrent injections have been beneficial in many patients.**

Some types of ulcers have responded well to trypsin therapy, as have some specific traumatic injuries, such as boxers' black-eye and a number of other injuries to athletes and others.

Streptokinase

It is a bacterial enzyme obtained principally from β-hemolytic streptococci. **It causes fibrinolysis and dissolution of clot. It is used in the treatment of haemothorax and haematoma.**

Hyaluronidase

It is prepared from mammalian testes. It acts by depolymerizing hyaluronic acid and increasing tissue permeability. **It is used in the treatment of traumatic or postoperative edema.**

Pepsin

It is obtained from hog stomach. It is used in the treatment of gastric achylia (congenitally undeveloped gastric glands).

Thromboplastin

This is prepared by lysis of blood platelets and is used for blood coagulation.

Urokinase

It is prepared from human urine and is used in the treatment of pulmonary embolism and in myocardial infarction to dissolve the clot.

Fibrinolysin

It is prepared by activating fibrinolysinogen by streptokinase and is used in the treatment of venous thrombosis, pulmonary and arterial embolism.

Rennin

It is obtained from the glandular layer of calf stomach and is used in the therapy of gastric achylia.

DIAGNOSTIC IMPORTANCE OF ENZYMES (AT A GLANCE)

The assay of serum enzymes is used as an important aid to diagnosis. The level of enzymic activity of a number of enzymes gets raised in different pathological conditions. With the advancement of 'Biochemistry', it is now preferable to take into account the level of serum enzymes in certain diseases before starting the treatment. Timely enzymic investigations are of great value and significance to the physicians/ surgeons.

Some enzymes of diagnostic importance with principal conditions involved are as follows: (in alphabetical order, Table 7.3).

The great significance of enzymes is that the thousands of chemical transformations going on continually in living matter would not be possible without enzymes, which are the most important tools of the living cell. For the hydrolysis or the oxidation of such substances like fats and proteins, in the laboratory we commonly employ strong acids or alkalies or oxidizing agents and high temperatures.

Enzymes are organic catalysts produced by living organisms. They are generally soluble and colloidal substances, characterized by great activity, specificity and susceptibility to the influence of pH, temperature, and other environmental changes.

All the enzymes which have been isolated in pure condition to date are proteins. (The converse of this statement, i.e., that all proteins are necessarily enzymatically active is, however, not true).

All enzymes are proteins in nature does not hold true 100% as now there do exist few enzymes that are made up of RNA; **such enzymes are called as ribozymes. Thomas Cech** and **Sidney Altman** discovered ribozymes for which they were awarded Nobel Prize in Physiology and Medicine in the year **1989.**

Table 7.3 : Enzymes of diagnostic importance with principal conditions involved

Enzymes	*Principal conditions in which level of activity in serum gets elevated*
Amylase	Acute pancreatitis
Acid phosphatase (optimum pH 5)	Prostatic carcinoma *
Alkaline phosphatase (optimum pH 10)	Diagnosis of liver diseases, especially biliary obstruction and detection of osteoblastic bone disease, e.g. rickets.
Aspartate transaminase (AST-previously GOT)	Myocardial infarction. Liver diseases, especially with liver cell damage.
Alanine transaminase (ALT-previously GPT)	Liver diseases especially with liver cell damage.
Lactate dehydrogenase (LDH or LD)	Myocardial infarction, but also increased in many other diseases (liver disease, some blood diseases).
Creatine phosphokinase (CPK) or Creatine kinase (CK)	Myocardial infarction and skeletal muscle diseases (muscular dystrophy, dermatomyositis).
γ-glutamyl transferase (γ-GT) * *	Diagnosis of liver diseases, particularly biliary obstruction and alcoholism.
Urinary Elevation N -acetyl glucosaminidase in Urine can be used to indicate renal transplant rejection.	

* *Determination by radioimmunoassay technique which gives good results, is the choice of estimation these days, therefore, it should be carried at least in cases of suspected* ***prostatic carcinoma.***

** *γ - GT is elevated in the plasma of* ***alcoholics****, and also of* ***epileptics*** *taking barbiturates. This is because consumption of alcohol or barbiturates causes considerable proliferation of the endoplasmic reticulum inducing high levels of the enzyme.*

CHAPTER 8

VITAMINS

FAT-SOLUBLE VITAMINS

1. Vitamin A
2. Vitamin D
3. Vitamin E
4. Vitamin K

WATER-SOLUBLE VITAMINS

5. Thiamine (B_1)
6. Riboflavin (B_2)
7. Niacin, Nicotinic acid, Niacinamide, B_3
8. Pantothenic acid, B_5
9. Pyridoxine, Pyridoxal, Pyridoxamine, B_6
10. Biotin (Vitamin H)
11. Folic Acid (Pteroylglutamic acid), B_9
12. Vitamin B_{12}, Cyanocobalamine
13. Ascorbic acid (Vitamin C)
14. Lipoic acid

VITAMINS

INTRODUCTION

It will not be wrong to say that **'necessity is the mother of invention'**. In the **Japanese Navy** a high proportion of the sailors suffered for many years from **beriberi,** a condition now known as a vitamin B_1 deficiency disease. Scientist Takaki, after many attempts was finally able in the 1880s to arrange certain reforms in the diet of the Japanese navy. Meat and vegetable allowances were increased and evaporated milk was added to the diet. The effects on the health of the men were so dramatic that extension of the reforms was undertaken and thereafter only few cases of **'beriberi'** were detected in Japanese navy.

Scurvy, another deficiency disease, was so widespread among various early sailing crews that long voyages were usually either victims of a high incidence of sickness or loss of life. It were the English who early introduced limes or lemons into the diet of their sailing men to help protect against Scurvy. The English sailors are still called as **'limeys';** the term supposedly originated from the fact that they carried crates of limes aboard the vessels.

Today, a number of vitamins are known to exist which have been studied thoroughly from every angle.

What are Vitamins?

Vitamins are chemical entities which are essential for maintaining the metabolic processes at a normal level in animals and some have important roles in the plant metabolism also. With some exceptions, all animal species require the major vitamins preformed in the diet for the obvious reason that they are unable to synthesize them from other food constituents. A large number of vitamins have been isolated, characterized and then synthesized.

Plants and various microorganisms synthesize vitamins; animals eat the plants and store certain vitamins and the animal tissues also serve as vitamin sources for other species.

Vitamins, on the basis of solubility, have been divided into two categories as shown below:

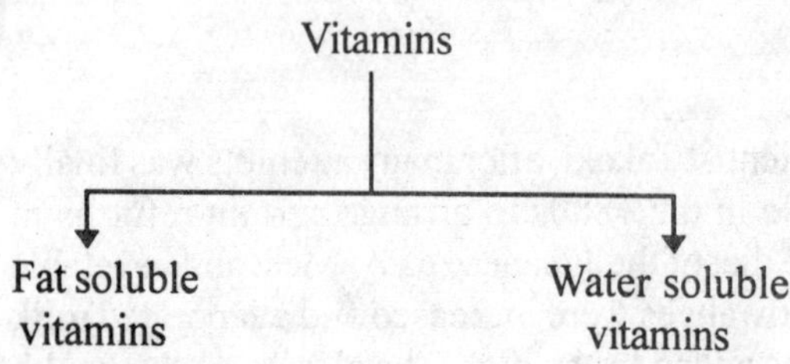

FAT SOLUBLE VITAMINS

These include vitamins A, D, E and K and are fat soluble as is evident from the name itself.

VITAMIN A

The discovery of vitamin A resulted from feeding experiments with rats and mice using purified rations. **McCollum is generally credited with the discovery of this vitamin.**

Vitamin A occurs in animal tissues only, but many plant tissues contain substances that, when fed to rats suffering from xerophthalmia, for instance, will relieve the condition. Thus, one must distinguish between vitamin A content and vitamin A activity. A number of carotenoid pigments of plants act as precursors of vitamin A. In other words, the animals can consume these pigments and bring about chemical alterations in them to produce vitamin A. **Remember, carrots and yellow corn contain no vitamin A, but since carotenes are present, they afford vitamin A activity to animals that eat them.**

Chemistry of vitamin A

A number of naturally occurring pigments can be converted into vitamin A (retinol) by animal tissues. These pigments known as the carotenoid pigments, are found primarily in green leafy plants and yellow vegetables. They are important sources of vitamin A for man and some animals.

Kuhn and Karrer showed that β-carotene is a symmetrical molecule containing two β-ionone rings connected by a carbon chain. It has the structure as given on next page.

Because of the marked chemical similarity of the carotenoid pigments, it is practical to show their differences without setting down the entire formulae. The two rings in β-ionone are marked A and B. The formula of α-carotene, for instance, can be indicated by showing the difference in the B ring of this pigment compared to the B ring of β-carotene. The remainder of the molecules are identical.

Since, the A ring in these pigments is a β-ionone ring, these compounds are vitamin A precursors. In **xanthophyll** (found in nature with the carotenes), each ring contains a hydroxyl group and thus this pigment does not yield vitamin A. **Licopene** has two open rings (as the B ring in γ-carotene) and hence, no activity is found in it.

The manner in which animals convert various precursor pigments into vitamin A is not understood; presumably it is an enzymatic process.

The relationship of insulin to vitamin A metabolism is not clear. It has been felt by various workers that diabetic individuals have impaired efficiency of carotene conversion to vitamin A.

Vitamin A_1 (retinol), $C_{20}H_{29}OH$ and vitamin A_2 (retinol$_2$), $C_{20}H_{27}OH$ are alcohols with the structures as given on the next page.

Vitamin A_2 contains one more double bond

A ring β-Carotene B ring

B ring in α-carotene shift in double bond

B ring in γ-carotene open ring

All trans vitamin A_1 (retinol$_1$)

All trans vitamin A_2 (retinol$_2$)

in the ring. It is a dehydrovitamin A_1 formed by the loss of two H atoms in the body. No carotenes are known from which the animal body can form directly.

Absorption of vitamin A

In the small intestine, the vitamin A esters of foods are hydrolyzed to fatty acids and the free vitamin. The vitamin is absorbed here mainly by the lymphatic system and appears in blood plasma as the ester, indicating reesterification in the intestinal wall. Carotene is absorbed in the small intestine. Bile salts help in the absorption of carotene and vitamin A but may not be essential for the latter.

Physiological functions of vitamin A

1. ***Growth.*** In the absence of a vitamin A source, animals fail to grow and may die before body stores are completely exhausted, and often before typical deficiency symptoms develop. The mechanism of vitamin A in the growth processes is not understood.
2. ***Epithelial tissue.*** The epithelium of a wide variety of organs in the body under goes changes in vitamin A deficiency. The changes have been demonstrated in the salivary glands, tongue and pharynx in the mouth, the respiratory tract, the genitourinary tract, the eyes and certain glands of internal secretion. The chemical and physiological functions of these lining tissues are thus altered.
3. ***Eyes.*** There are various eye conditions resulting from vitamin A deficiency. Early symptoms in rats (and other species) are enlargement of the eyelids and

Nightblindness is a common condition in man during famine and is prevalent in certain parts of the world continuously as a result of low vitamin A intake. **Xeroderma** is also common in adults.

In children one finds poor dark adaptation, xerosis, keratomalacia, growth failure and death.

inflammation of the conjuctiva. This is followed by corneal changes leading to blindness.

In man, **night blindness or nyctalopia,** is one of the early symptoms of deficiency. If the deficiency is slight, further changes may not be seen, but with a more severe deficiency, especially in children, xerosis and keratomalacia develop. The eyelids stick together as a result of a purulent discharge. Small ulcers may appear on the cornea and blindness may ensue. Metaplasia of the corneal epithelium and vascularization of the **substantia propria** are typical findings and generally lead to infection and obstruction of the ducts of the ocular glands.

The basis for the relationship of the dark adaptation test to vitamin A status lies in the work of scientists Hecht and Wald. The latter investigator pointed out a functional role of vitamin A in vision. As early as 1935, he indicated a mechanism, called as **visual cycle (Rhodopsin cycle),** involving vitamin A in the vision as mentioned below.

Visual cycle (Rhodopsin cycle)

The biochemistry of vitamin A in the visual process involves both types of photoreceptor cells in the retina. The rods provide black and white vision and respond to dim light. The cones provide colour vision and respond to bright light. Both these cells require vitamin A, also called retinol, for the formation of the visual pigments.

The 'Visual cycle' is summarized in Fig. 8.1.

The protein opsin, when complexed with 11-cis-retinal by the formation of a Schiff's base with a free amino group, produces the visual pigment rhodopsin. Under the influence of light, the retinal moiety is converted to all-trans-retinal. This isomerization is associated with a conformational change in the opsin. Such a change is transferred as a nerve impulse, possibly by alteration of the permeability to Na^+ or K^+ ions, from the photoreceptors to the optic nerve endings. Dissociation of the all-trans- retinal is followed by reduction of the aldehyde group to the primary alcohol to give all-trans-retinol. Retinol returns to the circulating blood pool of vitamin A that is stored in the liver.

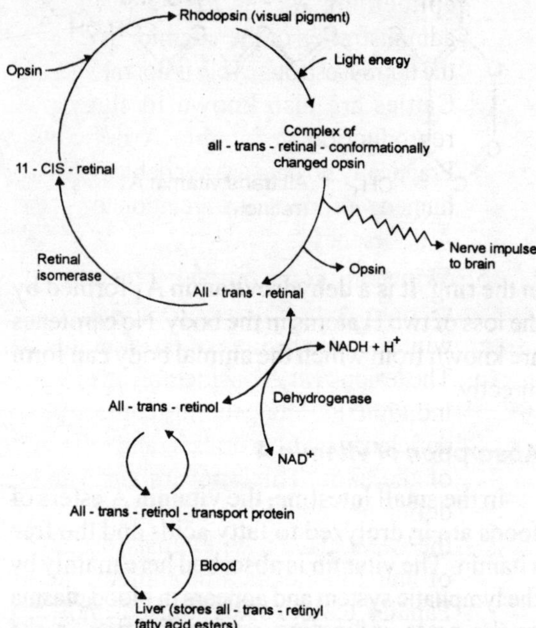

Fig. 8.1 : The Rhodopsin cycle (Visual cycle) and storage of Vitamin A

The retinol is then converted back to all-trans retinal in the retina where it is also isomerized back to 11-cis-retinal. The cycle is completed when 11-cis-retinal reacts with opsin to produce rhodopsin.

Colour vision

Similar photochemical events occur in both the rod and the cone cells. Each cone cell has one of three different colour sensitive pigments, blue (430 mμ), green (540 mμ), or red (575 mμ). The three pigments contain the same 11-cis-retinal moiety, but their opsins are different. Each pigment has a different wavelength of maximum absorbance, as noted above in parentheses and its photochemical reaction responds to one of the three primary colour components of the incident light. In each case the visual cycle is the same as that noted for rhodopsin.

4. ***Reproduction***. In rats, reproduction fails in vitamin A deficiency. Males develop rather rapidly an atrophy of the germinal epithelium; this is reversed after the administration of the vitamin. In females, the normal estrous cycle is not maintained. Cattles are also known to show poor reproduction in vitamin A deficiency. Practically no data are available regarding human reproduction in relation to vitamin A deficiency.
5. ***Skin.*** Only comparatively recently has a vitamin A deficiency been associated with specific lesions of the skin in man. The lesions vary considerably in different individuals. The general features of the deficiency involve dryness and roughness of the skin. This appears early in the deficiency and is due to a suppression of the sweat glands. A keratosis, especially of hair follicles is a prominent feature. Papules, masses of keratinized epithelium develop, which may be readily felt by rubbing a finger over the involved area.
6. ***Bones and teeth.*** Bone growth is markedly impaired in vitamin A deficiency.

   Teeth are derived from epithelial tissue, so, it is logical to expect a correlation between dietary vitamin A and tooth development.
7. ***Urolithiasis.*** In a long-standing vitamin A deficiency in rats, Higgins found that a high percentage of animals developed this condition.
8. ***Infection.*** **Vitamin A has been called the anti-infective vitamin.** The vitamin does help to establish and maintain a resistance to infection in the body.
9. ***Carbohydrate metabolism.*** A more specific function of vitamin A in metabolism involves its role in glucose synthesis from triose molecules.

Hypervitaminosis A

Excess vitamin A intake in humans leads to a number of untoward symptoms including in the acute phase, headache, nausea and vomiting, and drowsiness. In the chronic disease the findings include anorexia, dry itchy skin, alopecia, cracking of the lips and painful areas over various bones. **Often the serum alkaline phosphatase level is found to be elevated.**

Sources of Vitamin A

Many marine fish oils, especially the liver oils, have high concentrations of the vitamin. **Soupfin shark, ling cod, halibut and swordfish are among the species whose liver oils contain very high concentrations at certain seasons.**

Synthetic vitamin A preparations such as vitamin A palmitate, are now used in great quantity. Such products have no fishy taste and are preferred by many than the natural concentrates. .

Eggs, milk, cheese and the green leafy vegetables are good sources and many of the yellow crops such as corn and carrots are fair vitamin A sources for human beings.

Units and requirements of vitamin A

The USP (United States Pharmacopoeia) unit

There is some evidence that Vitamin A and retinoids protect an individual against cancer. The evidence appears to be strongest for lung cancer, but an inverse relationship between vitamin A intake and cancers of bladder, upper gastrointestinal tract and breast has also been proposed.

Vitamin A deficiency

1. Eye changes	1. Cell differentiation
(a) **Bitot's spot**	2. Epithelial metaplasia
(b) Corneal ulcer	3. **Keratin debris → kidney stones**
(c) Keratomalacia	
2. Blindness	4. **Increased Cancer?**

and the international unit (I.U.) of vitamin A are identical. The international standard is a specially prepared vitamin A acetate; and one unit of vitamin A is equal to the activity of 0.344 μg of this ester. This is equivalent to 0.3 μg of vitamin A and to 0.6 μg of β-carotene.

Recommended daily vitamin A intake for different categories is as follows:

1. For average men and women (age 18-75 years) : 5000 I.U./day
2. Boys (9-18 years) : 4500-5000 I.U./day
3. Girls (9-18 years) : 4500-5000 I.U./day
4. Children:
   - 1-3 years : 2000 I.U./day
   - 3-6 years : 2500 I.U./day
   - 6-9 years : 3500 I.U./day
5. Infants:
   - 0-1 year : 1500 I.U./day

Storage of vitamin A

Vitamin A is stored in the liver in large amounts ranging from 0.2 to 2.0 μmoles/g. Clinical problems do not arise so easily unless deprivation is extreme and is continued for relatively long periods i.e. for several months.

VITAMIN D

The disease rachitis (Figures 8.2, 8.6, 8.7 & 8.8), now popularly known as 'Rickets' is prevalent since ancient times.

HYPOVITAMINOSIS D : RICKETS AND OSTEOMALACIA

Both of these chronic conditions are basically same and characterised by a deficient calcification of bones caused by insufficient saturation of body fluids with calcium and phosphate, usually due to hypovitaminosis D. The age at which this occurs makes all the difference in their clinical, biochemical and pathological features. **Rickets occurs in the growing and osteomalacia in grown bones.**

CLINICAL FEATURES

A. Rickets

The name given by Ell is after an English bone setter named Rickets who around 1620 became famous for the diagnosis and treatment of the vitamin D deficiency. The affected infant may not look severely malnourished but is restless and irritable and has flabby toneless muscles. A 'pithed frog' position is usually adopted and abdomen is distended. There are also craniotabes, visible enlargement of epiphysis of lower end of radius and beading of ribs (Figs. 8.2, 8.7 and 8.8). There may be accompanying diarrhoea, respiratory infection and delayed milestones. In somewhat later stage there are frontal and parietal 'bossings' and chest deformities like Harrison's sulcus in untreated cases. By the age of 2-3 years, these signs become exaggerated and more severe deformities like **kyphosis** or **lordosis** of spine and low legs develop. Still later, the pelvic deformities develop which lead to serious obstetrical complications in women who had rickets in childhood. In more severe cases, infantile tetany may follow closely.

B. Osteomalacia

The patient suffering from osteomalacia is almost always a young mother, having been burdened with a rapid succession of pregnancies and lactations. Depending upon the severity of the condition she may present with anorexia, weight loss, bone pains, bony deformities (Fig. 8.6, 8.7 & 8.8), muscular weakness (myopathy), urinary tract infections, renal stones, chronic pyelonephritis and tetany. The gait is typically waddling. The sequence of postures adopted on trying to rise from squatting is also characteristic. The patient cannot suddenly rise, there is first extension of knees with hips remaining flexed. The trunk is straightened by the help of arms.

Chemistry of vitamin 'D'

This is a fat soluble vitamin. Two following anti-rachitic substances are active when taken by mouth:

(a) D_3 (cholecalciferol, Fig. 8.3), a derivative of cholesterol, and
(b) D_2 (ergocalciferol) (Fig 8.5), a synthetic derivative of plant sterol.

There is no vitamin D_1 but vitamin D_2 and D_3 are of great importance to human beings. Vitamin D_4 is activated 22-dehydroergosterol; whereas vitamin D_5 is activated 7-dehydrositosterol. A number of other products have been found to have some degree of antirachitic activity. Ergosterol and lumisterol are not antirachitic; however, tachysterol after reduction to dihydrotachysterol is used especially in the treatment of some types of **'tetany'** in human beings. The vitamins are not strictly sterols since ring B is open. The immediate precursor of D_3 is 7- dehydrocholesterol, which is found in the skin and sebum, and the agent promoting the change is ultraviolet light (Figs. 8.3 & 8.4). **If**

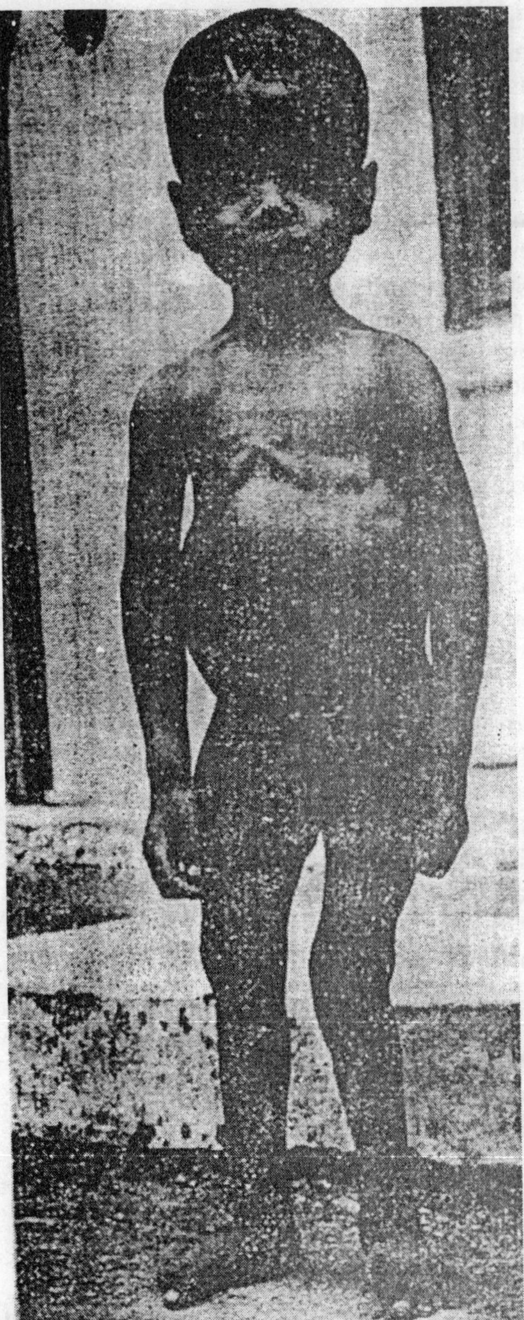

Fig. 8.2 : Rickets and osteomalacia, the puzzling quiz: Indians seem to be peculiarly susceptible to hypovitaminosis D (and calcium deficiency). This child from Darjeeling exhibits all the classical signs of rickets; big forehead, bent legs and swollen wrists ('cuffs'). (Picture by courtesy of WHO.)

the skin is exposed sufficiently to direct sunlight; sufficient vitamin will be formed, its intake in food is then unnecessary. There is indeed evidence that endogenously produced cholecalciferol derivatives are retained more efficiently in the body than those formed from ingested vitamin D. This evidence is based on the measurement of plasma levels of 25-OH-cholecalciferol, where it is associated with a specific vitamin-D-binding protein. Prolonged exposure of the whole body to ultra-violet light does not cause the 25-OH-D_3 levels to rise to more than double the normal level, whereas high doses of oral vitamin D may cause it to rise 10 fold. As 25-OH-D_3 is the metabolite most closely associated with toxic effects of hypervitaminosis D, it is now being suggested that supplementation of foodstuffs should not be regarded as adequate prophylactic, by comparison with UV irradiation of the skin.

The most important of the active substances, so far as the present knowledge goes is dihydroxycholecalciferol, which is formed from calciferol by two successive hydroxylations. (Fig 8.3). The first of these takes place in liver and the second in kidney. Thus cholecalciferol is taken up by liver from plasma, although it is not stored there, and 25-OH-D_3 is resecreted into plasma. The product of the second hydroxylation, 1,25-di-OH-D_3 has a short half-life. **It is now clear that production of 1,25-di-OH-D_3 is under hormonal control.** It is found that its concentration in plasma rises when the body's demand for Ca is high, as in

(a) Pregnancy, and
(b) Lactation

Regulation of Vitamin 'D'

It appears that its regulation is monitored through the action of parathyroid hormone on the renal cells, and not through direct feedback by plasma Ca^{++} or by calcitonin.

Owing to the regulatory action of the parathyroid gland, the serum Ca level in rickets is rarely low, even when the rickets is directly due to Ca deficiency in the diet. Instead, the inorganic phosphate level in serum is usually diminished.

PROVITAMINS:

(i) Ergosterol (plants, yeast)
(ii) 7-dehydrocholesterol (skin)
Vitamin D_2 is known as ergocalciferol
Vitamin D_3 is known as cholecalciferol

Physiological functions

Vitamin D is associated with a number of physiological processes in the body. Following are the established actions of vitamin D in the body:

(1) **Vitamin D is required for normal growth in mammals.** This is probably related to calcium and phosphorus absorption and their utilization, vis-a-vis it promotes minerals (mainly Ca and P) deposition in the skeleton.

(2) **It increases calcium and phosphorus absorption from the intestine.**

(3) It is antirachitic. Its deficiency causes rickets (Figure 8.6) which is a disease of young ones. The disease may involve a low blood calcium level or a low blood phosphorus level. In humans, the latter type is generally seen. **In infancy, the inorganic phosphorus level of blood is normally 4 to 6 mg per cent but in rickets this may be decreased to 1 to 2 mg percent.**

(4) Vitamin D has got a specific function on kidney tubular reabsorption of calcium and phosphate, thus inhibits their excretion via urine.

(5) It has got a general effect on the metabolism of citric acid which is a normal

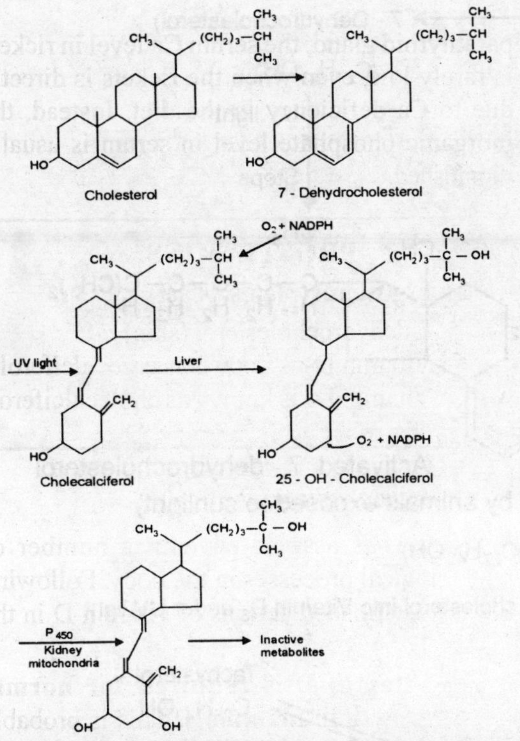

Fig 8.3 : The transformation of cholesterol into the major active metabolite 1 ,25-di-OH cholecalciferol.

constituent of many body tissues, including bone. Rachitic rats given vitamin D show increased urinary excretion of citric acid and increased levels in blood, bone, kidney, heart and small intestine with no elevation in liver.

In infants and children clinical symptoms of severe deficiency are readily seen on gross examination. Enlargement of the ankle, knee and wrist joints are noted. Other prominent features are bowed legs, delayed closure of the frontanelle, beading of the ribs at the costochondral junction (**"rachitic rosary"**), and delayed tooth eruption.

The mineral content of the bone decreases as the severity of the rickets progresses.

In adults osteomalacia occurs.

Absence of vitamin D causes rickets, a disease of infants. The bones become soft, the legs unable to support the weight, the flat bones deformed. The rib cage may become so deformed that death from respiratory failure occurs. The skeleton of the newborn child is always deficient in calcium and any derangement of Ca metabolism quickly makes the bones soft.

In adults, vitamin D deficiency causes osteomalacia, but the calcium reservoir in the adult is so large that the deficiency must be present for several years before the softening of the bones is present (it is usually only seen associated with pregnancy and lactation).

Hypervitaminosis

In human beings, it mainly causes:

(i) Hypercalcaemia,
(ii) Hypercalcinuria, and
(iii) Nephrocalcinosis

Daily requirements

Daily requirements for different categories of human beings are as follows:

(a) For infants : 400 IU/day
(b) During childhood : 400 IU/day
(c) During pregnancy and lactation : 400 IU/day
(d) Adults have apparently got little or no need of this vitamin

Serious overdosage is toxic which may cause calcification of the renal tubules. **Several deaths, mostly of children from vitamin D overdosage have been reported in last few years in several countries.**

Cholesterol ($C_{27}H_{45}OH$) → 7 - Dehydrocholesterol)

($C_{27}H_{43}OH$)

↓ UV light

↓ Steps

CH_3, CH_3, CH_2, HO

$-\underset{H}{C}-\underset{H_2}{C}-\underset{H_2}{C}-\underset{H_2}{C}-\underset{H}{C}(CH_3)_2$

Activated 7 - dehydrocholesterol

Vitamin D_3 (Synthesized by animals exposed to sunlight)

($C_{27}H_{43}OH$)

Fig 8.4 : Scheme to show the conversion of cholesterol into Vitamin D_3 under UV light

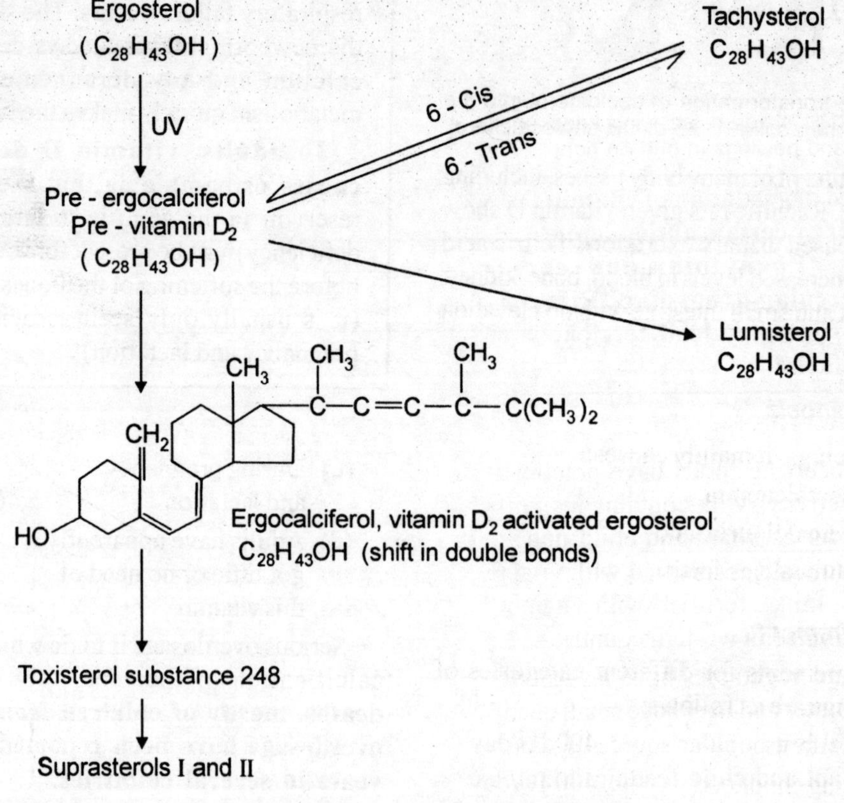

Fig 8:5 Scheme to show the conversion of erogosterol into Vitamin D_2 under UV light

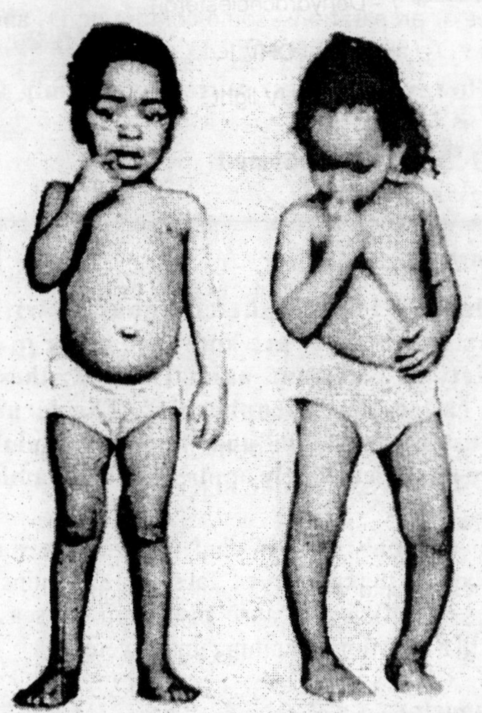

Fig 8.6 : Rachitic children, showing knock-knees in child on left and bowlegs in one on right.

Enhanced degradation of vitamin D and 25(OH) D by certain antiepileptic drugs such as 'Phenytoin' and certain antitubercular drugs like 'Rifampin' (Rifampicin) may lead to rickets and osteomalacia.

Sources

Naturally occurring foods have practically no vitamin D activity. Milk contains insignificant amounts as far as infant and child nutrition is concerned unless it is fortified with vitamin D. That is why, milk , fortified with vitamin D is widely distributed in western countries.

Grains and vegetables have less amount of vitamin D. Butter and liver have small quantities. Cod liver oil is a popular source of vitamin D (D_3) for infant and child feeding. Many other

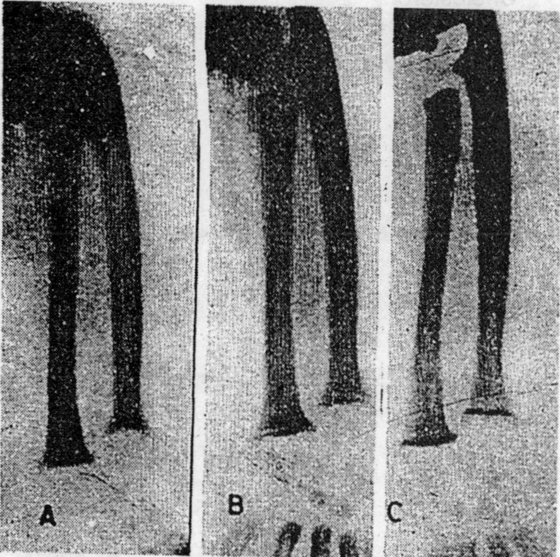

Fig 8.7 : X-ray films of forearm of a rachitic child, showing the effect of treatment A to C, views of the forearm. A, Before treatment: marked trabeculation of the radius and ulna is apparent, particularly in the cortical portion of the bone, with slight periosteal thickening. The *end* of the bone is slightly mushroomed *and* cupped and shows distinct fringing; the cartilage is swollen. The distal epiphyses of the radius are absent. There are two small centers of ossification in the wrists. B, One month after the treatment: a new centre of ossification has appeared in the distal epiphysis of the humerus. The centres of ossification at the wrists are still two in number but are larger *and* more distinct in outline. There is a fresh line of calcium deposition at the ends if the radius *and* the ulna, in the *zone* of provisional cartilage (line test). A clear area is present between this new calcification and the shaft (submetaphyseal rarefaction). Cupping, fringing *and* stippling are present; spur formation is also *noted,* outlining the swollen cartilage at the distal epiphysis of the ulna (beginning healing). C, *One* & a half months after the treatment. Healing is *now* advanced. The shaft shows calcification of subperiosteal osteoid at the outer aspect of the radius, giving the bone a greater width. Calcification of the provisional zone in the metaphyses is much more distinct *and* the submetaphyseal area is filling in.

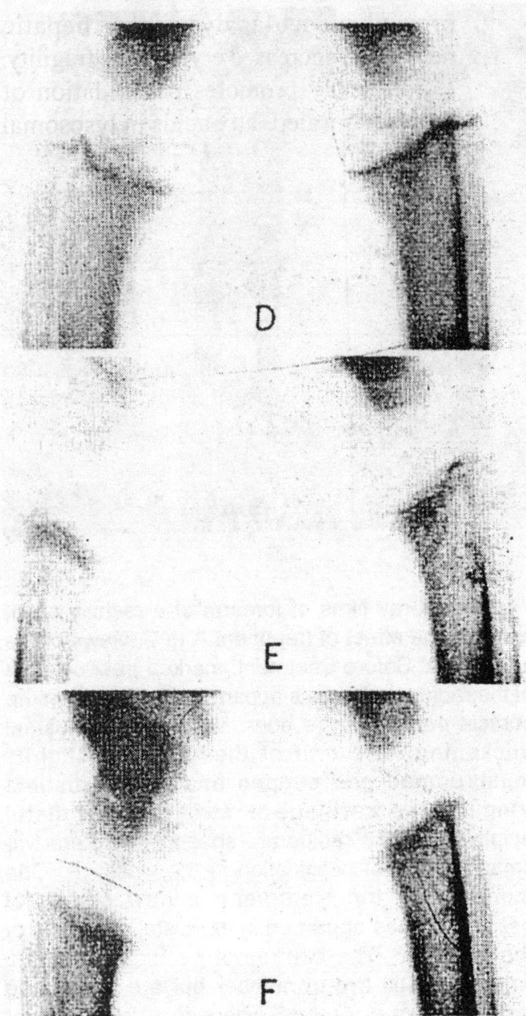

Fig 8.8 X-ray films of legs of a rachitic child A. Before treatment: cupping of the distal ends of both tibias and fibulas with compression and widening of the end of the shaft. B. One month after treatment: beginning healing of the distal ends of both bones (tibia and fibula) (line test). Submetaphyseal rarefaction. Periosteal hyperplasia at the distal third of both tibias. C. One and a half months after treatment: advanced healing. Submetaphyseal rarefaction is now well filled in. The ends of the bones are well calcified with marked stippling in the distal cartilage of the tibia and the beginnings of a centre of ossification in the distal epiphyseal cartilage of the tibia.

types of preparations, some containing D_2 and some D_3, are also marketed.

However, the best sources of vitamin D are as follows:

1. **Fish liver oils and**
2. **Margarine**

VITAMIN E

Today, at least eight compounds with vitamin E activity are known to occur in a variety of plant and animal tissues; these are called the "tocopherols". The terms "antisterility vitamin" and "fertility vitamin" have also been widely applied to the vitamin E.

It was only in 1977 that this vitamin was included in the category of 'fat soluble vitamins'. Does its deficiency cause any specific disease is still a question remaining unanswered?

Chemistry

Evans and co-workers prepared three crystalline derivatives of compounds from the nonsaponifiable fraction of wheat germ oil and showed that the original alcohol obtained by hydrolysis of one of them had high vitamin E activity. **These workers gave the active alcohol the name "α-tocopherol".**

There are eight naturally occurring tocopherol derivatives known. Six are toco derivatives and two are tocotrienol derivatives as given below:

toco derivatives:
- α - tocopherol (alpha)
- β- tocopherol (beta)
- γ - tocopherol (gamma)
- ζ_2 - tocopherol (zeta$_2$)
- η - tocopherol (eta)
- δ - tocopherol (delta)

tocotrienol derivatives:
- ε - tocopherol (epsilon)
- ζ_1 - tocopherol (zeta$_1$)

Pure tocopherols are oils and are fat-soluble.

The tocopherols are extraordinarily stable to heat in the absence of oxygen and they withstand acids at elevated temperatures. Ultraviolet light destroys the vitamin activity as does oxidation. **The tocopherols are excellent antioxidants.** This property is assuming great importance from a physiological standpoint. **α-tocopherol is biologically more potent than any other form,** the structure of which is as shown below:

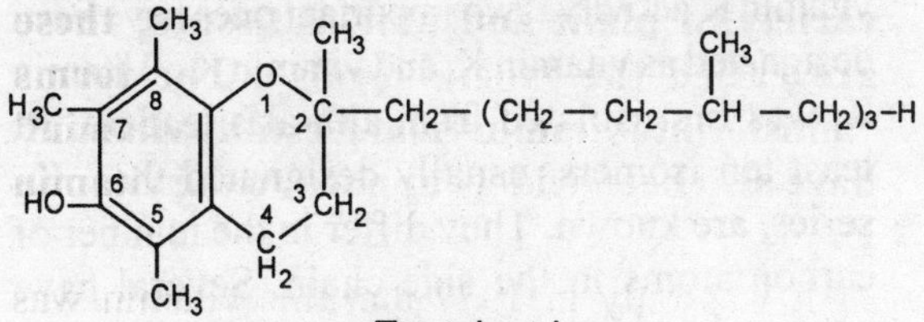

α - Tocopherol

(5,7, 8-Trimethyltocol)

> There is no evidence that large doses (mega doses i.e. in grams) of this vitamin provide any benefit to the human beings in the form of the maintenance of muscular activity or sexual vigour or the youthfulness of the skin.

Functions

Tocopherols act as antioxidants to prevent many undesirable oxidations in the body out of which some important ones are the following:

1. Scavenger of free radicals: By their antioxidant actions, tocopherols, function as scavengers of free radicals like free OH radical, superoxide anion (O_2), free halogen radicals (Cl), etc. to prevent their peroxidative effects on unsaturated lipids present in membranes, and thus are responsible for stabilizing the membranes.

   By reducing free radicals in this way, tocopherols preserve the integrities of membrane-bound organelles and thereby prevent muscular dystrophy, hepatic necrosis or increased erythrocyte fragility. E-deficiency promotes peroxidation of polyunsaturated fatty acids in lysosomal membrane.
2. Antioxidant action of tocopherols is very helpful in preventing the peroxidative effects of atmospheric pollutants like O_3, H_2O_2 and NO_2 on lipids of respiratory membranes.
3. Antioxidant action of tocopherol is also helpful in protecting selenide at the active sites of membrane selenoproteins against the harmful effects of free radicals.
4. Since, the tocopherols are responsible for preventing peroxidative changes in the mitochondrial membranes, therefore they maintain the translocation of phosphate ions into mitochondria; in this way, **they may increase the rate of oxidative phosphorylation.**
5. Antisterility factor: It has been proved that tocopherols prevent sterility in lower animals like rodents etc. but it has yet to be established in human beings.

Vitamin E deficiency

In man, deficiency symptoms are not well established, primarily because known cases of deficiency are rare. It is agreed that man requires vitamin E. **Red blood cells are subject to hemolysis by hydrogen peroxide or dialuric acid to a greater degree in vitamin E deficiency.** In some newborn infants, the red

> **Deficiency of vitamin E causes anaemia in premature infants.**
>
> Hypervitaminosis has been reported to induce blurred vision, headache, dizziness, fatigue, acne, vasodilation, gastrointestinal symptoms, prolonged clotting time and rise in serum cholesterol and fats.

blood cells are readily hemolyzed by hydrogen peroxide. Gyorgy found that administration of vitamin E by mouth prevents this hemolysis.

Sources

The most potent natural sources of tocopherols are the vegetable oils; of these, wheat germ oil has the highest concentration. Corn oil, cottonseed oil and safflower oil contain considerable amount. Fish oils are poor sources. Lettuce and alfa-alfa are good sources of the vitamin. Other foods have little activity. Of the animal tissues, liver is usually the highest in vitamin E although the level is generally low in other animal tissues.

Requirement of Vitamin E

Although animal requirements for vitamin E are fairly well established, there are no acceptable experimental data on human requirements.

It has been opined that the adult human requirement may vary from 10 to 30 mg per day; whereas for infants an intake of 0.5 mg per kg body weight has been suggested.

VITAMIN K

History

In 1929, Dam reported that chicks developed a hemorrhagic condition and prolonged blood clotting time when grown on specific synthetic rations. In 1935, he proposed the term vitamin K (Koagulation-vitamin) for a factor in certain foods which protected chicks against this haemorrhagic syndrome. Many foods were tested by Dam for vitamin K activity, who later on concluded that hog liver was very high, cod liver oil practically devoid of activity, whereas egg yolk as a poor source. **Among the vegetable material tested, hemp seed was found to be an excellent source.** The factor was found to be fat soluble.

Dam, Karrer and their co-workers isolated the vitamin from alfa-alfa in 1939. In the same year Doisy and associates isolated the principle from both alfa-alfa and fish meal. It was evident that the vitamin from alfa-alfa was clinically different from the product obtained from fish meal. Vitamin K_1 was used to designate the former one and K_2 the latter one.

Chemistry

There are several compounds that exhibit vitamin K activity. Two important ones have been designated as vitamin K_1 and vitamin K_2. Vitamin K_1 was first isolated from alfa-alfa leaf oil. At least ten isomers, usually designated the K_2 series, are known. They differ in the number of carbon atoms in the side chain. Several have been isolated from natural sources.

Vitamin K_1 is 2-methyl-3-phytyl-l, 4-naphthoquinone. The original K_2 contains two farnesyl units in the side chain at position 3 which is equivalent to 6 isoprene unit or 30 carbon atoms. Other K_2 molecules contain 7 isoprene units and 9 isoprene units in the side chains (35 and 45 carbon atoms). To simplify naming of these compounds, it was suggested that they be designated as vitamin $K_{2(30)}$, vitamin $K_{2(35)}$ and $K_{2(45)}$.

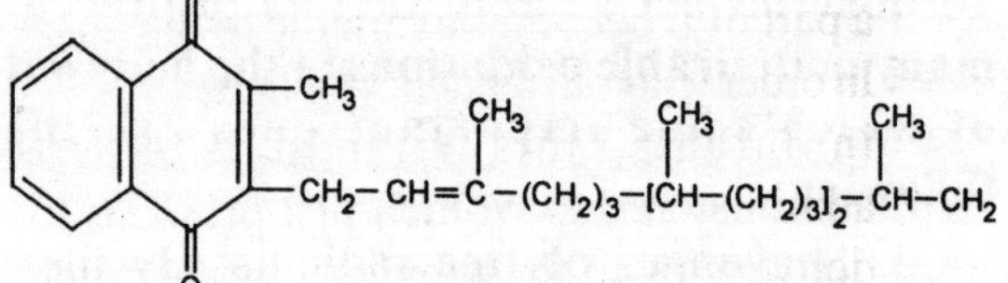

$-CH_3$; $-CH_2-CH=C(CH_3)-(CH_2)_3-[CH(CH_3)-(CH_2)_3]_2-CH(CH_3)-CH_2$

Vitamin K_1

(2 - methyl - 3 - phytyl - 1, 4 - naphthoquinone)

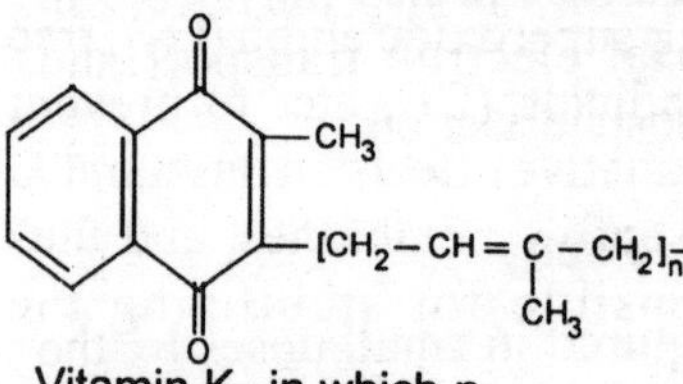

$-CH_3$; $-[CH_2-CH=C(CH_3)-CH_2]_n-H$

Vitamin K_2 in which n can be 6, 7, 9,

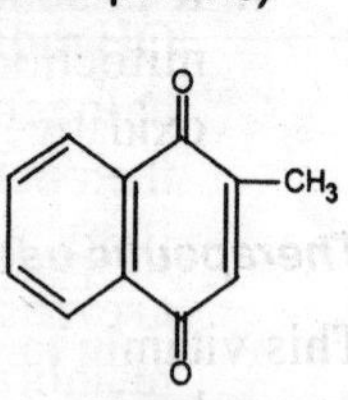

$-CH_3$

Menadione (Vitamin K_3)

A number of vitamins of both the K_1 and K_2 series have been synthesized. A simple molecule,

2 - methyl - l, 4 - naphthoquinone, is known as vitamin K_3 or menadione and is readily obtainable in pure form.

Physiological Aspects

1. The specific function of vitamin K is to stimulate the production of prothrombin by the liver. Since the clotting process depends on the conversion of fibrinogen to fibrin by the action of thrombin, a deficiency of prothrombin prolongs the clotting time of the blood by slowing the rate of formation of fibrin threads. The action of thrombin is enzymic; prothrombin is, therefore, a zymogen or inactive form.
2. It is also involved in the manufacture or preservation of other blood-clotting factors, including proconvertin, Christmas factor and Stuart factor.
3. The newborn infant is subject to an alimentary vitamin K deficiency because of the fact that vitamin K is not readily passed from the mother to the foetus. The disease is characterized by low prothrombin levels and consequently, a tendency to hemorrhage. Many common intestinal flora synthesize the vitamin, and a part of it becomes available to the host. In order to avoid tendency of haemorrhage in infants, this vitamin is either administered to women just previous to delivery or to the newborn infant; such kind of practice is now common.
4. It is believed that it also plays role in mitochondrial electron transport and oxidative phosphorylation.

Therapeutic uses; toxicity

This vitamin is required in small doses by the human beings. Since, it is found in abundance in the foods which a man commonly consumes daily, hence dietary supplementation is rarely necessary in adult humans. It is of value, however, in treating cases of congenital hypoprothrombinernia or in minimizing the decrease in prothrombin concentration, often seen in newborn infants.

Vitamin K_1 is also administered to patients where prothrombin time has been deliberately increased (clotting slowed) by the use of vitamin K antagonists such as **dicumarol.** When a thrombus (blood clot) is formed in a coronary artery, the portion of the heart muscle being supplied by that artery becomes necrotic and the person usually has symptoms of **'heart attack'**. The rationale of administering an antagonist of vitamin K is to slow the clotting time of the blood to minimize the possibility of the formation of additional clots; since an excessive amount of such antagonists will cause spontaneous haemorrhages by inhibiting the clotting mechanisms, the dosage must be carefully controlled and vitamin K_1 administered if the prothrombin time becomes too long.

Requirements and sources

Official requirements for human beings have not yet been set, but the minimal amount for adults has been estimated as 2 mg of menadione, injected intravenously. Microgram quantities are required to prevent the decrease in prothrombin concentration that usually takes place in the blood of infants a few days after birth; **this can be administered either to the new born infant**

Green leafy vegetables, such as alfa-alfa, spinach, cabbage are the best sources of vitamin K. Roots, tubers, seeds and fruits contain only small amounts.

Certain microorganisms found in the intestinal tract are able to synthesize vitamin K_2 and undoubtedly provide an important source of this vitamin for the human beings.

or to the mother shortly before delivery. Because of the termination of supply from the maternal circulation with the cutting of the umbilical cord, the concentration of the several blood-clotting factors are low in the circulatory system of newborn infants; supplements of vitamin K often prevent haemorrhage by stimulating synthesis of prothrombin in the liver.

As regards sources of this vitamin; they include both plants and animals, a list of which is as shown in Table 8.1.

Table 8.1: Major sources of vitamin K

Sl. No.	Source	Vitamin K (mg/100g edible portion)
1.	Alfa-alfa	425-850
2.	Spinach	334
3.	Cauliflower	275
4.	Cabbage	250
5.	Soyabean	190
6.	Wheat bran	80
7.	Wheat germ	37
8.	Wheat, whole	36
9.	Liver, pork	115-230

Vitamin K activates blood clotting factors II, VII, IX and X
Its deficiency causes in:
Infants : haemorrhagic disease of newborn
Adults : defective blood clotting

WATER SOLUBLE VITAMINS

As is evident from the title itself, vitamins included in this group are soluble in water which include well established members of the B complex group i.e. thiamine (B_1), riboflavin (B_2), niacin, pantothenic acid, pyridoxine (B_6), biotin, folic acid, cyanocobalamine (B_{12}), choline, inositol, lipoic acid and p-aminobenzoic acid have also been included in this category. Ascorbic acid (Vitamin C) and compounds with related activity, such as citrin **(Vitamin "P")**, are also water-soluble vitamins.

Since the vitamins of this category are soluble in water, therefore, their absorption remains unaffected by malabsorption states except severe diarrhoea in which it certainly gets affected. Various members of this group function as coenzymes in intermediary metabolism and thus play very important roles in the human body, particularly in energy-releasing mechanisms and haematopoiesis (formation of erythrocytes and other blood cells).

THIAMINE (VITAMIN B_1) (ANTI-BERIBERI OR ANTI-NEURITIC VITAMIN)

History

The term **'deficiency disease'** was first applied to a condition known as beriberi, which was found to be common in south-eastern Asia and the islands of the Pacific Ocean. The similarity in pathology between this disease and polyneuritis noticed in chickens given a restricted diet of polished rice only, both of which could be cured by feeding the **"silver skin" (i.e., pericarp and germ) of the grain,** prompted scientist Eijkman to investigate the subject thoroughly from the nutritional standpoint. Eijkman, then was able to produce beriberi by feeding a diet of polished rice and prevented the syndrome by dietary means. He reported his classic studies in 1896-97. Besides those oriental countries where polished rice is the main item of diet, **other places in which beriberi has been observed include prisons or asylums, localities where the diet is faulty, war-stricken countries, etc.**

The vitamin was finally crystallized from rice polishings by Jansen and Donath in 1926 in the same laboratory where Eijkman conducted his original studies. **Eijkman was able, after thirty years, to confirm the antineuritic activity of the crystalline vitamin hydrochloride.** A

A deficiency of this vitamin primarily involves the following two important systems of the human body namely:

(i) Nervous system, and

(ii) Circulatory system

In the absence of thiamine, peripheral neuritis develops, resulting in paralysis (Fig. 8.9). Cardiovascular symptoms like edema and loss of appetite also appear.

Its deficiency in man leads to the condition known as **beriberi;** in animals the syndrome is referred to as polyneuritis.

Beriberi is widespread amongst low-socioeconomic groups of South-East Asia, where due to poverty B_1-deficient polished rice forms the main food item of their diet.

Nausea, vomiting, anorexia, loss of body weight, lassitude and rise in blood pyruvate level are found in all types of 'beriberi'.

decade later the structure and synthesis of the vitamin were announced by R.R. Williams and his co-workers.

The cause of Beriberi was proved beyond doubt to be in the finding that the highest concentration of hitherto unknown intrient in cereals was in the germ and pericarp and high milling and polishing removed the same with resultant deficiency. **A discovery that won Nobel Prize for Eijkman.**

Clinical cases of thiamine deficiency in the western hemisphere are rare today. In the United States, U.K. and other advanced countries, foods are readily available to provide an adequate dietary intake of thiamine for all ages. Prior to the distribution of enriched foods of this vitamin, the neuritis in chronic alcoholics was shown to be the result of insufficient thiamine. **However, these days, it is difficult to find the cases of the deficiency of this vitamin even among alcoholics.**

Physiological and Clinical Aspects of Thiamine

This vitamin is essential for the growth and metabolism of all animals as well as of many plants and microorganisms. Deficiencies are characterized by a variety of symptoms and clinically are often complicated by the effects of lack of other nutrients.

In thiamine deficiency (avitaminosis B_1), a form of peripheral neuritis is manifested affecting both the sensory and motor nerves. During the early stages, neuralgia and cramps of the calf muscles are common; as the condition advances, the thigh muscles become weak and toe and foot -drop develop with hypesthesia. **The acute disease, beriberi, may be of following five types:**

(i) Dry beriberi

(ii) Wet beriberi

(iii) Acute cardiac beriberi

(iv) Infantile beriberi and

(v) Wernicke-Korsakoff encephalopathy

Onset of Beriberi

Both dry and wet beriberi have a similar, usually insidious onset in the form of anorexia,lassitude and weakness in the legs making walking difficult. Some patients may have a little pain in the pericardium, palpitation and edema, usually of face or legs. There is associated paresthesia and/or anesthesia of limbs. **Such patients, mostly belonging to labourer class usually ignore such symptoms and keep working.** A bout of undue exertion or fever may precede the above symptoms, or if they are already present, may drag the patient into more severe stages as described below.

(i) Dry Beriberi

This is usually a chronic condition and the patient as a markedly wasted or bedridden one with some superadded infections like tuberculosis or dysentery which overshadow the basic nutritional disorder. The diagnostic feature is polyneuropathy and the history is characteristic of progressively increasing weakness and wasting of muscles leading to correspondingly deteriorating walking capacity. Flaccid paresis, wrist drop and foot drop also are present.

In this type cachexia, numbness, and paralysis are the primary symptoms.

(ii) Wet Beriberi

As the name implies, this condition is marked by presence of **anasarca (generalized edema).** In contrast to dry beriberi, onset is marked by pain and tenderness in leg muscles after walking. **There are also palpitation, dyspnoea and congestive heart failure and a risk of passing into acute cardiac failure and death.**

It is associated with marked edema ('pitting') and paresthesia of the extremities.

(iii) Acute Cardiac Beriberi

The patients of acute cardiac beriberi present with suddenly appearing, fulminating cardiac failure, which if untreated results in death within a few hours.

(iv) Infantile Beriberi

This presents as a syndrome and is at times quickly fatal. **It affects infants within the first six months (mostly between one to four months and babies on breast).** Of the two forms, viz., acute and chronic, the former is more lethal and less likely to be correctly recorded because of the abrupt onset of cardiac failure leading to cyanosis and dyspnoea associated with convulsions, coma and death within 24-48 hours. **The whole thing may be over just in a few days.** The infants affected are pale, oedematous and ill tempered; have loss of appetite, **vomiting and green coloured diarrhoeic stools.** There is a characteristic thin whining cry, at times even aphonia (loss of voice). The involvement of cranial nerves predominates in contrast to that of the spinal in adults. The picture may be confused with encephalitis due to convulsion and coma. The other form, the chronic, is less common and presents a picture resembling marasmus, due to general poor nutrition associated with anorexia, vomiting and diarrhoea, and is less likely, to end fatally.

(v) Wernicke-Korsakoff Encephalopathy

This extremely rare presentation in India is found more in the Western countries and is usually superimposed upon conditions like alcoholism, chronic gastrointestinal disease, carcinoma of stomach, prolonged diarrhoea, hyperemesis gravidarum or, irregularly controlled diabetes. The patient presents with an acute picture of a psychiatric nature- the **Korsakoff's psychosis**, and may progress rapidly to coma and death.

This is characterized by lesions and haemorrhages near the third cerebral ventricle, paralysis of eye movements, depression, severe loss of memory and mental confusion, etc.

In animals, the symptoms are loss of muscular coordination, spastic movements, retraction of the head (opisthotonos), and paralysis (Fig. 8.9). Recovery from the symptoms of **'polyneuritis'** is very rapid when this vitamin is administered, especially by injection.

Debility and progressive decline in weight are observed early in thiamine deficiency due to **anorexia** (loss of appetite). This is one of the most striking symptoms of this deficiency which is due to reduced food intake, ultimately leading to failure of growth. The depression of appetite is related to the failure to metabolize carbohydrate at the point of pyruvic acid decarboxylation (see carbohydrate metabolism, glycolysis - TCA cycle).

In polyneuritis pathological changes in the

Thiamine deficiency in man leads to the condition known as beriberi, in animals the syndrome is referred to as **polyneuritis.**

Beriberi is not found in advanced countries but is widespread amongst low socioeconomic groups of South- East Asia, where due to poverty B_1 deficient polished rice forms the main food item of their diet.

Nausea, vomiting, anorexia, loss of body weight, lassitude (weariness, heaviness) and rise in blood pyruvate level are found in all types of 'beriberi'.

The vitamin has a characteristic yeasty odour and taste. It is a basic substance and forms insoluble compounds with picric, phosphotungstic and tannic acids. As the pH increases beyond neutrality, thiamine becomes unstable, especially at elevated temperatures. In foods, this is stable at cooking temperatures, though a considerable function gets extracted into the cooking water and may be lost if this is discarded.

The principal ester of thiamine is the pyrophosphate, known as cocarboxylase or diphosphothiamine.

tissues and organs of the body include cardiovascular and neural disturbances, atrophy of the endocrine glands and other vital organs and hypertrophy of the adrenals. **Prolonged deficiency leads to cardiac failure and death.**

Free thiamine is phosphorylated in vivo to a coenzyme known as cocarboxylase i.e., thiamine pyrophosphate by liver and kidney; the phosphorylating agent is ATP i.e., adenosine-5'-triphosphate. In animal tissues, **cocarboxylase** plays a role in various reactions involving principally the decarboxylation of pyruvic and other keto acids. In erythrocytes, transketolase, an enzyme of HMP shunt of glucose metabolism, requires the participation of cocarboxylase. In the brain, cocarboxylase plays a role in the reduction of pyruvate to lactate and the dismutation to CO_2 and acetate, and their subsequent oxidation to carbon dioxide and water. In liver and other tissue cells, cocarboxylase is involved in the conversion of pyruvate to oxalacetate which combines oxidatively and irreversibly with another molecule of pyruvate to enter the citric acid cycle. The oxidative decarboxylation of ketoglutarate to succinate and of pyruvate to acetoacetate, and the conversion of pyruvate to the acetyl group of acetyl coenzyme- A are additional examples of the reactions found to be mediated by cocarboxylase.

It has been shown by controlled studies in a number of experimental animals, and in man, that the activity of erythrocyte transketolase gets progressively decreased as the thiamine deficiency develops. In man, the addition of cocarboxylase to haemolyzed red cells which were obtained from a thiamine deficient person, restores the transketolase activity towards normal. **Therefore, thiamine occupies a key position in carbohydrate metabolism.** In advanced thiamine deficiency both pyruvate and lactate accumulate in the blood whereas glycogen concentration increases in the liver and heart muscle.

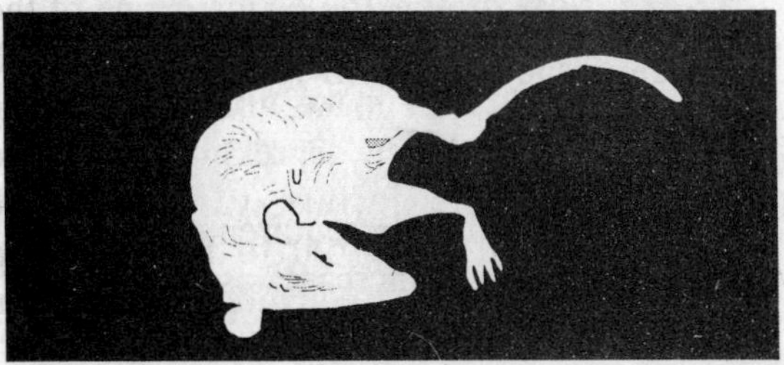

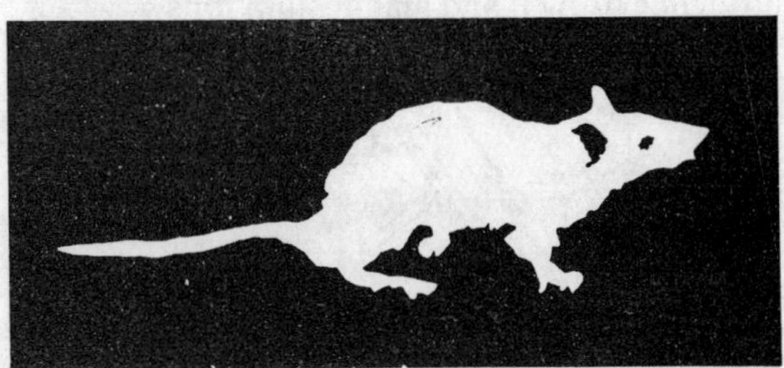

Fig. 8.9 Effect of thiamine deficiency and subsequent change after an adequate diet.

Storage and synthesis of thiamine

It is found to be stored in animal tissues in a very low concentration, meaning to say, it's storage capacity is small. It occurs both in free and phosphorylated form. It is found to be present in somewhat higher concentration in the heart, liver, and kidneys than in muscles and brain. It is possible to increase the thiamine content of the tissues by dietary means, however, total storage capacity is so limited that even under these circumstances only a few weeks' reserve can be maintained. It is, therefore, important that the daily diet should include an adequate supply of thiamine. **In man, this is synthesized by intestinal form, the nutritional importance of this contribution is not known.**

Chemistry

For the first time, it was isolated in crystalline form by Williams. Its structure was elucidated by Williams, Clarke and their co-workers. It consists of a pyrimidine and a thiazole ring system joined by a methylene bridge as shown below:

In acidic medium it may withstand prolonged heating at 120°C; whereas it is rapidly destroyed in alkaline medium. It is not oxidized by atmospheric oxygen under ordinary conditions. Mild oxidizing agents convert it to a pigment known as thiochrome which has got no vitamin activity.

Physiological actions of this vitamin are due to its pyrophosphoric ester, popularly known as cocarboxylase (TPP), which is formed by the phosphorylation of the vitamin under the influence of ATP and magnesium ions.

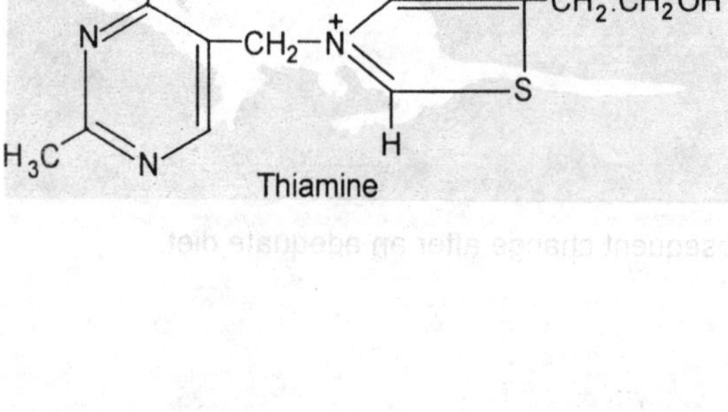

Thiamine

Coenzyme activity of thiamine

An important derivative of thiamine is the pyrophosphate. This molecule is known as cocarboxylase and is the coenzyme or prosthetic group of the enzyme decarboxylase, which is involved in the decarboxylation of α-ketoacids in the body. The structure of thiamine pyrophosphate is shown below.

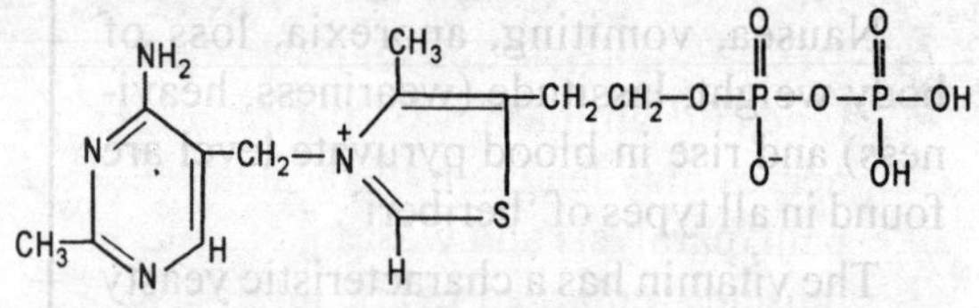

thiamine pyrophosphate (cocarboxylase)

$$CH_3COCOO^- + Pi \longrightarrow CH_3COCOOP + HCOO^-$$

pyruvate inorganic phosphate acetylphosphate formate

TPP is also involved as a coenzyme in a phosphoroclastic cleavage of α-keto acids.

In such a reaction the acyl of the acid is converted through acyl CoA to acylphosphate and the carboxyl group may become formate.

Deficiency

In humans its deficiency causes a disease called as **'beriberi'**. This disease is rare in the Western world because of food habits and food enrichment. Initially, in this disease, anorexia (loss of appetite), weight loss, fatigue and gastrointestinal-disturbances are noted; whereas in the later stage, cardiac impairment is seen. Administration of the vitamin or foods rich in it is the quick answer of the disease. Most thiamine deficiency states in human beings get aggravated by the deficiency of other B vitamins.

Daily Requirement

The recommended daily requirement is nearly 1 mg (333 IU), but it increases as the intake of carbohydrate increases.

- Its deficiency is generally encountered amongst **'chronic alcoholics'** because alcohol interferes with the absorption of thiamine by intestine.
- Principal tissues which are affected by its deficiency include the heart, central nervous system and the peripheral nerves.
- Beriberi is of five types; viz.,
  (a) **Dry or neuritic beriberi:** In this type, inflammation of peripheral nerves may lead to hyperaesthesia, pain, paralysis and wasting of limb muscles, enlarged heart, inflammation of ophthalmic nerve leading to blindness, etc.
  (b) **Wet or edematous beriberi:** Extensive edema in the extremities and heart, congestive heart failure and cardiac enlargement are encountered.
  (c) Acute cardiac beriberi
  (d) Infantile beriberi
  (e) **Wernicke-Korsakoff syndrome:** Characterized by lesions and haemorrhages near the third cerebral ventricle, paralysis of eye movements, abnormal gait, depression, insomnia, disorientation, extreme anxiety, severe loss of memory and mental confusions etc. **This syndrome is produced by B_1-deficiency in patients genetically deficient in transketolase activity.**

Sources

The vitamin is widely distributed in both plant and animal tissues. In plants, the seeds generally contain the highest concentration.

Dry peas, beans and soyabeans are excellent sources. This vitamin is concentrated in the outer layers of the grain kernels. Bran and rice polishings are, thus, good sources. Whole wheat bread and white bread made from enriched flour contain a good supply of thiamine. Yeast is an outstanding source of thiamine and of certain other members of the B complex. Many nuts have a high concentration of the vitamin. Peanuts contain a good supply, whereas Brazil nuts have still more.

Thiamine deficiency causes 'Beriberi' in human beings. Symptoms are anorexia, weight loss, fatigue and GIT disturbances.

Good sources are:

1. Dry peas, beans, soyabeans
2. Bran and rice polishings
3. Whole wheat flour
4. Nuts, yeast
5. Gooseberries and dried prunes, oranges
6. Pork chops and fat ham

Milk contains only one tenth, the amount of thiamine that is found in peanuts, but because the milk is consumed in larger quantity by an individual, therefore, milk is by far considered to be a very good source. Cheese also contains this vitamin.

Among fruits, gooseberries and dried prunes are the richest source of B_1. Oranges have around half the quantity found in figs or prunes.

Many animal tissues are also excellent sources of this vitamin for example pork chops, fat ham, beef cuts, etc.

RIBOFLAVIN (B_2)

Lactoflavin (name rarely used)

This vitamin is also called as B_2 or vitamin G. Pure riboflavin was isolated from milk and other foods in 1933 by scientist Kuhn and his co-workers. Lactoflavin (milk), hepatoflavin (liver), ovoflavin (eggs) and verdoflavin (grass) proved to be chemically identical with riboflavin. In nature, this vitamin is synthesized by all green plants and by most microorganisms.

Chemistry

The flavins are widely distributed in nature. Many derivatives have been studied. Structure of vitamin B_2 is as given below:

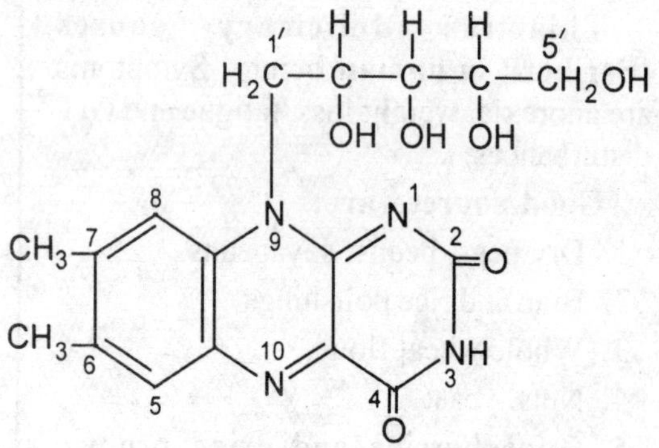

Riboflavin

(6,7 - dimethyl - 9 - (D - 1′ - ribityl) - isoalloxazine)

> Secondary deficiency of vitamin B_2 may occur with diffuse intestinal disease or by the prolonged use of psychotropic drugs that interfere with the production of FMN and FAD or by chronic alcoholism; extensive injuries (trauma, burns) and severe chronic debilitating (weakening) diseases. If the deficiency is of very severe nature then, the bone-marrow may become hypoplastic which induces a marked normocytic, normochromic anaemia.

The D in the chemical name of riboflavin indicates that the ribityl group is related to the D series of sugars. The one prime (1′) indicates attachment of the ribityl group at the first carbon atom, and the 9 that this attachment is to position 9 of the isoalloxazine ring system.

Deficiency

In human beings, the deficiency is generally associated with abnormal ectodermal tissue maintenance, the usual signs of which are:

(i) In human beings, the deficiency affects primarily the ectodermal tissues, producing lesion of the skin, eye and nervous system. One of the earliest symptoms is **cheilosis,** manifested at first by transverse fissures at the corners of the mouth, raw and scaly lips, and finally by many vertical, deep fissures.

(ii) Inflammation of the tongue **(glossitis)** : The tongue assumes a purplish or magenta tinge and glossitis (flattening of the papillae) is observed.

(iii) A seborrheic dermatitis: It occurs at the body folds e.g., at the alae nasi, and in the scrotal and vulvar regions.

(iv) The ocular manifestations i.e., corneal vascularization: They include dryness, burning and itching, photophobia and lacrimation, and vascular invasion particularly at the scleral junction of the cornea.

Coenzyme activity

The enzymes containing riboflavin are called flavoproteins. Two coenzymes viz; riboflavin phosphate, or flavin mononucleotide **(FMN)** and flavin adenine dinucleotide **(FAD).** The first flavoprotein isolated was **Warburg's yellow enzyme** which is composed of FMN and apoenzyme (specific protein). The enzyme can be separated into protein and FMN by dialyzing against dilute HCl. No enzyme activity resides in the individual constituents, but upon recombining them activity reappears.

FAD and FMN combine with different apoenzymes to form a large number of oxidation-reduction enzymes. FAD, for instance, is found in xanthine oxidase, D-aminoacid oxidase, aldehyde oxidase and fumaric dehydrogenase. FMN is associated with Warburg's yellow enzyme, cytochrome C reductase, L-amino acid reductase and others. **These enzymes operate in electron transport system.**

The structures of FMN and FAD are shown herewith.

Sources

It is found both in plant and animal sources. Plant seeds synthesize the vitamin during germination, hence germinating seeds are rich in this vitamin. **A few bacteria and the yeasts are very good sources. Other good sources are liver, kidney, eggs, cheese, peanuts, milk, ham, soyabean flour, white bread, dry peas, dry beans, etc.**

Polished rice, cereal foods and potatoes are not good sources but daily consumption of potatoes in the refreshment preparations and lunch or dinner contributes a lot and thus, potatoes are considered to be a very good source of this vitamin.

Daily requirement

Daily requirement ranges from 1.0 to 2.0 mg. During pregnancy and lactation, this allowance should be increased a little.

NIACIN - NICOTINIC ACID, NIACINAMIDE (B_3)
(Pellagra-Preventing (P-P) factor)

The terms niacin and niacinamide have replaced the older terms nicotinic acid and nicotine acid amide (nicotinamide). The latter

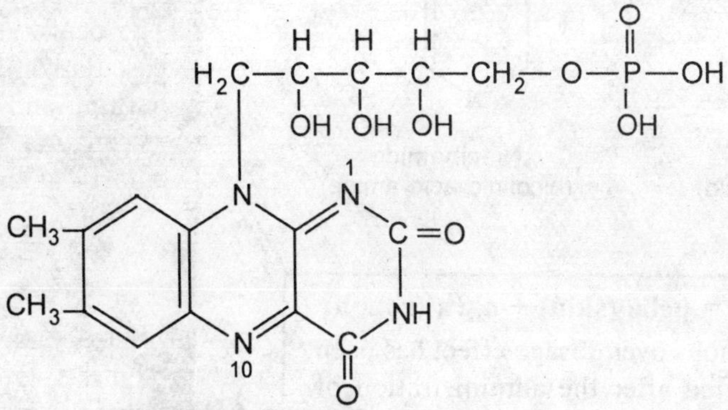

Riboflavin phosphate,
Flavin mononucleotide, FMN

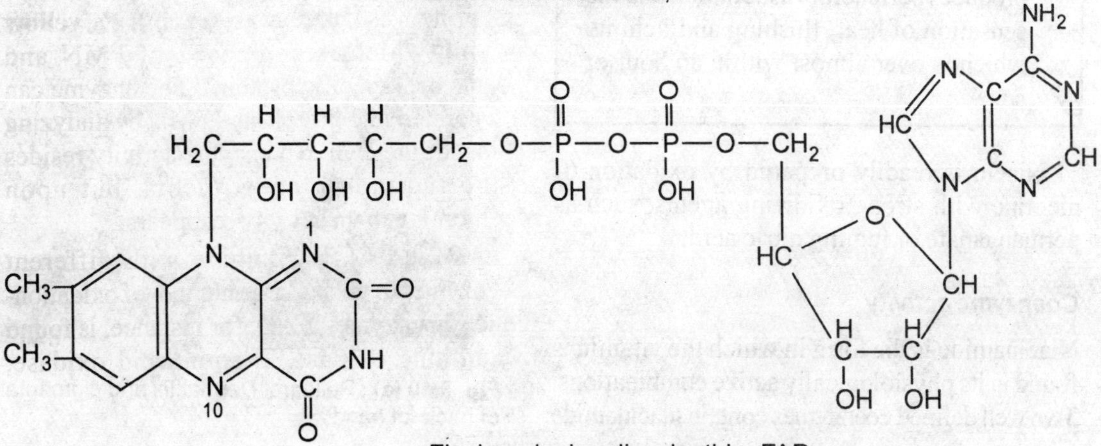

Flavin adenine dinucleotide, FAD

names were found to be undesirable because of the confusion and the unwarranted belief by many that they were physiologically related to nicotine.

The deficiency of this vitamin in human beings causes a disease named as **pellagra** {Fig 8.10 (a & b)} (from the Italian **pelle agra, rough skin**). Funk was the first to isolate the vitamin from rice polishings in 1914.

Chemistry

Niacin or nicotinic acid is pyridine 3-carboxylic acid. Niacinamide or nicotinic acid amide is the acid amide; the structure of these are given below.

O
C— OH
N

Niacin
(nicotinic acid)

O
C— NH_2
N

Niacinamide
(nicotinic acid amide)

> **Pellagra = pelle (skin) + agra (rough)**
>
> No serious over dosage effect has been identified after the administration of niacin. Parenterally (not orally) it produces peripheral vasodilation and the sensation of heat, flushing and itching, which is over almost within an hour or so.

Niacin is readily prepared by oxidation of nicotine with strong oxidizing agents, such as permanganate or fuming nitric acid.

Coenzyme activity

Niacinamide is the form in which the vitamin is found in its physiologically active combinations. Two well defined coenzymes contain niacinamide which act with a large group of hydrogen-transport enzymes (oxidation-reduction system).

The first is **NAD** (nicotinamide adenine dinucleotide, coenzyme I (Co I), or diphosphopyridine nucleotide **(DPN).** It contains nicotinamide-ribose-phosphate-phosphate-ribose-adenine.

The other coenzyme containing niacin is triphosphopyridine nucleotide **(TPN),** also called as coenzyme II (Co II) or **NADP** (nicotinamide adenine dinucleotide phosphate). This is composed of nicotinamide- ribose-phosphate-phosphate-ribose-2'-phosphate-adenine. It

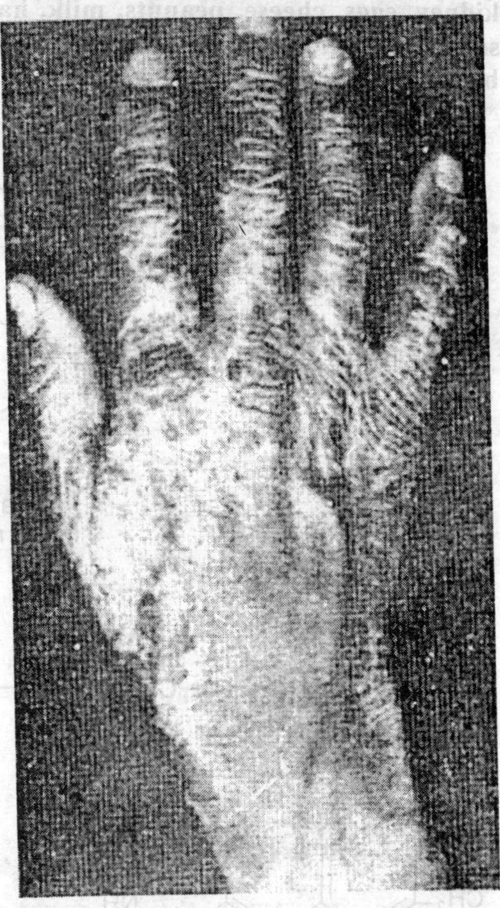

Fig. 8.10 (a) : Pellagra. Dermatitis and pigmentation of back of hand

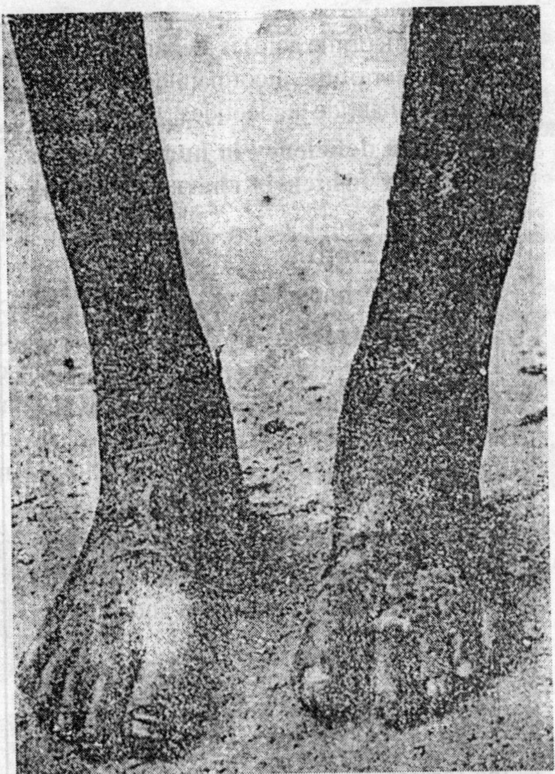

Fig. 8.10 (b): Pellagra, a changed concept: Considered a maize eaters' disease in other parts of the world, **it has been found in jowar eaters in India**, a finding that has almost radically changed the concept of its pathogenesis. This patient shows well marked skin lesions sharply limited to the areas exposed to sun.

> **The prevalence of pellagra is high in areas of the world where the diet is limited to maize (corn), molasses and salt pork, with very little lean meat or other sources of animal protein.**
>
> **In body, niacin may be synthesized in sufficient quantities by tryptophan, therefore, sufficient intake of tryptophan will never allow the deficiency symptoms of niacin to develop.**

differs from NAD only in the presence of a third phosphate group on carbon 2 of the ribose attached to adenine. It is synthesized from NAD and ATP.

The primary action of the two coenzymes is to remove hydrogen from substrates as part of dehydrogenase enzymes and transfer hydrogen and/or electrons to the next coenzyme in the chain or to another substrate which then becomes reduced. These enzymes are, thus, alternatively oxidized and reduced. NADH represents the reduced form. Many metabolic processes utilize one or other of these coenzymes. The structures of NAD and NADP are as shown below.

Deficiency

Pellagra is especially frequent among people eating corn as a large part of the diet. In some degree this may be explained by low tryptophan content of corn.

The flushing syndrome is well known in human beings taking nicotinic acid either by

NAD or DPN or Co I where R = H
NADP or TPN or Co II where R = $PO(OH)_2$

mouth or parenterally. The amide does not produce these symptoms. It is the niacinamide which is found in natural sources of the vitamin. Some individuals flush with only a few milligrams of niacin, while others are able to take 100 mg without untoward effects. Many people flush on the intravenous administration of 5 or 10 mg of niacin.

Serum cholesterol is lowered in human beings after the ingestion of large doses of nicotinic acid. In young adults the basal metabolism is also increased. The mechanism by which blood cholesterol is lowered has not yet been resolved.

Sources

In natural sources the vitamin occurs as free nicotinic acid, bound nicotinic acid, or nicotinamide in coenzyme form.

The vitamin is found to be present both in plant and animal tissues. Certain animal organs, e.g. liver, kidney, heart, lean meat and some fish flesh are outstanding sources.

As regards plant sources, peanuts, wheat germ, dried legumes and yeasts are also outstanding sources. Fresh legumes and a few green vegetables are good sources whereas milk, eggs and most fruits are poor sources. Niacin, like other B vitamins resides in wheat primarily in the bran and middling fraction.

Requirement

A diet providing 60g of mixed protein contains around 600 mg of tryptophan or 10 niacin equivalents from the amino acid. Recommended daily allowance for an average adult weighing 70 kg is 19 mg niacin equivalents and upto 22 for boys of the age group of 15-18 years (68 kg).

Role of Diet

It is a disease of those whose staple diet is maize. Maize actually contains more nicotinic acid than oats, rye and white wheaten bread. Pellagra is not found in those who consume besides maize, wheat and rice also. Maize has 6.7 niacin equi-

---

Niacin (nicotinic acid) is a vitamin used as a precursor of the nicotinamide moiety of the nicotinamide nucleotides.

Niacin deficiency in humans causes 'Pellagra' which is characterized by 3D's i.e.

(a) Dermatitis

(b) Diarrhoea and

(c) Dementia

In 1926, Goldberger and co-workers demonstrated that foods rich in 'water soluble B' were effective curing the symptoms of pellagra in man and black tongue in dogs. In 1937, Elvehjem and co-workers were able to isolate nicotinic acid amide from liver, which they found to be a cure for black tongue in dogs and pellagra in man.

Both nicotinic acid and its amide are active, the latter being preferred in medical practice because of its better tolerance than the former. In order not to confuse these compounds with nicotine they have been given the names niacin and niacinamide.

Pellagra is generally common in low-socioeconomic group. The disease starts with inflammation of the skin on the back of the hands {Fig 8.10 (a)}, forearms and neck. The skin becomes brown and scaly and finally open sores develop. The tongue becomes red and swollen and ulcers develop beneath it. Gastrointestinal disturbances, nausea, diarrhoea, intestinal ulcers are common. Nervous symptoms like insomnia and headache appear and in advanced stage, mental deterioration is also seen.

60 mg of tryptophan = 1 mg of niacin

---

valents per 1000 Kcal and levels less than 4.4 are needed to produce pellagra.

Besides occurring primarily in maize eaters, pellagra **has been reported in India in jowar eaters though,** there is no deficiency of nicotinic acid in that cereal.

Milk administration cures pellagra, though it contains very little nicotinic acid.

Pellagra is not encountered in populations who consume appreciable quantities or proteins of animal origin with nicotinic acid content not necessarily high.

The curative value of milk (and other animal proteins) has been found to be in its tryptophan content. Body can evidently synthesise nicotinic acid from tryptophan

Pellagra is not found in people who treat maize with lime (Mexico and Central America). This has been explained on the basis of the fact that in maize, niacin is found in a bound form and lime treatment releases it.

PANTOTHENIC ACID (B_5)

[Filtrate factor; chick antidermatitis factor (name rarely used)]

In 1933, Williams and co-workers demonstrated the widespread distribution of a substance that acted as a growth factor for yeast and other microorganisms. At that time these workers gave the name as pantothenic acid (Greek, from every where) to the active principle.

Chemistry

Chemically, pantothenic acid is α, γ-dihydroxy-β, β-dimethylbutyryl-β'-alanide. Its structure is as shown below:

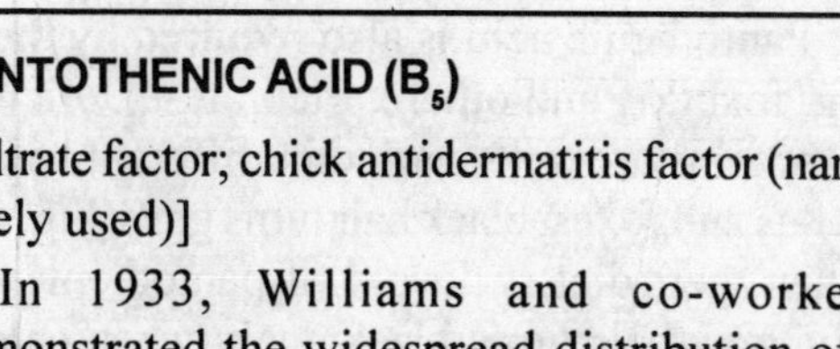

```
H2   CH3  OH   O    H    H2   H2
|    |    |    ||   |    |    |
C  – C  – C  – C  – N  – C  – C  – COOH
|    |    |
OH   CH3  H
```

Pantothenic acid

It is a condensation product of β-alanine and a hydroxyl-and methylsubstituted butyric acid. It is a pale yellow, unstable, viscous oil. The natural or vitamin active form of pantothenic acid is the dextrorotatory isomer. Commercially, it is synthesized as the calcium and sodium salts, in either dextrorotatory or racemic form, the latter having half the potency of the former. Pantothenic acid is soluble in water, ethyl acetate, dioxane and glacial acetic acid and is slightly soluble in ether and amyl alcohol and insoluble in chloroform and benzene. Being water-soluble, much of the pantothenic acid of a food may be lost in cooking if the cooking water is poured off.

Biochemical functions of pantothenic acid

Identification of pantothenic acid as part of the coenzyme A molecule has given this vitamin tremendous value in biochemistry i.e., biochemical reactions. **Scientist Lipmann and associates studied in depth about the role of coenzyme A vis-a-vis pantothenic acid.** Coenzyme A is the only known functional form of pantothenic acid in plant tissues, animal tissues and microorganisms, meaning by this vitamin is component of coenzyme A, the cofactor required for the metabolism of two-carbon compounds, notably acetyl groups. **In addition to the main contribution in acetylation reactions, it is also required for adrenocortical activity i.e., for the biosynthesis of cortical hormones.**

The physiologically active form of pantothenic acid in the animal organism appears to be coenzyme A (CoA) whose molecule contains pantothenic acid, mercaptoethylamine, adenine, ribose and phosphoric acid. CoA is readily synthesized by animal tissues provided pantothenic acid is supplied in the diet. **CoA participates in a wide variety of reactions involved in:**

(a) Carbohydrate metabolism,

(b) Fatty acid synthesis and metabolism,

(c) Propionate metabolism, and

(d) Branched chain fatty acids metabolism

Coenzyme A is found in larger quantities in liver if compared to the adrenals and other tissues where it is found in lesser quantities. There may be as much as 400 mg of CoA per kg. of liver. Lipmann has summarized many reactions in which CoA gets involved:

Acetyl Transfer

1. ATP - CoA - acetate:
   ATP+CoA+Ac→Ac-CoA+AMP+PP
2. Phosphotransacetylation:
   Ac - P + CoA → Ac - CoA + P
3. Formotransacetylation
   Pyruvate + CoA → Ac - CoA + formate
4. Transacetylation
   Ac-CoA+butyrate→butyryl CoA+Ac
5. Acetoacetate
6. Citrate
7. Acetaldehyde+CoA+NAD→Ac-COA
8. Pyruvate + CoA + NAD → Ac - CoA + NADH + CO_2

These reactions are examples of donor systems. The examples of acceptor systems may be: acetokinases (for aromatic amines, choline, histamine, amino acids and glucosamine) and condensation reactions (for acetoacetate, citrate and pyruvate).

Succinyl Transfer

As a donor system,

α-Ketoglutarate+NAD+CoA→Succinyl CoA + NADH

and as an acceptor system, the example may be the role of succinyl CoA in the synthesis of heme.

Benzoyl Transfer

Hippuric acid synthesis is an example.

Complex Synthesis

CoA is also involved in complex systems like fatty acid synthesis, butyrate and fatty acid oxidation, fat synthesis, steroid synthesis, etc.

Effects of Deficiency

The effects of deficiency are:

- growth failure in chick,
- dermatitis in chick,
- graying of the hair in rats and other animals,
- adrenal necrosis in the rat, and
- haemorrhage in the rat.

Pantothenic acid is essential in the diet of poultry. If it is deficient in the diet of hens, they produce eggs of low hatchability. If it is deficient in the diet of chicks, they develop dermatitis. Scales appear at the corners of the mouth and the neighbouring skin becomes inflammed. The chick dies in two or three weeks. Feeding calcium pantothenate cures this condition.

Pantothenic acid is also required by the rat, pig, fox, dog and other vertebrates. Deficiency symptoms are quite varied in different species. In rats and foxes, black hair turns gray (Fig. 8.11) when their diet is devoid of pantothenic acid. The gray hair turns black again when calcium pantothenate is fed to them. In dogs, the symptoms include respiratory disturbances, degeneration of kidneys and liver, and inflammation of the digestive tract.

Besides being widely distributed in plant and animal sources, this vitamin is also synthesized by intestinal microorganisms in humans, therefore, deficiency symptoms in them are rarely met with. However, its deficiency symptoms may include neuromotor disorders.

Cardiovascular instability, gastrointestinal distress, susceptibility to infections and mental depression - all these signs of deficiency disappear when pantothenic acid or its salts are added to the diet.

Distribution

It is widely distributed, and remains present in all living tissues whether of plant or animal origin. Excellent sources include:

(a) liver (b) kidney
(c) egg yolk (d) peas
(e) peanuts (f) rice bran
(g) molasses (h) yeast
(i) skimmed milk (j) butter milk
(k) cabbage (l) cauliflower etc.

It is also found in appreciable amount in sweet potatoes, wheat, barley, oats, rye and broccoli. Wheat germ is a rich source, but the content of milled white flour is rather low.

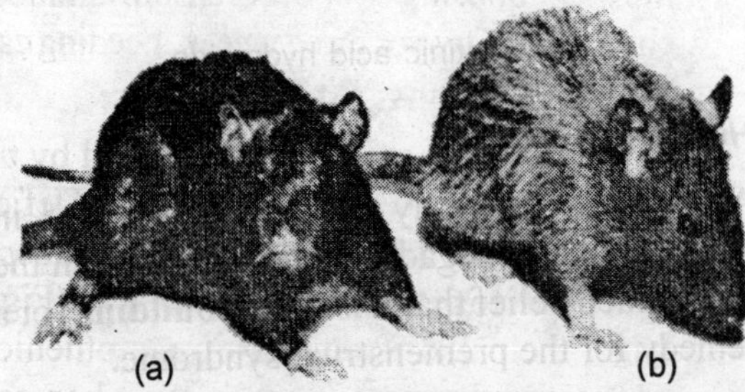

Fig.8.11 Pantothenic acid deficiency in a rat. These rats were litter mates, both originally black. Their diet, after weaning contained no pantothenic acid but the one on the left side (a) received 100 micrograms of this vitamin daily. After three weeks on this diet, the animal (b) on the right side showed evidence of graying which gradually became more pronounced. Other deficiency symptoms included scaly dermatitis, inflammation of the nasal mucosa and hemorrhages in various organs, particularly in the adrenal cortex.

Its poor sources include beets, turnips, egg white, prunes, raisins, canned peaches, canned peas, beans and apples.

Tea contains significant amount of vitamin B_3 (Pantothenic acid).

Daily Requirement

For human beings, the daily requirement is generally accepted as 10 mg, which is the amount usually consumed daily by an individual with approximately 2,500 calories of an adequate diet.

PYRIDOXINE GROUP (B_6)

Vitamin B_6 includes pyridoxine (which was the first one to be isolated), as well as pyridoxal and pyridoxamine, which were discovered later on by microbiological assay. The structures of them are as given below:

Pyridoxine — Pyridoxal — Pyridoxamine

Any of the three members of this group are active biologically.

Biosynthesis

A limited amount of pyridoxine can be synthesized by the bacterial flora of the gut.

Biochemical functions

1. It plays a very important role as a coenzyme in the intermediary metabolism of amino acids and complex glycolipids.
2. The active coenzyme form of vitamin B_6 is known as pyridoxal phosphate.
3. The enzymes which require pyridoxal phosphate as a coenzyme are:

(a) **Amino acid decarboxylases.**

(b) **Transaminases.** Among the several transaminase reactions, only those between glutamate and pyruvate to form alanine and between glutamate and oxaloacetate to form aspartate are reversible. In the deficiency of B_6, naturally, the activity of transaminase becomes slow.

(c) **Racemases.** These are the enzymes that catalyze the formation of an equilibrium mixture of DL-alanine from either D-or L-alanine.

(d) **Enzymes** involved in tryptophan metabolism e.g. tryptophanase, which converts tryptophan to indole, pyruvate and ammonia.

(e) **Cystathionase.** This enzyme is involved in the conversion of cystathionine to serine and homocysteine.

- Pyridoxine exists in the form of pyridoxal phosphate in the cells and functions as a coenzyme for a variety of chemical reactions concerned with the amino acids and protein metabolism.
- Its important role is that of coenzyme in the transamination process for the synthesis of amino acids.
- It is also believed to facilitate the transport of some amino acids across the cell membranes.

Distribution

It is widely distributed in vegetables, fruits, grains, meats and other foodstuffs; therefore its dietary deficiency is not at all common.

Deficiency States:

However, secondary deficiency states may be produced by long-term use of a variety of drugs such as isoniazid (**used in the treatment of tuberculosis**).

Alcoholism may also lead to its deficiency. In addition, there is a group of uncommon inborn errors of metabolism known as pyridoxine-dependency syndromes, which require massive doses of this vitamin.

However, a lack of vitamin B_6 has been associated with dermatitis, glossitis, cheilosis, and in infants and children diarrhoea, anaemia, peripheral neuropathy and sometimes convulsions. In rats several symptoms are observed as shown in Figure 8.12.

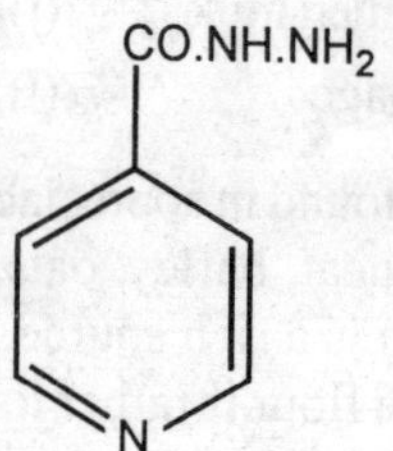

Isonicotinic acid hydrazide

Hypervitaminosis

A severe neuropathy has been described in patients taking megadoses of pyridoxine in the ill-founded belief that it is **'body building'** or a remedy for the premenstrual syndrome.

Antagonist

Isonicotinic acid hydrazide is a potent antagonist of B_6 which is extensively used as a potent antitubercular drug.

BIOTIN (VITAMIN H, NAME RARELY USED)

Biotin is known by a variety of names i.e. bios, vitamin H, coenzyme R and **the antiegg-white injury factor.**

As early as 1916, the toxicity of diets rich in egg white was observed. Later on, scientist Boas described egg white injury in those rats which were fed a diet containing raw egg white as the source of protein. She described muscle incoordination, dermatitis, loss of hair and

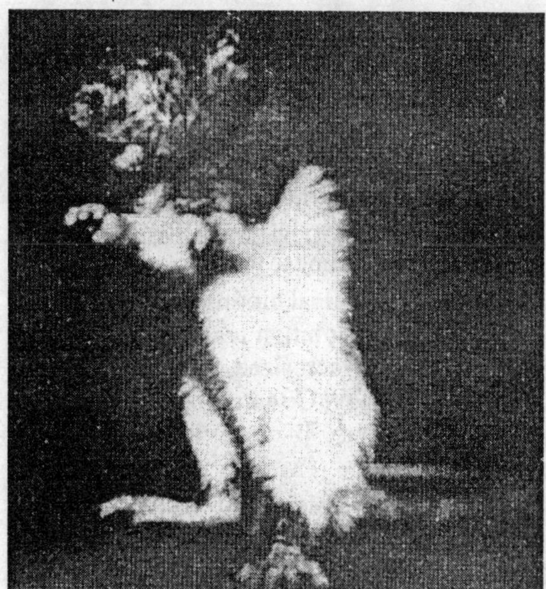

Fig. 8.12 : Pyridoxine (vitamin B deficiency in a rat, characterized by dermatitis of the extremities, beginning with swelling of the ears, nasal region, and paws and followed by crust formation on these areas.

nervous manifestations as the symptoms of this syndrome. She observed that cooked egg white was not toxic and that liver, yeast and certain other foods apparently contained a substance that protected rats against the toxicity of the raw egg protein; this protective substance was called vitamin H by Gyorgy. Lease and Parsons showed that chicks were subject to egg white injury. Williams and co-workers some six years later demonstrated that egg white injury in rats and chicks was actually due to an antivitamin in egg white; this substance is a basic protein and is known as **avidin**, and its ability to inactivate biotin was later on confirmed in 1941.

Biotin was isolated as crystalline methyl ester from egg yolk, yeast, liver and milk. Its structure was established by du Vigneaud and his associates as 2-keto-3, 4-imidazolido-2-tetrahydrothiophene-n-valeric acid.

Chemistry

1. Biotin is a monocarboxylic acid, only slightly soluble in water and alcohol.
2. Its colourless crystalline needles melt between 231° - 232°C.
3. The vitamin is destroyed by acids and alkalies only on rigorous treatment and by oxidizing agents such as peroxide and permanganate.
4. It is soluble in dilute alkali and hot water and practically insoluble in organic solvents.
5. In natural products it occurs mainly in bound form. One of the simple biotin compounds isolated is: **biocytin which can be hydrolyzed by an enzyme known as biotinidase.**
6. It is a cyclic compound containing two rings, i.e., a cyclic ureid and the other a reduced thiophene ring. A valeric acid side chain remains attached to the reduced thiophene ring.

It structure is as shown below:

```
          O
          ||
          C
        /   \
     HN       NH
      |        |
     HC       CH
      |        | /H
    H2C       C – CH2 – CH2 – CH2 – CH2 – COOH
        \   /
          S
```

Biotin

Physiological and biochemical properties of Biotin

It appears to be necessary for certain biochemical reactions. It may serve as a coenzyme. It may also be necessary for enzyme synthesis. Its main roles are as mentioned below:

1. The role in carboxylation and decarboxylation reactions.

It plays a key role in carboxylation reactions involving CO_2, fatty acids and various dicarboxylic acids. Thus, it participates in such reactions as the interconversion of pyruvic and oxaloacetic acids, of propionic and succinic acids and of oxalosuccinic and α-ketoglutaric acids; in the synthesis of citrulline from ornithine, of serine from CO_2 and of fatty acids from acetyl CoA.

In 1958, Wakil and Gibson provided the evidence that biotin is required for carboxylation reactions by first observing that CO_2 was required for fatty acid synthesis and that use of the enzymes of fatty acid synthesis contained large amount of biotin. Biotin remains tightly bound to the enzyme. The biotin-enzyme catalyzes the carboxylation of acetyl CoA to malonyl CoA according to the following reaction:

$$\underset{\text{Acetyl CoA}}{CH_2COS.CoA} + CO_2 + ATP \xrightleftharpoons[\text{Carboxylase}]{\text{Mn++ Acetyl CoA}} \underset{\text{Malonyl CoA}}{HOOC.\,CH_2COS.CoA} + ADP + Pi$$

Now a days, several biotin-enzymes that are involved in carboxylation reactions have been isolated and characterized, the examples of which are propionyl CoA carboxylase, pyruvic acid carboxylase, β-methylcrotonyl CoA carboxylase, etc.

2. It plays a role in the deamination of certain amino acids, and
3. It also plays a role in the synthesis of oleic acid by certain lactic acid-producing bacteria.

- Deficiencies of this vitamin are difficult to produce experimentally because it is synthesized by intestinal flora in higher animals.
- Biotin is an essential food factor and is coenzyme for carboxylation.
- Biotin is the prosthetic group in a number of carboxylation reactions, and functions as a carrier of CO_2
- **The protein material from egg *white,avidin* is denatured and inactivated by heating, therefore, egg should not be taken in raw state.**
- Avidin, if not denatured by heating, then forms a stable complex with biotin, resulting in inactivation of the biotin.

Deficiency

1. Deficiencies of this vitamin are difficult to produce experimentally because it is synthesized by intestinal flora in higher animals. However, deficiency symptoms may be induced by feeding either materials (such as avidin) which combine with the biotin to form non absorbable complexes or sulfa drugs which interfere a lot with bacterial synthesis of this vitamin in the intestines.
2. One of the first symptoms of biotin deficiency in young animals is cessation i.e. check of growth which is followed by a typical dermatitis (Fig. 8.13). Scales develop around the mouth and between the toes and the eyelids may become granular and stick together.
3. Rats, chicks and human beings develop a dermatitis as mentioned above when fed large quantities of raw egg white. This so-called **'egg white injury'** may be

easily prevented by boiling the egg before feeding. Raw egg white contains a protein called **'avidin'**, which combines with biotin and thus prevents its absorption, as a result of which symptoms of biotin deficiency develop.

4. In human volunteers, raw egg-white feeding leads to low urinary biotin level, depression, nausea, easy fatigue, incoordination of movements, dermatitis, etc.
5. Clinical cases of its deficiency in man are very rare. **In a rare genetic deficiency of holocarboxylase synthase** which makes helpful the utilization of biotin in several metabolic roles, the affected child is unable to utilize biotin, as a result of which he/she suffers from dermatitis, loss of hair, incoordination of movements, poor growth and high urinary lactate, β-hydroxypropionate and β-methyl-crotonate.

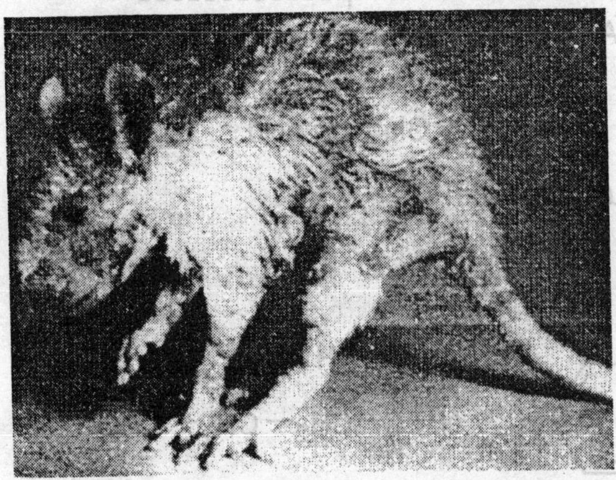

Fig. 8.13 : Biotin deficiency in a rat. This animal had been on a diet containing 35% uncooked dried egg white as the sole source of protein. Alcoholic extract of yeast supplied vitamin B complex. Although not biotin-free, the uncooked egg white combines with the biotin, making this unavailable to the animal. This deficiency is characterized by swelling and redness of the lips, denuded areas and brown scaliness of the skin with extensive dermatitis. Later, the eyes become gummed shut, the edema of the paws increases and nerve involvement is shown by progressive spasticity. In advanced cases, the rat exhibits the so-called "kangaroo posture" as seen here.

Sources

Biotin remains present in a variety of foodstuffs. It is found in abundance in liver, kidney, peas, yeast, cauliflower, egg yolk, milk etc. It is found in lesser amount in other foodstuffs i.e. a variety of vegetables, cereals and nuts.

For man and some other animals, synthesis by bacteria in the intestinal tract is an important source.

Requirement

150 to 300 μg per day for man.

FOLIC ACID (PTEROYLGLUTAMIC ACID), VITAMIN B_9 OR VITAMIN M (NAME RARELY USED)

Sources

Folic acid is found abundantly in nearly all natural foods which include fresh or fresh-frozen, uncooked vegetables and fruits. Good sources are green leafy vegetables and yeast. Grain also, contains this vitamin. Sufficient amounts may also be obtained through bacterial synthesis in the intestine or the rumen.

Daily requirement

Adult man or woman: 0.1 mg; pregnant women: 0.3 mg; lactating women: 0.15 mg; infants and children: 0.05 - 0.1 mg.

Chemistry

Folacin or folic acid or pteroylglutamic acid (PGA) is composed of one molecule each of p-aminobenzoic acid, glutamic acid and the pigment pteridine. It is a yellow crystalline substance and is slightly soluble in water. It is soluble in dilute alcohol. Its structure is as shown below:

Functions

1. **Folic acid helps in the transfer and metabolism of one-carbon compounds.** It is firstly reduced to H_4 folate (5, 6, 7, 8-tetrahydrofolate) by the enzyme dihydrofolate reductase in the presence of NADPH. H_4 folate is the active form of folic acid which may receive C_1 groups such as the formyl, methyl, methenyl, methylene and formimino groups on its N^5 and/or N^{10} from different substrates during their catabolism: H_4 folate then acts as a carrier and donor of these C_1 groups to other substrates as the coenzyme for many one-carbon group transferases.
2. Role as a coenzyme: Various coenzyme

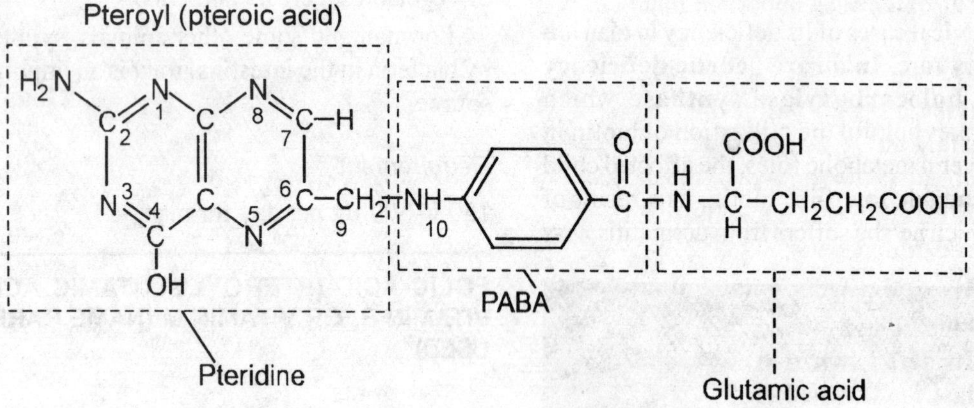

Pteroyl (pteroic acid)

Pteridine

PABA

Glutamic acid

Folic acid, pteroylglutamic acid (PGA)

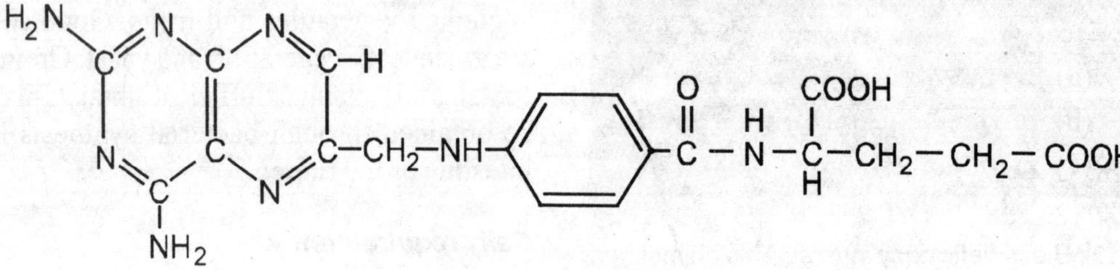

Aminopterin (4 - Amino PGA)

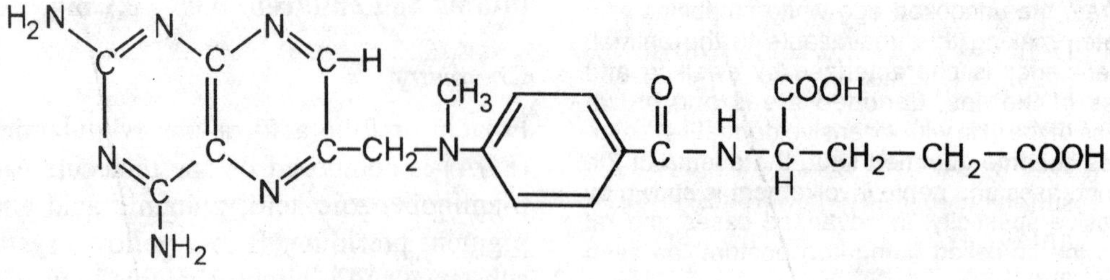

Amethopterin

— It functions as a carrier of hydroxymethyl and formyl groups.

— **Perhaps its most important use in the body is in the synthesis of purines and thymine,** which are required for the formation of deoxyribonucleic acid i.e. DNA. Therefore, this vitamin i.e., folic acid, like vitamin B_{12} is also required for the replication of cellular genes. This, probably explains one of the most important functions of the folic acid - that is to promote growth.

— If it is absent from the diet, the animal shall not grow properly i.e., very unsatisfactory growth will take place.

— **It is required for the maturation of red blood cells.**

— **Its deficiency causes macrocytic anaemia.**

— **Its deficiency also causes megaloblastic anaemia.**

forms of folic acid play an important role in a variety of important metabolic reactions as shown below:

(a) **serine-glycine interconversion,**

(b) **purine acid pyrimidine synthesis,**

(c) **methionine-homocysteine relations i.e., methyl synthesis,**

(d) **histidine synthesis,**

(e) **formiminoglutamate formation, etc.**

Deficiency

1. Deficiency of folic acid is difficult to produce in most of the animals unless intestinal bacterial growth is inhibited by feeding certain types of drugs, such as sulfonamide drug or antibiotics. Folic acid antagonists like aminopterin and amethopterin have also got a tendency to produce its deficiency.
2. In man, its deficiency causes macrocytic anaemia, which resembles pernicious anaemia except that the nervous involvement of the latter condition is absent.
3. Folic acid deficiency occurs most commonly among pregnant women because of their increased need for this nutrient.
4. Its deficiency symptoms have also been observed in chronic alcoholics and drug addicts; such people generally belong to the affluent society and do not believe in the consumption of green fresh vegetables and fruits.
5. Its deficiency also causes megaloblastic anaemia.
6. Its deficiency is also responsible for diarrhoea, gastrointestinal lesions and other related symptoms.
7. Folic acid is also effective in treating pernicious anaemia, although it is without effect on the nervous symptoms, which respond to vitamin B_{12}.
8. The **sprue syndrome** and some other types of anaemia in humans also respond to folic acid therapy.

Determination of the absorption of folic acid

For determining the absorption of folic acid-folic acid labelled with tritium is given by mouth to the patient and then the radioactivity is determined in the serum three hours later.

Folic acid antagonists

There are two well known antagonists of folic acid named as **aminopterin and amethopterin** whose structures are as given over here :

Folic acid antagonists namely aminopterin and amethopterin bear a striking resemblance to folic acid.

Aminopterin has been used with some success to obtain temporary relief in some cases of **acute leukaemia** in children.

These antagonists inhibit the enzymatic reduction of folic acid to tetrahydrofolic acid (FH_4) by binding very tightly to the enzyme. Such kind of inhibition results in blocking a number of reactions involving FH_4 and its derivatives - e.g.

(a) amino acid synthesis
(b) methyl group synthesis and
(c) purine synthesis from formate

VITAMIN B_{12} (COBALAMINE)

(**Cyanocobalamine,** cobamide, antipernicious **anaemia factor, 'extrinsic factor' of Castle**)

Antipernicious anaemia factor from liver extract was isolated in 1948 by Rickes and co-workers and by Smith. This factor is known as **'animal protein factor'** and has got the capability to cure pernicious anaemia and is now termed as vitamin B_{12}. It is found in animal tissues in the form of a conjugate with a polypeptide.

For the first time, **pernicious anaemia** was treated successfully by Minot and Murphy in 1926. In 1929, Castle suggested that gastric mucosa forms a carbohydrate-rich protein known as **intrinsic factor** which, together with a factor present in the food (**extrinsic factor**), forms a system responsible for the proper maturation of the erythrocytes. **People with pernicious anaemia do not make this protein. Pernicious anaemia turned out to be a genetic defect of the stomach, rather than a dietary deficiency disease.** With the isolation of vitamin B_{12} and its dramatic action in cases of pernicious anaemia, the extrinsic factor has been identified. Vitamin B_{12}, when injected, restores the red cell count to normal and also improves the functioning of central nervous system as well.

It has been suggested that the commercial vitamin cyanocobalamine does not normally occur in nature, but is an artifact of the isolation procedure.

Chemistry

1. **Vitamin B_{12} is a dark red compound containing one atom of cobalt which remains linked to four reduced pyrrole rings, forming a macro ring. The structure of vitamin B_{12} is given in Fig. 8.14.**

The central portion of the molecule is composed of four reduced and highly substituted pyrrole rings namely A, B, C and D around cobalt atom; this structure bears a close, but not complete resemblance to the porphyrins. The

— B_{12} is known to act as a coenzyme in the methylation of homocysteine, and in a reaction in which methyl malonyl CoA is converted to succinyl CoA. Both of these reactions involve methyl group transfer.
— In pernicious anaemia, the maturation of erythrocytes is greatly delayed.
— Intramuscular injection of B_{12} induces a rapid increase of peripheral blood.
— Biochemical action of the B_{12} in the process of red blood cell production is unknown.
— **Plant tissues are devoid of B_{12}**
— It is abundant in animal tissues, especially in the liver, kidney, pancreas, adrenal and pituitary and as well as in fish and oysters. **Milk and eggs are also good sources.**
— Microorganisms in the digestive tracts of ruminants have got the capability to synthesize vitamin B_{12}

central structure is referred to as a **'Corrin'** ring system. Below the corrin ring system, there is a 5, 6-dimethylbenzimidazole riboside, which remains connected at one end to the central cobalt atom and at the other end from the ribose moiety (Fig. 8.14).

Addition of cyanide forms **'cyanocobalamine'** which is identical with the originally isolated vitamin B_{12} and the removal of cyanide group results in the formation of the compound known as **'cobalamine'. Cyanide group if substituted by a hydroxy group forms** 'hydroxycobalamine'; replacement by a nitro group accordingly forms 'nitrocobalamine' and

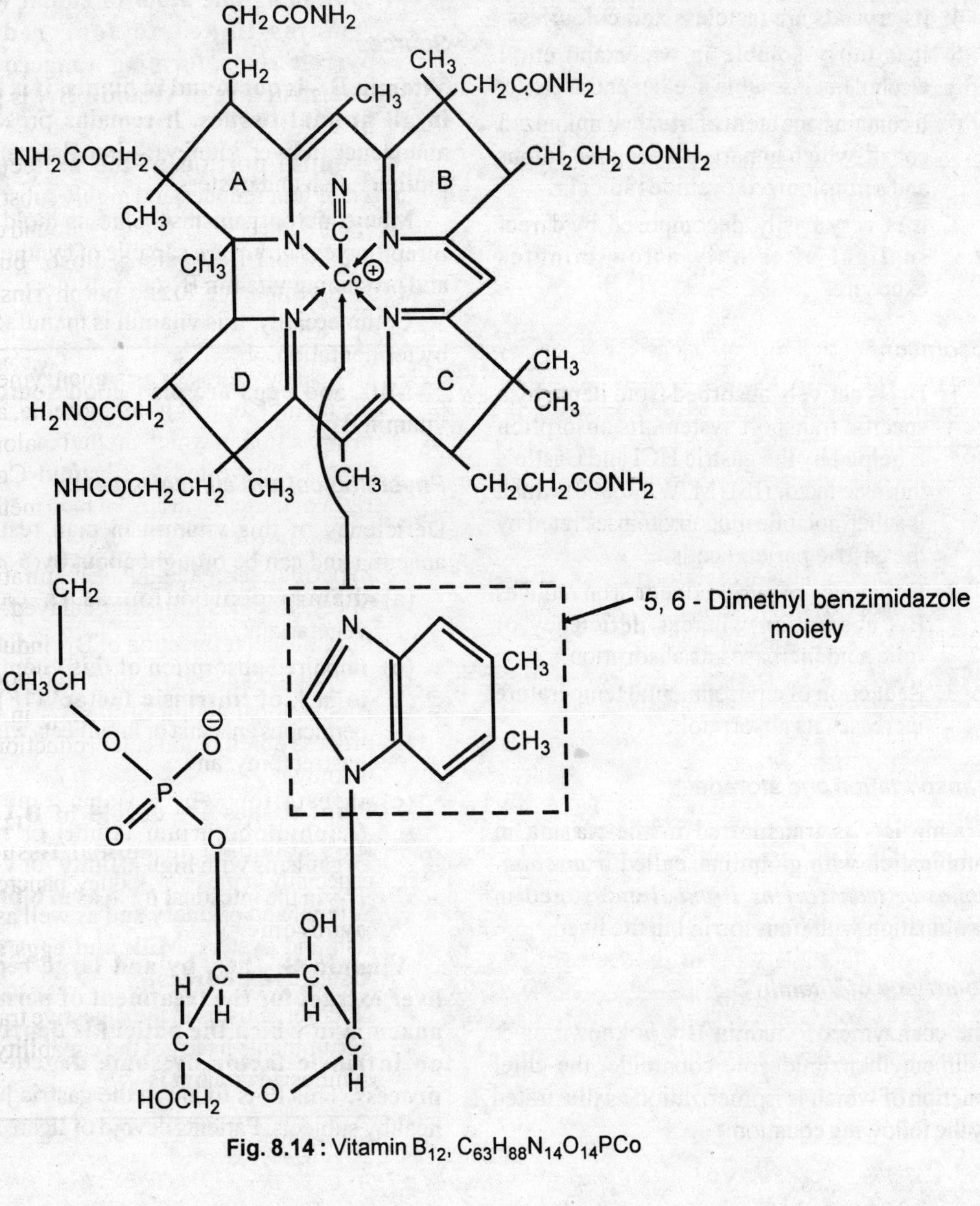

5, 6 - Dimethyl benzimidazole moiety

Fig. 8.14 : Vitamin B_{12}, $C_{63}H_{88}N_{14}O_{14}PCo$

by a methyl group forms 'methylcobalamine'. It contains nearly 4.35 per cent cobalt in its molecule.

2. Cyanocobalamine has a net charge of one.
3. Its molecular weight is 1490 ± 150 and its empirical formula is $C_{63}H_{88}N_{14}O_{14}PCo$.
4. Its crystals are tasteless and colourless.
5. It is fairly soluble in water and ethyl alcohol but insoluble in ether and acetone.
6. It contains one atom of trivalent unionized cobalt, which imparts it a deep red colour and a non-ionized cyanide radical.
7. It is very easily decomposed by direct sunlight after only a few minutes exposure.

Absorption

1. B_{12} is actively absorbed from ileum by a specific transport system. Its absorption is helped by the gastric HCl and Castle's intrinsic factor (IF) (M. W. 50,000) which is a thermolabile mucoprotein secreted by the gastric parietal cells.
2. Deficiency of pyridoxine or iron reduces B_{12} absorption whereas deficiency of folic acid increases its absorption.
3. Reduction of environmental temperature increases its absorption.

Transportation and storage

Vitamin B_{12} is transported in the plasma in combination with globulins, called *transcobalamins or transcorrins I and II* and stored in combination with transcorrin I in the liver.

Coenzyme of Vitamin B_{12}

The coenzyme of vitamin B_{12} is known as 5, 6-dimethylbenzimidazole cobamide, the chief function of which is isomerization as illustrated by the following equation:

$$\begin{array}{c} \quad CH_3 \\ \quad | \\ COOH - CH - CHNH_2 - COOH \\ \Big\Updownarrow \text{Glutamic isomerase} \\ COOH - CH_2 - CH_2 - CHNH_2 - COOH \end{array}$$

Sources

Vitamin B_{12} is not found in plants. It is found in all animal tissues. It remains present in abundance in liver, kidneys, adrenals, pancreas, pituitary, fish and oysters.

Many microorganisms including mold of the Streptomyces group are capable of synthesizing and producing vitamin B_{12}.

Commercially, this vitamin is manufactured by fermentation.

Milk and eggs are also good sources of vitamin B_{12}.

Physiological and clinical aspects

Deficiency of this vitamin in man results in anaemia and can be brought about by:

(a) dietary deprivation as in case of vegetarians
(b) impaired absorption of this vitamin due to lack of **'intrinsic factor' (IF)** as in pernicious anaemia or in subjects with total gastrectomy, and
(c) infestation by fish tapeworm (Diphyllobothrium latum) or microorganisms with high affinity for vitamin B_{12} in the intestinal tract, **as in blind loop syndrome.**

Vitamin B_{12} has, by and large replaced liver extract for the treatment of pernicious anaemia in which the patient is deprived of an intrinsic factor by some degenerative process. This IF is found in the gastric juice of healthy subjects. Patients devoid of IF are unable to absorb orally administered vitamin B_{12} in physiological doses unless IF is given to them simultaneously. The disease is marked by macrocytic anaemia, leukopenia, megaloblastic changes in the bone marrow and degeneration of the spinal cord. In this disease, the level of B_{12} in serum falls far below the normal range of 14-98 mcg per 100 ml, **a value below 8 mcg is considered diagnostic of pernicious anaemia.** The symptoms are reversed by the parenteral administration i.e. intramuscular injection of cyanocobalamine. A daily dose of one or two micrograms given intramuscularly for one week produces a therapeutic response, whereas 5 mcg daily by mouth with intrinsic factor (gastric mucopolysaccharide) or a single dose of 5,000 mcg orally without IF will be effective.

Metabolic functions

This vitamin participates in a number of metabolic functions as described below:

1. Purine biosynthesis: **It plays a role in the formation and synthesis of nucleic acid.**
2. Synthesis of labelled methyl group: Vitamin B_{12} increases the biosynthesis of the methyl group from precursors such as the α-carbon of glycine and β-carbon of serine. The α-carbon of glycine and the β-carbon of serine or formate are utilized less efficiently in the absence of vitamin B_{12}.
3. Its deficiency impairs transmethylation.
4. It plays an important role in the stimulation of protein synthesis, especially incorporation of amino acids into proteins.
5. **Vitamin B_{12} plays a role in the conversion of carbohydrate to lipid.** Vitamin B_{12} deficiency can be corrected by the parenteral administration of glutathione (GSH) or by the injection of vitamin B_{12}. Dietary deprivation of vitamin B_{12} results in a decrease in the reduced glutathione content and in the enzyme which degrades glucose to ribose, in the red blood cells and in the hepatic $NADH_2$ and in the increase of CoA. Be it known that hepatic $NADH_2$ is necessary for the maintenance of the activity of enzymes involved in lipid metabolism.

Effects of deficiency

Symptoms of vitamin B_{12} deficiency are those of pernicious anaemia as mentioned below:

1. **achlorhydria (no HCl in gastric juice)**
2. **severe macrocytic and megaloblastic anaemia**
3. **neurological degeneration and**
4. **glossitis**

Animal proteins are the sole source of this vitamin. The animals, in turn, acquire the vitamin from microorganisms growing in soil, water and their intestinal tract.

Requirement

Daily requirement is as follows:

(a) Adult man/ woman: 1 μg

(b) Pregnant or lactating woman: 1.5 μg

(c) Infants and children: 0.2-1 μg

ASCORBIC ACID (VITAMIN C)

(The Antiscorbutic Vitamin)

This is one of the water-soluble vitamins. This is also known as Vitamin C, whose absence gives rise to **scurvy.** At one time 'scurvy' was supposed to be the most common disease amongst sailors whose foods were found to be devoid of green fresh vegetables and citrus fruits because of the fact of their nonavailability during such long voyages. **This disease is characterized by a tendency of bleeding and pathological changes in the teeth and gums. Supplementation of their diets by lime and**

lemon juice cured all the symptoms of 'scurvy'.

Dietary deficiencies of this vitamin are sometimes encountered in chronic alcoholics, the very elderly people who live on a 'tea and toast' diet and the neglected underprivileged poor of the world who are generally unable to afford citrus fruits and fresh green vegetables.

Chemistry

In its chemical properties, it is quite strongly acidic, owing to the ionization of the two hydroxyl groups separated by the double bond. **Szent-Gyorgi** isolated the crystalline compound from paprika plant and named it hexuronic acid. It was later on isolated by **King** from lemon juice. The true configuration of the molecule was established by **Haworth** in his laboratory in 1933 in England.

The pure substance is optically active and is soluble in water. It is a very strong reducing agent. It is easily oxidized by air, especially in the presence of traces of metal ions like Cu^{++} or Fe^{+++}

It is also oxidized even by dissolved oxygen at room temperature, particularly if Cu^{2+} ions are present. **The first oxidation product is dehydroascorbic acid.**

It melts at 190 - 192°C and is stable for years

O = C
HO — C
HO — C
O
H — C
HO — C — H
CH_2OH

L-Ascorbic acid, $C_6H_8O_6$

in crystalline form. Its taste is sour. It is insoluble in most organic solvents. It readily forms salts of several metals. It takes up iodine at the double bond and can be reduced by hydrogenation.

Synthesis

Plants and all animals except pigs, man and other primates have an ability to synthesize ascorbic acid. The rat, for instance, is resistant to scurvy. In animals, probably the main sites for its synthesis are the liver and adrenals (cortex). In plants, all tissues contain vitamin C except woody tissues or seeds, although it remains present in the early stages of germination.

On the basis of many studies in recent years, the following scheme is presented for the biosynthesis of ascorbic acid in non-primates, which probably is also applicable to plants:

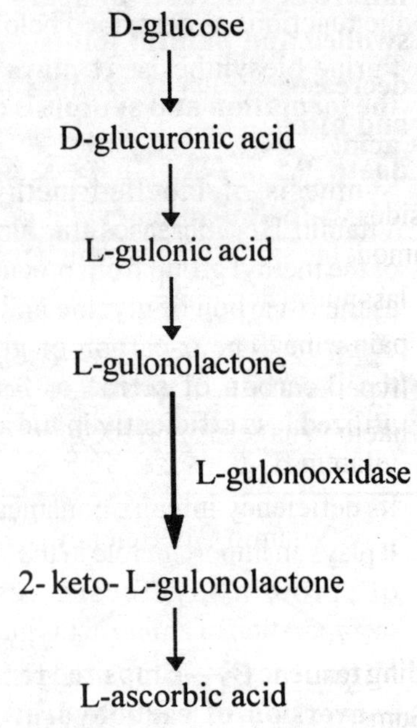

The defect in man that prevents the synthesis of ascorbic acid is the absence of the enzyme L-gulonooxidase.

Ascorbic acid can also be synthesized from another sugar i.e. D-galactose via D-galacturonic acid, L-galactonic acid, L-galactono-γ-lactone, and 2-keto-L-galactonolactone.

Deficiency Symptoms

Deficiency of this vitamin causes a disease named 'Scurvy' (Fig. 8.15). In its extreme form it is characterized by:

(a) **weakness**
(b) **loss of teeth and shrinkage of gums**
(c) **weakened blood vessels, particularly microvessels** having the least muscular support
(d) **peripheral haemorrhages**
(e) **defective synthesis of osteoid (a derivative of collagen)**
(f) **failure of wounds to heal**
(g) **failure of fractures to heal**
(h) **swollen and painful joints**
(i) **decreased ability to combat infections and often**
(j) **death**

Besides, **'subclinical scurvy'** is perhaps not uncommon; the symptoms of which include:

(a) lassitude (heaviness)
(b) pain in back
(c) hyperkeratosis of the hair follicle
(d) haemorrhage around the hair follicles

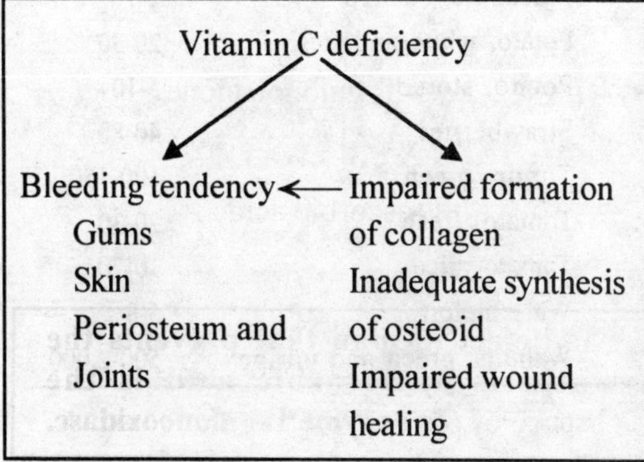

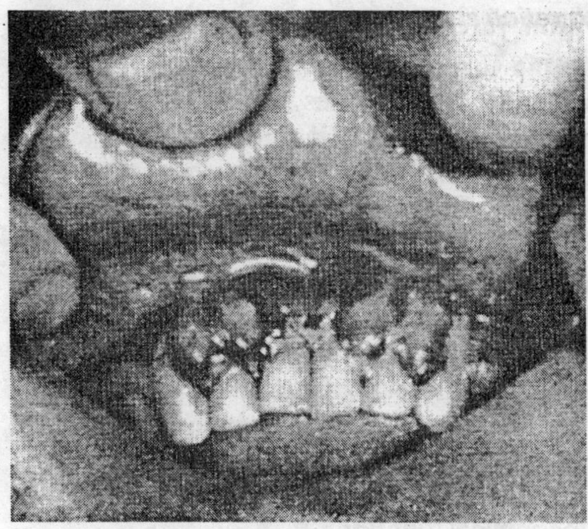

Fig 8.15 : Scurvy. Gingival swelling and petechiae

Diagnosis

Diagnosis of scurvy is made by X-rays which reveal skeletal abnormalities and sometimes microfractures, low plasma levels of vitamin C, urinary excretion measurements following administration of vitamin C (saturation test) and increased capillary fragility test (positive tourniquet test). Bleeding time (BT) and coagulation time (CT) are usually normal.

Test for Ascorbic acid deficiency

Inflate a blood pressure cuff over the upper arm and observe the red blotches (eruptions upon the skin) in the skin of forearm which is due to severe deficiency of ascorbic acid.

Cause. On inflating the cuff, venous return of blood gets occluded as a result of which, the capillary pressure rises which leads to the rupture of capillaries because of the fact that blood vessels become fragile in 'scurvy' and as a result many small petechial haemorrhages beneath the skin cause purpuric (pertaining to skin disease) blotches which may be seen easily in the forearm.

Excretion and storage

Vitamin C is not excreted by the kidneys until the body tissues are saturated and the concentration in the blood exceeds a certain level. Vitamin C is not stored, as are vitamins A and D in the body fat. Deprivation of this vitamin results in a gradual decrease of the tissue levels. The decrease in vitamin C levels is reflected in the blood, particularly in the leucocytes. Replacement cf vitamin C in the diet brings the patient back to health quite rapidly. Saturation, shown by excretion of the vitamin in the urine occurs in less than two weeks.

Biochemical functions

1. **The major function of vitamin C appears** to be in the formation of normal collagen.
2. In the formation of hydroxyproline from proline.
3. In the formation of hydroxylysine from lysine.
4. In the oxidation-reduction reactions. This property is concerned with the hydroxylation of aromatic compounds and thus in the metabolism of tyrosine and is also possibly involved in the hydroxylation of the steroid nucleus.
5. Absorption and utilization of iron: Vitamin 'C' helps in the intestinal absorption ,of iron by reducing Fe^{3+} to Fe^{2+} and by forming water soluble iron-ascorbate chelates. Besides this, it also increases the utilization of iron by reducing Fe^{3+} of tissue ferritin to Fe^{2+} for its release into plasma.
6. Hydroxylaion of dopamine to norepinephrine: In adrenergic neurons and chromaffin cells of adrenal medulla, a Cu^{2+}-protein known as dopamine β-hydroxylase utilizes L-ascorbate as an electron donor in hydroxylating dopamine to norepinephrine.

Daily requirement

1. It is established that the minimum amount of ascorbic acid required to prevent or cure scurvy in an otherwise healthy adult is about 10 mg daily or less. It has been argued, however, that the daily intake should be sufficient to saturate the body tissues. This amount is 60 to 100 mg daily depending upon the age, size and associated stressful conditions, such as wound healing or whether a woman is pregnant or lactating.
2. Studies of Hodges and associates have indicated that **in a healthy, normal adult, 45 mg daily is quite satisfactory.**

Ascorbic acid content of various routine food items are as mentioned in Table 8.2.

Table 8.2 : Ascorbic acid content of some routine food items

Sl. No.	Food	Ascorbic acid (mg per 100 g)
1.	Apple	3-10
2.	Beans, green (canned)	2-5
3.	Cabbage, fresh	40-70
4.	Cabbage, cooked	15-20
5.	Lemon juice	40-60
6.	Lettuce, head	5-10
7.	Orange juice	40-70
8.	Pineapple, fresh	20-30
9.	Pineapple, canned	2-10
10.	Potato, white and fresh	20-30
11.	Potato, stored	5-10
12.	Strawberries	40-80
13.	Turnip, green	100-150
14;	Tomato, fresh	20-30
15.	Tomato juice	10-20
16.	Watermelon	5-8
17.	Walnuts, green and unripe	500-2,000

MAIN PHYSIOLOGICAL/BIOCHEMICAL FUNCTIONS OF VITAMIN C

1. Collagen biosynthesis
2. Antioxidant property
3. Formation of hydroxyproline
4. Formation of hydroxylysine
5. Absorption and utilization of iron
6. Synthesis of chondroitin sulfates
7. Maintenance of the folate pool
8. Synthesis of neurotransmitters

MAJOR SOURCES

1. Fresh fruits (especially citrus)
2. Vegetables

MEGADOSE CONTROVERSY OF VITAMIN C

Some physicians are of the opinion that the intake of Vitamin C in large doses (nonphysiologic quantity of Vitamin C) helps in curing the attack of common colds and as well as advanced cancers, but the controlled scientific studies do not prove these above myths. An occasional individual may experience some slight alleviation of symptoms, probably because large doses of vitamin C have got a mild antihistaminic effect. In cases of metastatic cancer, megadose of vitamin C has been proved to be of no value in either way.

Contrarily, in large doses it predisposes to oxalate and urate urinary tract stones, may be responsible for aspirin-induced gastric erosions, interacts with the metabolism of some drugs, **unnecessarily increases intestinal absorption of iron and may lead to iron overload and may be responsible for various other side-effects.**

LIPOIC ACID (THIOCTIC ACID)

This vitamin for the first time was isolated from yeast and later from various animal tissues like liver, etc. This is treated to be an essential growth factor for various microorganisms but not for mammals.

It is a cyclic disulfide containing a carboxyl group which is attached to a protein by means of an amide linkage, probably to lysine. Its structure is as shown below:

```
      CH2
     /   \
 H2C      CH . CH2 — CH2 — CH2 — CH2 — COOH
  |        |
  S ────── S
```

Lipoic acid or thioctic acid

Main biochemical function of this vitamin is that it participates in the enzymatic oxidative decarboxylation of α-keto acids at a stage between thiamine pyrophosphate and coenzyme A. In oxidative decarboxylation, loss of CO_2 is accompanied by oxidation of an aldehyde to an acid. Important examples of the oxidative decarboxylation reactions are the ones involving enzymes like pyruvate dehydrogenase, oxoglutarate dehydrogenase, etc. as shown below:

$$\text{Pyruvate} + \text{CoA} \xrightarrow[\text{pyruvate dehydrogenase}]{\text{NAD} \;\rightarrow\; \text{NADH}} \text{Acetyl CoA} + CO_2$$

The pyruvate dehydrogenase enzyme has a complex mechanism, which involves binding sites for pyruvate, NAD^+, thiamine pyrophosphate and lipoic acid. Acetyl Co A thus formed now enters the tricarboxylic acid cycle as discussed in the chapter of carbohydrate metabolism.

MAKE VITAMINS WORK FOR YOU

- Children between eight and 16 years should have adequate vitamin A which helps in vision improvement and boosts the immune system.
- **Pregnant women should take vitamin B Complex with folic acid, which is good for foetal growth.**
- **Menopausal women should have vitamins C, E and B Complex.These will check excessive bleeding and restore elasticity of skin.**
- People who work out should have vitamins C, E and A post-exercise. The body is low on energy at this time and hence susceptible to easy attacks from the free radicals that are deadly for our constitution.
- People who are constantly on the computer are exposed to the danger of **Carpel Tunnel Syndrome,** which affects the region between the elbow and the index finger, which is active while using the mouse. Vitamin B Complex works as both, a preventive as well as a curative device.
- During PMS syndrome, vitamin B_6 reduces irritability.
- Vitamin B_{12} helps in depression.
- Vitamins C, E and A are antioxidants and are helpful in fighting dangerous free radicals that can threaten a post-operative surgery patient.
- Those above the age of 50 can take a daily tablet of vitamin B Complex, containing vitamin B_{12} and folic acid.
- Vegetarians, who do not consume milk and milk products, should take vitamin B_{12} daily.

WAYS TO MAXIMISE VITAMIN ABSORPTION

- Do not refrigerate vegetables and fruits (raw and uncut) **for more than two days.**
- Don't go by the advertisements that show refrigeration not slowing down loss of nutrients from fruits. It can't stop the process altogether and fruits certainly do not get any fresher by refrigerating them for a long time.
- **Eat your fruits whole rather than cutting them into pieces.** When exposed to air (oxygen), vital vitamins are lost. **By that logic, raw fruits are better than fruit juices and pies.**
- Take a sunbathe around 9 A.M. for 15-20 minutes and you do not need to pop any vitamin D supplements, except if otherwise advised by a medical practitioner.
- Give full attention to food while eating rather than sharing the meal with your favourite soap on TV, so that your parasympathetic nervous system is dominant and the digestive system works to its optimum level.

DANGER: OUR DAILY DIET DECONSTRUCTED

Today there are more reasons why one should have vitamin tablets/ tonics daily. The increased consumption of processed foods like **pizza, pastries, fried chips and burgers** (basically foods that do not have any nutrients) make it essential to supplement the diet with pills. Caffeinated products like tea, coffee, all types of aerated drinks and chocolates should be minimised, if not abstained from, as they prohibit the absorption of vitamins. Alcohol and tobacco products are even worse.

CHAPTER 9

HUMAN NUTRITION/BALANCED DIET

(Longer the belt, shorter the life; few people die by taking less calories but many times more from excess; check the obesity from the very begining of life, do not depend upon fast foods, do atleast moderate exercise/yoga daily and enjoy the life till the last respiration)

Nutrition deals with the needs of the organism for sustenance. Food is the basic requirement for all the living beings whether microorganisms or plants or animals, without which the existence of life is not possible. The modern science of nutrition deals mainly with the requirement of the body, both in kind and amount, and the choice of food to meet these needs. **Main three functions of food are to:**

(a) supply energy

(b) form (or maintain) body tissues and

(c) preserve a suitable internal environment so that enzymes bringing about hundreds of metabolic reactions and the hormones regulating various processes might function properly.

Following is the nutritional requirement of human beings:

(a) **carbohydrates** (b) **lipids**

(c) **proteins** (d) **minerals**

(e) **vitamins, and** (f) **sufficient amount of water**

Excess intake of such foods should be taken care of which contain various food toxins (Table 9.1).

* *a south american plant with thick roots that is grown for food; its roots are used as food; synonym: tapioca*

Table 9.1 : Various food toxins found in routine edibles.

Sl. No.	Food toxin	Source(s)
1.	5-dehydroxytryptamine	Banana and some other fruits
2.	Tyramine	Some cheeses
3.	Cyanide	Almonds, cassava* and other plants
4.	Cycasin	Cycad nuts
5.	Nitrosamines	Some fishes, meat or cheese
6.	Sanguinarine	Mustard oil
7.	Hemagglutinins	Legumes
8.	Oxalate	Rhubarb
9.	Solanine	Green potatoes
10.	Various mycotoxins	Fungi
11.	Aflatoxin B_1	Produced by the species of fusarium
12.	Aflatoxin G_1	

ENERGY REQUIREMENT

The energy requirement of the animal body may be divided into two functional classifications, viz., **that for basal metabolism and that for active work. (Table 9.2). Basal metabolism includes the energy expended in respiration, blood circulation, intestinal contractions, activities of various organs, maintenance of muscular tonus, thermal**

Table 9.2 : Energy requirement for basal metabolism and active work.

Energy Requirement	
Basal metabolism	**Active work**
(It covers involuntary actions like respiration, blood circulation, intestinal contractions, activities of various organs, maintenance of muscular tonus, thermal equilibrium, etc.)	(It covers voluntary actions like playing, running, swimming, walking, pulling rikshaw, ploughing fields manually, wood-cutting manually, etc.)

equilibrium, etc. The basal metabolic rate is influenced by the amount of active protoplasmic mass (hence by height, weight, surface area, age, sex, composition of the tissues, etc.) and is governed by endocrine organs, particularly the thyroid and pituitary glands.

The energy consumed in work, play and indeed all forms of voluntary activity, imposes an additional requirement for fuel over the basal which depends upon the nature and extent of the muscular work. Whereas an average man expends about 100 Cal per hour while sitting at rest, his/her metabolism may increase to as high as six times this value with extreme physical effort.

Mary, Swartz and Rose summarised the hourly expenditure of calories of an average 70 kg man under various conditions as follows :

1. Sleeping : 65
2. Awake lying still : 77
3. Sitting at Rest : 100
4. Standing relaxed : 105
5. Dish washing : 144
6. Light exercise : 170
7. Walking slowly to moderately fast : 200-300
8. Carpentry or painting : 240
9. Active exercise : 290
10. Walking down stairs : 364
11. Sawing wood : 480
12. Swimming : 500
13. Running 5.3 miles per hour : 570
14. Very severe exercise : 600
15. Walking up stairs : 1100

From the above estimates one may predict the calorie requirement of the individuals. **The total energy requirement for different types of workers ranges from:**

(a) a minimum of **2000 to 2500** Cal per day (White - collar workers)

Break-up of calories per day by a normal adult individual may be considered as:

(i) Carbohydrates
(400 g) x 4 = 1600 Calories

(ii) Lipids
(80 g) x 9 = 720 Calories

(iii) Proteins
(45 g) x 4 = 180 Calories

2500 Calories

(b) **to a maximum of 4000 to 6000 (lumbermen, excavators, etc),** of which about 1400 to 1900 Cal are consumed in basal metabolism and the balance in various forms of activity.

Calorie intake must be adjusted to specific needs. The proper allowance is that which will maintain body weight and rate of growth at the desired levels over extended periods. **When disease is present, calorie supply must provide energy for tissue repair, for the immunological mechanisms and for the wasting effects of fever.**

The Food and Nutrition Board, National Research Council, recommended daily calorie intake as given in Tables 9.3 (a & b) The calorie allowances apply to the individual normally engaged in moderate physical activity, under usual environmental stresses.

For a long time, emphasis in the study of nutrition was laid on calorie requirements. **Animal calorimeter was developed by Atwater, Rosa and Benedict. Human calorimeter developed by Du Bois revealed that a normal 70 kg man expends, on an average, energy equivalent to about 3,000 calories per day.** There is yet another calorimeter which is known as Bomb calorimeter; this can be used to determine the caloric value of various foods. Composition and energy content of various common food stuffs are as given in Table 9.4.

On the basis of the definition of a large calorie (Cal or kcal), the quantity of heat necessary to raise the temperature of 1kg of water through 1°C, the following values are obtained:

1 gm of carbohydrate = 4.1 kcal
1 gm of fat (lipid) = 9.4 kcal
1 gm of protein = 5.6 kcal

However, in the body, protein is not completely utilized, although carbohydrates and lipids are. On this basis, the following round figures are commonly used in Medicine/Science.

1 gm of carbohydrate = 4 kcal
1 gm of fat = 9 kcal
1 gm of protein = 4 kcal

Daily Requirement

The average normal man needs 2,,500 to 3,000 calories (see above break-up of calories) per day and the normal woman somewhat less, usually, 1,700 to 2,100 calories per day. Recommended daily- dietary allowance for various categories of human beings is given in Table 9.3 (a and b)

Following is the nutritional requirement of human beings:

(a) carbohydrates
(b) lipids
(c) proteins
(d) minerals
(e) vitamins, and
(f) sufficient amount of water

High fat consumption has been found to be associated with **cancer of breast and colon.**

The main sources of saturated fat in the human diet are the meat of ruminants, dairy products and hard margarine. Cholesterol is found only in foods of animal origin, particularly in egg yolk.

Carbohydrates

Principal carbohydrates in the human diet are the starches and the sugars. Grains and vegetables constitute the primary sources of the starches, while fruits of sugars. Carbohydrates make up some 40-80 per cent of total calories furnished by the diet. Less than 1 percent of the carbohydrate intake is found in the tissues, emphasizing its ready utilization as a source of energy or its conversion to fat stores in adipose tissues as a potential energy source.

When ingested in amount in excess of that required to produce energy, carbohydrate is converted to fat, e.g., glycogen, a principal carbohydrate of the human body, gets firstly converted to pyruvic acid **via 'glycolysis' and then to acetyl CoA which is the precursor for the biosynthesis of fatty acids vis-a-vis fats in the human body.**

No definite amount of the intake of carbohydrates is known today but it has been established so far that at least **100 grams of carbohydrates are required per day by a normal healthy adult in order to avoid ketosis, excessive protein catabolism and other undesirable responses.** These carbohydrates remain confined to almost all kinds of foodstuffs which we consume daily in a normal course i.e., all types of vegetables (potatoes, carrots, chillies, arums, beans, pumpkin etc.), spices, condiments, corns (wheat, maize, oat, millet, gram, etc.), pulses, meat, egg, milk, fish etc.

The paper with which we come across daily

Table 9.3 (a) : Recommended daily calories intake and other dietary allowances for different categories

	Age years	Weight kg (lbs)	Height cm (In)	Calories	Protein 'g'	Calcium 'g'	Iron 'mg'	Vitamin 'A' 'I.U.'	Thiamine 'mg'	Riboflavin 'mg'	Equiv. Niacin 'mg'	Vitamin 'C''mg'	Vitamin 'D''I.U.'
Men	18-35	70(154)	175 (69)	2906	70	0.8	10	5000	1.2	1.7	19	70	
	35-55	70(154)	175 (69)	2600	70	0.8	10	5000	1.0	1.6	17	70	
	55-75	70(154)	175 (69)	2200	70	0.8	10	5000	0.9	1.3	15	70	
Women	18-35	58(128)	163 (64)	2100	58	0.8	15	5000	0.8	1.3	14	70	
	35-55	58(128)	163 (64)	1900	58	0.8	15	5000	0.8	1.2	13	70	
	55-75	58(128)	163 (64)	1600	58	0.8	10	5000	0.8	1.2	13	70	
Infants	0-1	8 (18)		kgx11.5 ± 15	kgx2.5 ± 0.5	0.7	kg x 1.0	1500	0.4	0.6	6	30	400
Children	1-3	13 (29)	87 (34)	1300	32	0.8	8	2000	0.5	0.8	9	40	400
	3-6	18 (40)	107 (42)	1600	40	0.8	10	2500	0.6	1.0	11	50	400
	69	24 (53)	124 (49)	2100	52	0.8	12	3500	0.8	1.3	14	60	400
Boys	9-12	33 (72)	140 (55)	2400	60	1.1	15	4500	1.0	1.4	16	70	400
	12-15	45(98)	156(61)	3000	75	1.4	15	5000	1.2	1.8	20	80	400
	15-18	61 (134)	172(68)	3400	85	1.4	15	5000	1.4	2.0	22	80	400
Girls	9-12	33 (72)	140 (55)	2200	55	1.1	15	4500	0.9	1.3	15	80	400
	12-15	47 (103)	158 (62)	2500	62	1.3.	15	5000	1.0	1.5	17	80	400
	15-18	53 (117)	163 (64)	2300	58	1.3	15	5000	0.9	1.3	15	70	400

Table 9.3 (b) : Important daily allowances of nutrients for expectant and nursing mothers

Nutrient	Normal Women			Pregnant	Lactating
	Sedentary	Moderately active	Very active		
Calories (Cal)	1900	2200	3000	+ 300	+ 500 to 700
Proteins (g)	45	45	45	55	65
Calcium (g)	0.4-0.5	0.4-0.5	0.4-0.5	1.0	1.0
Iron (mg)	30	30	30	40	30
Vitamin 'A' as					
(i) retinol (μg)	750	750	750	750	1150
(ii) carotene (μg)	3,000	3,000	3,000	3,000	4,600
Thiamine (mg)	1.0	1.1	1.5	+ 0.2	+ 0.4
Riboflavin (mg)	1.0	1.2	1.7	+ 0.2	+ 0.4
Folic acid (μg)	100	100	100	150-300	150

Table 9.4 : Composition and energy content of various common foodstuffs

Sl. No.	Foodstuff	Food energy (calories/ 100 gm)	Composition of foods, 100 gm. edible portion					
			Water %	Protein 'gm'	Fat 'gm'	Carbohy-drate 'gm'	Calcium 'mg'	Phosphorus 'mg'
1.	Bread, white	275	34.7	8.5	3.2	51.8	79	92
2.	Bread, toasted	313	25.5	9.7	3.7	59.0	90	105
3.	Whole wheat	240	36.6	9.3	2.6	49.0	96	263
4.	Barley	349	11.1	8.2	1.0	78.8	16	189
5.	Millet	350	9-13	7-13	2.2 ±	73.0	-	-
6.	Rice (brown, raw)	360	12.0	7.5	1.7	77.0	39	303
7.	Rice (milled, cooked)	119	70.5	2.5	0.1	26.2	8.0	45
8.	Wheat flour (whole)	333	12.0	13.3	2.0	71.0	41	372
9.	Wheat germ	361	11.0	25.2	10.0	49.5	84	1096
10.	Butter	720	15.5	0.6	81.0	0.4	20	16
11.	Cheese	398	37.0	25.0	32.2	2.1	725	495
12.	Milk (cow's whole)	69	87.0	3.5	3.9	4.9	118	93
13.	Milk (cow's skimmed)	36	90.5	3.5	0.1	5.1	123	97
14.	Eggs, fresh, whole	165	74.0	12.8	11.5	0.7	54	210
15.	Eggs, fresh, white	50	87.8	10.8	0	0.8	6.0	17
16.	Eggs, fresh, yolk	361	49.4	16.3	31.9	0.7	147	586
17.	Apple	66	84.1	0.3	0.4	14.9	6.0	10
18.	Banana	88-132	74.8	1.2	0.2	23.0	8.0	28
19.	Orange	45	87.2	0.9	0.2	11.2	33	23
20.	Peach	46	86.9	0.5	0.1	12.0	8.0	22
21.	Carrots, raw	42	88.2	1.2	0.3	9.3	39	37
22.	Poatoes, peeled, boiled	83	77.8	2.0	0.1	19.1	11	56
23.	Tomatoes, raw	20	94.1	1.0	0.3	4.0	11	27
24.	Almonds	600	4.7	18.6	54.1	19.6	254	475
25.	Groundnuts (roasted)	560	2.6	26.9	44.2	23.6	74	393
26.	Walnuts	650	3.3	15.0	64.4	15.6	83	380

is a form of cellulose, which, chemically has got as much glucose in it as starch has, but this paper can not be digested by the human beings because of the lacking of the corresponding enzyme i.e. **'cellulase'** in the digestive tract. On the other hand, this enzyme remains present in ruminants, therefore, they are able to digest cellulose which is found in abundance in their diet. Be it known that the main food of the ruminants is different types of grasses.

Potato consists of starch granules surrounded by an envelope of cellulose. If a raw potato is eaten, even if it is chewed thoroughly, it will pass as such through the digestive tract without yielding any calories and appear undigested in the faeces. **A raw potato, therefore, has got no food value. On the other hand, if the potato is heated, then the cellulose**

envelope will burst, and the content is then available for digestion. This is an example of a food which has got no food value in the raw state, but has a very high food value in the cooked state. Calorie values of some of the important routine items (foods) are as mentioned in Table 9.5.

Table 9.5 : Calorie values of some important common foods

1. Cow's milk	: 69 Cal/100 ml
2. Buffalo's milk	: 109 Cal/100 ml
3. Human milk	: 67 Cal/100 ml
4. Butter	: 720 Cal/100 g
5. Desi ghee	: 830-890 Cal/100g
6. Fishes	: 50-150 Cal/100g
7. Meats	: 100-450 Cal/100g
8. Egg	: 165 Cal/100g
9. Curd (cow's)	: 69 Cal/100 ml
10. Curd (buffalo's)	: 109 Cal/100 ml
11. Apple, one medium size	: 66 Cal
12. Banana, one	: 88-132 Cal
13. Potato, boiled, 1 medium size	: 83 Cal
14. Tomato, raw, 1 medium size	: 20 Cal
15. Peas, green, cooked, 1/2 cup	: 56 Cal

Lipids

Lipids are the principal energy yielding substances and the per unit heat production from lipids (fats) is more than double in comparison to carbohydrates and proteins which are other two major food stuffs for the human beings. Fat is rather slowly digested and the large amounts of it in a meal tend to slow down the digestion process of other foods as well.

There is no rule for the proportion of fat and carbohydrate in a diet. For a normal person, 80gm fat is recommended. Of course, the essential fatty acids(Table 9.6) must be supplied, the requirement of which is small and these fatty acids are found in many food oils. The deficiency of the so called essential fatty acids in the diet of rats causes retarded growth, scaly skin, kidney lesions, and bloody urine formation (haematuria). **These fatty acids are also believed to control the rate of cholesterol biosynthesis in animals.**

Linoleic, linolenic and arachidonic acids are considered to be essential fatty acids (EFA) in the mammals as they are not synthesized in them, hence, must be supplied in the diet. They all are polyunsaturated fatty acids.

Although, the synthesis of fatty acids from intermediates in the catabolism of carbohydrates and amino acids has been demonstrated in many species of animals and plants, most mammals are unable to synthesize in adequate amounts fatty acids containing more than one double bond in the carbon chain. When rats are fed a diet not containing polyunsaturated fatty acids for two to three months, they develop deficiency symptoms, characterized by scaliness of the skin, desquamation and sloughing of the tail, lesions in the kidneys, and ultimately death. All these symptoms can be prevented or cured by the addition of 10 drops of lard oil or a small amount of linoleic acid to the diet. Other polyunsaturated fatty acids are also curative, **but linoleic acid is considered to be the essential fatty acid, since it cannot be synthesized but is the precursor for the biosynthesis of other polyunsaturated fatty acids.**

Table 9.6: Essential fatty acids

Sl No. Name	Sources
1. Linoleic acid	linseed oil, cottonseed oil, peanut oil, corn oil, soyabean oil, egg-yolk, etc.
2. Linolenic acid	linseed oil, rapeseed oil, soybean oil, fish viscera, etc.
3. Arachidonic acid	lecithin*, cephalin*

* these are phospholipids which are found both in plants and animal tissues, viz; plant seeds (soyabean etc.), egg yolk etc.

Although the deficiency of linoleic acid in the diet of humans is very rare, there have been reported some cases of dermatitis in infants and animals that responded to the addition of a few drops of lard oil to the diet (Fig. 9.1).

Polyunsaturated fatty acids also decrease the biosynthesis of cholesterol from either saturated fatty acids or nonfat sources. As little as 2 to 3

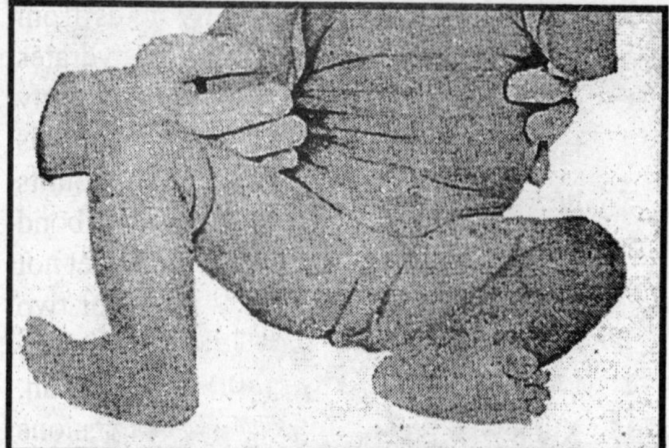

Fig 9.1 : Essential fatty acid deficiency

grams of fats per day like cottonseed, corn, and safflower (Kusumbh) oils will inhibit the cholesterol-promoting effect of 1 gram of fat consisting of saturated fatty acids, such as beef tallow (animal fat melted down) or butter.

The hydrogenation of fats, which is carried out extensively in order to convert liquid oils into a more solid state, **results into considerable reduction in the amount of essential unsaturated fatty acids.**

An outstanding problem of lipid nutrition these days is the relationship of dietary fat to hyper-cholesterolaemia and that of hypercholesterol-aemia to atherosclerosis which remains unclear even to day.

Atherosclerosis is a disease primarily concerned with the integral layer of the artery and is characterized by the thickening and loss of elasticity of the arterial wall by the excessive deposits of cholesterol and other lipids. When narrowing of a vessel occurs (Figures 9.2, 9.3, 9.4 and 9.5), serious impairment of the blood supply to important structures may result. **Atherosclerosis, for instance, in the coronary arteries, is responsible for angina pectoris (pain in the heart i.e., heart attack), and in the cerebral arteries for many mental changes in the old age.** In the vessels of the legs it may be responsible for intermittent claudication (limping, lameness). Complete obstruction of blood flow, usually due to thrombosis results in cardiac infarction, hemiplegia or senile gangrene.

Streptokinase and urokinase are the enzymes being used to disintegrate thrombus (clots) in the cardiac arteries and elsewhere.

Normal amount of the cholesterol in serum is in the range 0f 150-250 mg. It's still on safer side if the level of cholesterol is maintained between **150 to 200 mg%** in blood as per the latest recommendations of the Nutrition Board

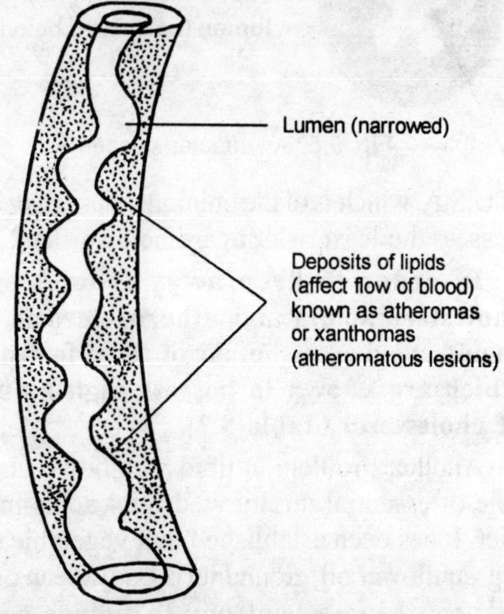

Fig 9.2 : A vessel in which lumen has become narrow due to haphazard deposit of lipids (cholesterol, TG etc.). Sick artery / vessel.

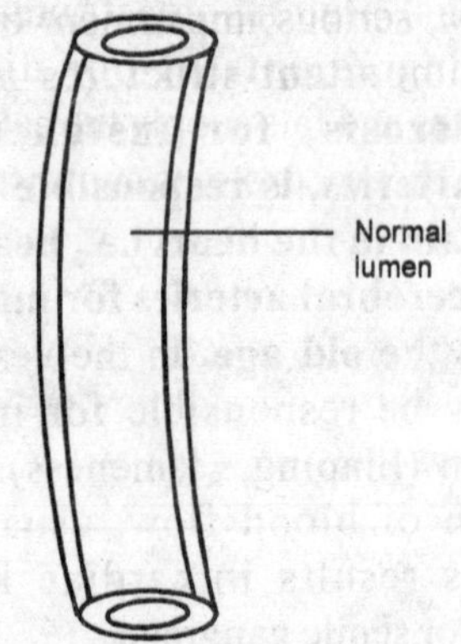

Fig 9.3 : A vessel in which blood flow is normal

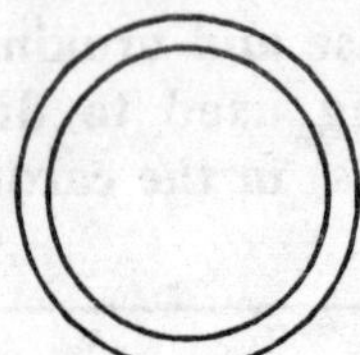

Fig. 9.4 : A normal vessel in which blood flow is normal

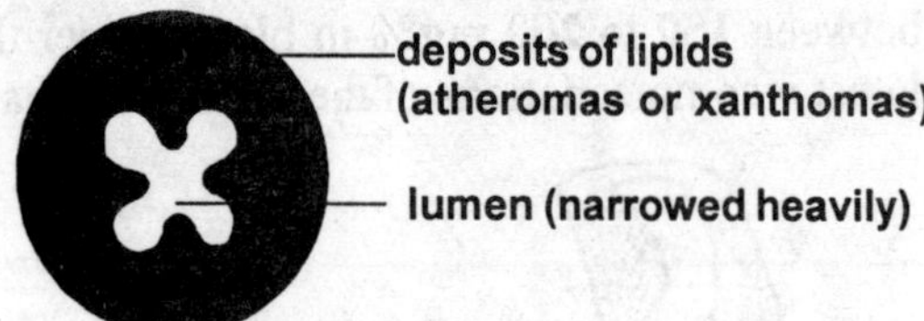

Fig. 9.5 : An affected vessel

of U.S.A. which is of the opinion that such people possess the least risk of cardiac disorders.

In order to keep away from hyper-cholesterolaemia and atherosclerosis one should avoid excess intake of those foodstuffs which are known to possess high amount of cholesterol (Table 9.7).

Another problem in lipid metabolism is the role of essential unsaturated fatty acids in the diet. It has been established that vegetable oils, e.g. sunflower oil, groundnut oil, soyabean oil, til oil, etc. have a tendency to reduce serum cholesterol level in human beings in contrast to the effect of dietary animal fat i.e. desi ghee

Table 9.7 : Cholesterol content of some important human foods

Sl. No.	Food	Cholesterol (mg per 100 gm edible portion)
1.	Vegetable oils	nil
2.	Margarine (imitation butter)	nil
3.	Milk, cow's skimmed	3
4.	Milk, cow's whole	11
5.	Chicken	60
6.	Fish	70
7.	Pork	70
8.	Beef	70
9.	Cheese	100
10.	Butter	250
11.	Liver	300
12.	Kidney	375
13.	Egg, whole	550
14.	Egg, yolk	1,500
15.	Brain	2,000

etc.

Habitual consumption of too much mustard oil is also not good for the heart, according to the researches conducted by the Indian Council of Medical Research (ICMR) as it causes myocardial fibrosis(growth of fibrous tissue). The mechanism by which mustard oil leads to **'myocardial fibrosis'** is not clear but the agent suspected is erucic acid, which is a major component of mustard oil. The ICMR bulletin says, it may be necessary to cultivate mustard varieties with low levels of erucic acid or no erucic acid. Consumption of too much coconut oil and mustard oil can lead to an increase in the level of blood cholesterol; contrarily gingily oil (til oil) can actually reduce cholesterol content.

Percentage of linoleic acid, the so called essential fatty acid in fats and oils of plant and animal origin is as follows :

1. Safflower oil (Kusumbh)	80%
2. Sunflower oil	70%
3. Corn oil	55%
4. Soyabean oil	50%
5. Cottonseed oil	45%
6. Sesame oil (Til oil)	45%
7. Peanut oil	30%
8. Coconut oil	5%

Those having a tendency of obesity/family history of obesity or hypercholesterolaemia should avoid the food items summarised in 'box'.

FAT CONTROLLED DIET: FOODS TO BE AVOIDED

Whole milk, ice cream sour cream, cheese, commercial biscuits, beef, pork, chicken, lamb, kidney, brain, liver, butter, lard, coconut oil, olive oil, chocolate, custards, puddings, etc.

Lipids play an important role in the diet by helping in the absorption of fat soluble vitamins i.e. A,D, E and K. Lecithins prevent development of fatty livers. **Nutritional cirrhosis of liver is caused due to the deficiency of dietary choline which remains present in lecithin.**

Lipids serve as the more important source of energy in the diet of the hard workers such as wrestlers, athletes, labourers, wood-cutters, etc. Ordinarily, excess fat intake should be avoided because this causes an increase in adiposity, hypercholesterolaemia, ketosis, etc. which all are undesirable.

Proteins

Nature of Proteins and their role in nutrition

Proteins are complex nitrogenous substances present in all living tissues. They are built up of simpler molecules called **'amino acids'**. There are **22** different amino acids which occur in an infinite variety of combinations in proteins.

Together with carbohydrates, fats, minerals and vitamins, proteins constitute one of the essential ingredients of our diet. While, carbohydrates and fats supply the calorific needs of the body, dietary proteins supply the building blocks for the formation of blood and tissue proteins, enzymes, antibodies, and certain hormones. They are essential for body growth and maintenance of normal physiological processes. **Recent researches have indicated that protein deficiency in infancy and early childhood (upto 5 years) impairs not only physical growth but also mental development, the damage being permanent and irreversible.**

Protein is required by every cell and is the basis of protoplasm. Moreover, it is the most expensive of the foodstuffs.

Protein's Quality

Now, the chemists have reached the fact that the quantity of protein alone does not solve the entire purpose but the quality of a protein has got more significance, hence, one must give emphasis on the quality of a protein. By the quality of a protein, we mean that it must comprise of essential amino acids in it. This came about with the realization by chemists that proteins from various sources differ widely in their amino acid make up and that their value in nutrition depends largely upon the presence of specific amino acids.

It should be known that the requirement of animals and man is not for proteins, but for specific amount of specific amino acids, the so called essential, or indispensable amino acids.

Casein of milk has been respected as a complete biological protein. It supplies sufficient quantity of all the amino acids required for growth and other needs of the body (Table 9.8). Proteins have been classified into two categories i.e. adequate and inadequate (Table 9.9).

The adult human body can maintain nitrogenous equilibrium on a mixture of eight pure amino acids as its sole source of nitrogen. These eight are as given in Table 9.7. **For growth in infants, histidine is also needed.**

Are all dietary proteins equally good?

No, it is a common fallacy to consider all dietary proteins to be equally good. Actually, proteins differ widely in their nutritional value. The variations are due to differences in digestibility and more particularly the amino acids' composition (Figures 9.6 and 9.7). The nutritive value of a protein is largely determined by the relative concentrations of the **'essential amino acids'** it contains.

Studies of various investigators have shown that an intake of about 0.9 gm of protein per kg body weight is adequate for all ordinary needs in the normal adult. In childhood, this allowance must be increased considerably to permit growth of new tissues. The same applies in pregnancy and lactation. The recommended daily dietary allowance for protein for an average man weighing about 70 kg is 70 g and for an average woman 58 grams.

What are 'essential' amino acids?

The human organism has the ability to synthesize all except **eight** amino acids, utilizing the available sources of nitrogen. The **eight** amino acids should be supplied ready- made by the diet and are, therefore, called **'essential amino acids'. They are the following: Tryptophan, Lysine, Methionine, Threonine, Phenylalanine, Leucine, Isoleucine and Valine (Table 9.8).**

Table 9.8 : Nutritive classification of the amino acids

Essential (Indispensable)	Semi-essential (semi-indispensable)	Non-essential (dispensable)
1. Lysine	1. Arginine	1. Glutamic acid
2. Leucine	2. Tyrosine	2. Aspartic acid
3. Isoleucine	3. Cystine	3. Alanine
4. Methionine	4. Glycine	4. Proline
5. Valine	5. Serine	5. Hydroxyproline,
6. Phenylalanine	6. Histidine*	etc.
7. Tryptophan		
8. Threonine		

* It's treated to be an essential amino acid for the infants

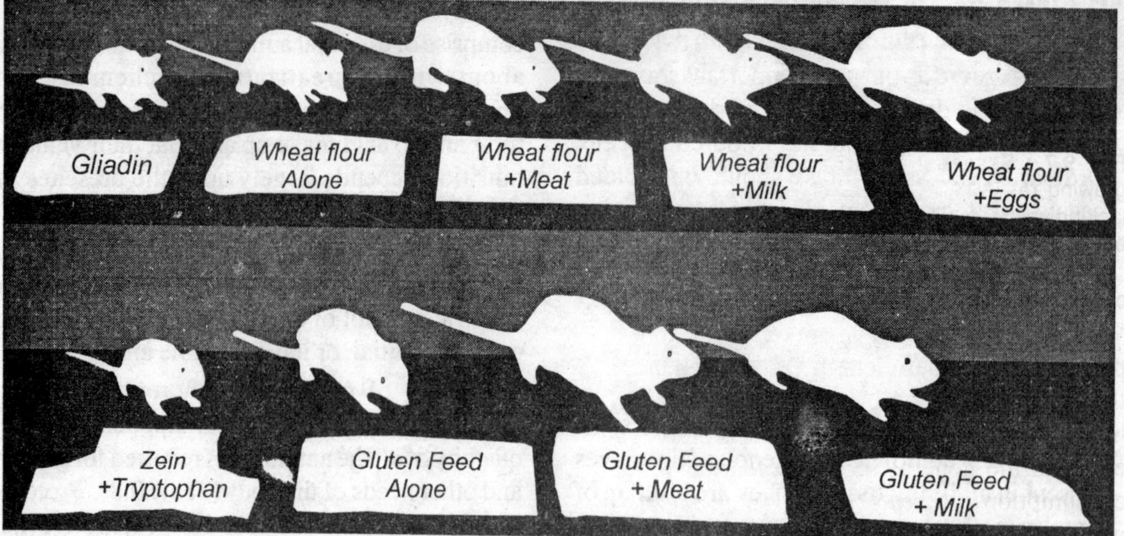

Fig. 9.6 : These rats were all of the same age and had been fed for the same length of time on diets containing the same proportion of protein. The variation in size is due to differences in the chemical constitution of the proteins eaten.

Table 9.9 : Proteins for the growth of rats

Sl. No.	Adequate (Sufficient)	Sl. No.	Inadequate (insufficient)
	Animal Proteins		
1.	Casein of milk	1.	Gliadin of wheat
2.	Lactalbumin of milk	2.	Legumin of pea
3.	Ovalbumin of egg	3.	Zein of corn
	Vegetable Proteins	4.	Hordein of barley
4.	Globulin of cottonseed	5.	Gelatin of horn
5.	Glutenin of wheat	6.	Legumelin of soyabean
6.	Edestin of hempseed		
7.	Excelsin of Brazil nut		

Can the deficiency of one protein be made good by another?

Yes, this is known as mutual complementation between proteins. Although one protein is deficient in one essential amino acid 'X', it may

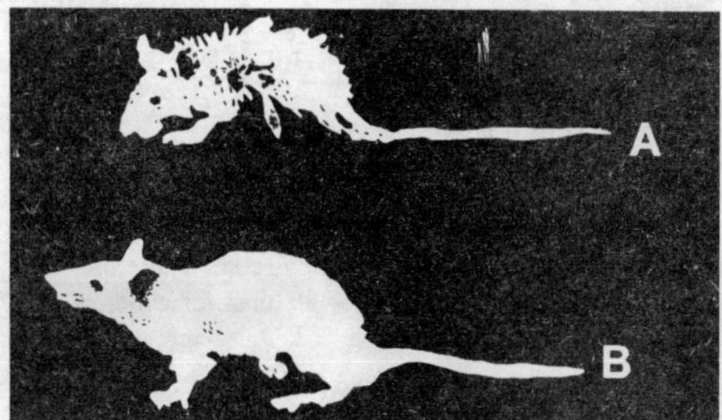

Fig. 9.7 : Essential amino acid deficiency in the growing rat. A. A rat fed a mixture of amino acids lacking valine. B. The same rat after receiving valine added to the amino acid mixture.

contain an excess of another essential amino acid 'Y'. If such a protein in mixed with another protein which is deficient in 'Y' but rich in 'X', the NPU of the combination is considerably higher than that of either individual protein. This explains the general recommendation for the consumption of cereals (low in lysine but rich in methionine) together with pulses (rich in lysine but low in methionine).

Relation between calorie intake and protein utilization

Carbohydrates and fats are the main sources of energy (i.e. calories). Proteins are primarily of value in the formation and regeneration of tissues but they too can serve as a source of energy. When the calorie needs of the body are not adequately met from the intake of carbohydrates and fats, part of the dietary protein is diverted towards energy production. To prevent such wastage of proteins, therefore, care should be taken to raise the intake of carbohydrates and fats to the required levels when offering protein supplements to cover a dietary protein gap.

1. Protein content of the product should be sufficiently high to facilitate the administration of atleast 10-20 grams of protein daily.
2. Nutritive value of the protein should be high. Adequate (first class proteins) are given in table 9.9.
3. Product should be palatable enough to enable the easy administration of the required quantity of protein.
4. Product should not have been baked or toasted at high temperature which damages the nutritive value of the protein.
5. Its protein should preferably be in intact condition and not predigested, i.e. not in the form of protein hydrolysate or mixture of amino acids.
6. It has been established that amino acids mixture cannnot be utilized as efficiently as equivalent amount of proteins.
7. Abnormally high concentration of amino acids in the intestines may also provoke diarrhoea while the elevated blood amino acids levels may cause nausea and vomiting.

Protein foods in slimming regimens

The sheet anchor of any weight reduction course consists in reducing the carbohydrates' content of the diet and limiting the calorie intake by restricting the quantity of the diet. As protein has a high satiety value, protein-rich foods with low carbohydrate content find an important place in slimming regimens.

Daily Protein Requirements

The protein requirements of an individual depend upon the age, sex and body- weight. Primarily, it is expressed in terms of the **"ideal reference protein"**. Infants, whether breast-fed or bottle-fed, receive only the reference protein (NPU = 75-100) until they are weaned. But the mixed proteins of the diets of children and adults are of lower quality and, therefore, due allowance should be made for this factor in calculating the protein requirements. For instance, if the requirement of an adult, in terms of the ideal reference protein, is 0.5 g. per kg bodyweight, it will be 1 g per kg in terms of a dietary protein with an NPU of 50. This is the basis of the official recommendations made recently regarding the dietary allowances for Indian subjects.

Recommended Dietary Protein Allowances for Indians

The following are the daily protein allowances for Indians recommended by the Expert Group of th Indian Council of Medical Research.

Category	Description	Daily protein allowance (g)	Nature of diet
Man	Body weight 55 kg	55	Mainly cereals and pulses NPU = 65*
Woman	Body weight 45 kg	45	
Woman	2nd half of pregnancy	55	
Woman	Lactation upto 1 year	65	
Infants	0-3 months	2.3/kg	Entirely milk NPU = 75-100
Infants	3-6 months	1.8/kg	
Infants	6-9 months	1.8/kg	Milk, cereals and pulses;NPU= 65
Infants	9-12 months	1.5/kg	
Children	1 year	17	Mostly cereals and pulses NPU = 50*
Children	2 years	18	
Children	3 years	20	
Children	4-6 years	22	
Children	7 -9 years	33	
Children	10-12 years	41	
Adolescents:	Boys 13-15 years	55	
Adolescents:	Boys 16-18 years	60	
Adolescents:	Girls 13-18 years	50	

* The essential amino acid requirements of adults are less exacting than those of infants and children. Therefore, the same diet has a higher NPU for adults than for children

Nature of the "Protein Gap" in India

The considered opinion of nutrition authorities is that the protein content of the average Indian diet is adequate but the actual quantity of food consumed by the majority is insufficient. An increased consumption of the normal diets would serve to make up the calorie deficit and also ensure a satisfactory level of protein intake. However, this does not apply to some cases, e.g. weaned infants, pre-school children and pregnant or lactating mothers, whose protein needs in both quality and quantity are considerably higher than those of the general adult population. For such vulnerable groups, the average diets consisting mostly of cereals and pulses cannot satisfy the needs, as the persons find it inconvenient or physically difficult to eat enough of such diets. Therefore, they need more concentrated sources of proteins as dietary supplements.

Effect of Heat on Protein Quality

Under normal condition of cooking, the digestibility of food proteins is generally improved and no damage occurs to the availability of the amino acids. **In the raw state, some vegetable foodstuffs, e.g. peas and beans, contain trypsin- inhibitors which lower the**

digestibility of their proteins. Mild heating destroys these inhibitors and improves the protein digestibility and thereby the nutritive value.

However, proteins suffer serious damage in nutritive value when they are subjected to drastic conditions of heating, especially in presence of sugars and other carbohydrates in the dry state, as in the baking of biscuits. **The damage is due to the formation of an indigestible linkage between the essential amino acid lysine and a reducing sugar.** The deterioration can be detected only by biological tests but not by chemical analysis. As lysine is the most limiting essential amino acid in cereal proteins, even a slight reduction in its availability results in a conspicuous fall in the nutritive value af cereal-based products. It is, therefore, imperative to avoid any drastic process of heating such as baking or toasting in the manufacture of protein foods.

How Useful are Protein Hydrolysates and Amino Acid Preparations for Oral Administration?

The practical value of 'oral" amino acid preparations (predigested proteins) has been seriously overemphasized. Their use was originally based on a misconception, concerning the digestive capacities of the human gastro-intestinal tract. **Actual feeding trials have proved that, even in extreme starvation or diseases like peptic ulcer, ulcerative colitis or regional enteritis,** protein digestion and amino acid absorption are normal and the use of hydrolysed protein seems unnecessary. **It was observed that being unpalatable, protein digests were often rejected and vomited by the patients.** It is also established that amino acid mixtures cannot be utilized as efficiently as equivalent amounts of proteins. The main reason for such poor utilization seems to be the extremely rapid absorption of free amino acids and the consequent flooding of the tissues with excessive amounts af amino acids which cannot be utilized equally rapidly and are therefore partially wasted. The abnormally high concentration of amino acids in the intestines may also provoke diarrhoea while the elevated blood amino acid levels may cause nausea and vomiting. On the other hand, in the course of normal protein digestion, the amino acids are released in a slow and regulated manner, keeping pace with absorption and utilization, there being neither accumulation of amino acids in the intestines nor unduly high level in the blood.

The recent craze for the addition of lysine to multivitamin and mineral preparations intended as supplement to children has no rational basis. Being in the free form, it is rapidly absorbed but is largely wasted as the other essential amino acids are not supplied simultaneously. Further, although lysine content of cereals is low, **the most limiting essential amino acid in the average mixed diets consumed in our country may be either methionine, threonine or tryptophan but not lysine.**

Increased Protein Needs of Diabetics and the Elderly

Additional protein upto 0.5 g per kg body weight per day is recommended to diabetics because it has a more sustained effect in maintaining blood sugar than carbohydrate. A protein rich snack at bed time serves as a precaution against morning hypoglycaemia.

In old age, the calorie requirements are considerably reduced but not those of proteins and other nutrients. **Owing to the increased proneness to illness with the resulting tissue break-down and negative nitrogen balance, speedy recovery demands a higher protein intake than that provided by the normal diet. Therefore, the elderly should receive, protein-rich foods fortified with minerals and vitamins:**

Conclusion

In view of the scientific data presented in the earlier pages, the following consideration should be borne in mind while selecting a protein food as a dietary supplement.

1. The protein content of the product should be sufficiently high to facilitate the administration of at least 10-20 grams of protein daily.
2. The nutritive value of the protein should be high equivalent to a Net Protein Utilization of at least 60.
3. The product should be palatable enough to enable the easy administration of the required quantity of protein.
4. The product should not have been baked or toasted at high temperatures which damage the nutritive value of the protein.
5. Its protein should preferably be in the intact condition and not predigested, i.e. not in the form of protein hydrolysate of mixture of amino acids.

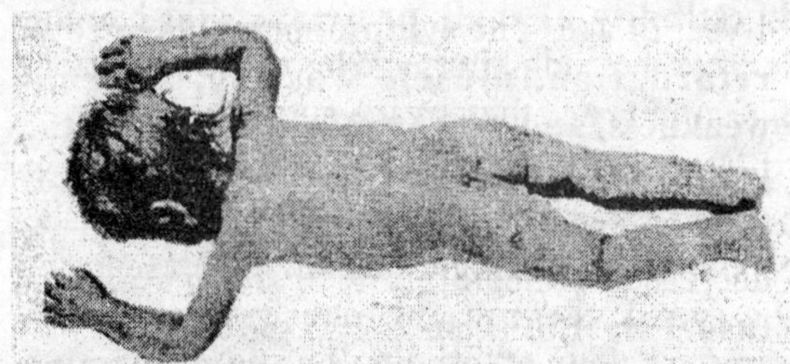

Fig. 9.8 : Symptoms of protein deficiency : Boy, 2 years 1 month old on admission. Note widespread distribution of skin lesions and edema.

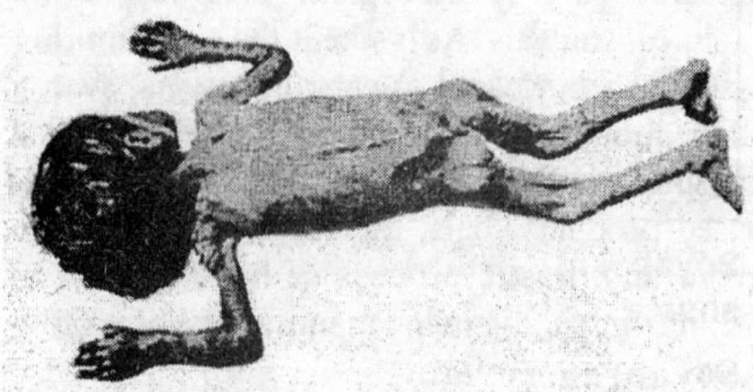

Fig. 9.9 : Same child two weeks after starting the treatment, showing disappearance of the edema and improvement in the skin lesions. Note the degree of muscular wasting, which had been concealed by the edema.

Kwashiorkor

It is mainly a disease of rural areas, occurring in the second year of life. It occurs most commonly in the infants after weaning (breast feeding) when the diet which replaces the mother's milk is markedly deficient in protein (Figures 9.8 & 9.9) but high in carbohydrate. Kwashiorkor disease has its highest incidence between the age group of **1 to 4 years** when the need for essential amino acids for tissue synthesis is great. No age is immune, but in elders, clinical manifestations not so obvious and usually less severe, because both protein and energy requirements are relatively reduced as age advances.

The disease is characterized by growth failure, retarded development, loss of appetite, mental apathy, hypoalbuminemia leading to edema, diarrhoea, pellagrous skin lesions, low plasma amino acids, lipids, glucose and potassium. Gastrointestinal disturbances, dermatosis, fatty liver infiltration and mental disturbances are also frequent. The condition is usually complicated by dietary deficiencies other than protein and calories. It has been observed in children that protein malnutrition causes a reduction of the circumference of the head which may lead to impaired growth of the brain and its development and mental retardation. Malnutrition may likewise reduce resistance to infection. Treatment consists in instituting more adequate diet, with special reference to protein and correction of electrolyte and water balance.

Marasmus

Marasmus literally means **"to waste"**. It results from a continued severe deficiency of both **dietary proteins** and the **calories** i.e. **energy.** It generally occurs in the children below

1 year of age. **The symptoms include growth retardation, muscle wasting, anaemia, weakness, and repeated infections. Attitude is irritable.** Skin is shrunken, dry and atrophic.

A marasmic child does not show edema on decreased concentration of plasma albumin **(usual level in them is 2 to 3g/dl whereas in kwashiorkor cases it is always less than 2g/dl)** and the level of cortisol in serum gets increased in marasmic child whereas decreased in kwashiorkor.

> Marasmus is predominantly due to the **deficiency of calories.** This is usually observed in children given watery gruels (of cereals) to supplement the mother's breast milk.

Soyabean (Glycine hispida - a very good source of proteins for vegetarians).

Soyabean is being eaten in China for several thousands of years. The whole dry grain contains about **40-43 percent of protein** (twice as much as in most other pulses) and also upto **20% fat.** Soyabean forms the basis of the great variety of the sauces and pastes with which Chinese cooks garnish their food. Contrarily, in India and Europe the people have not yet been attracted by it because of its peculiar bitter flavour.

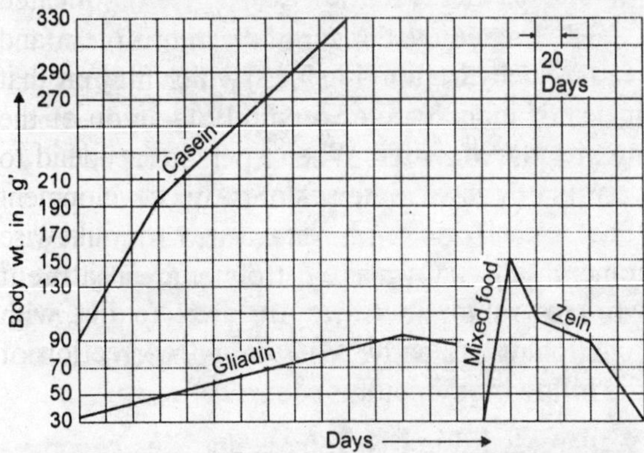

Fig. 9.10: Growth curve of rats maintained on diets containing a single protein. Poor growth is observed with gliadin as the protein (lysine deficient), and with zein (lysine and tryptophan deficient). Excellent growth is obtained with a casein diet.

It has been observed that the nutritive value of the wheat flour is increased by several folds if the soyabean flour is mixed with it in the ratio of 50:50. Such a flour has been proved to be very useful for the growing children. Effect of a single protein on the growth of rats has been shown in figure 9.10, whereas supplementation effect (supplemented with amino acids and protein) has been shown in Figures 9.11 and 9.12 respectively.

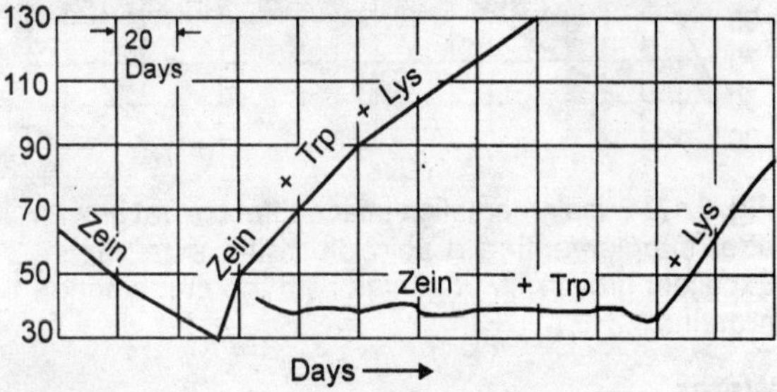

Fig. 9.11: Graph showing supplementation effect. When zein supplemented with tryptophan and lysine, excellent growth is obtained. With tryptophan as the only supplement, body weight alone is maintained, there is no remarkable gain in body weight; growth takes place only after further addition of lysine.

Minerals

These have equally important role in the human body for proper growth and maintenance. Living organisms contain at least 29 elements. among these, **13 are non metals** i.e. C, H, O, N, S, P, Cl, F, Br, I, B, Si and As. The metals are Ca, Mg, Na, K, Fe, Cu, Zn, Ni, Co, Mn, Al, Pb, Sn, Mo, V and Ti.

Among the elements needed in quantities **greater than 100 mg daily are** Ca, Mg, Na, K, P, and Cl; these are called the **macroelements.** The others are needed in very minute quantities (less than 100 mg daily) and are termed as **microelements or oligoelements or trace elements.**

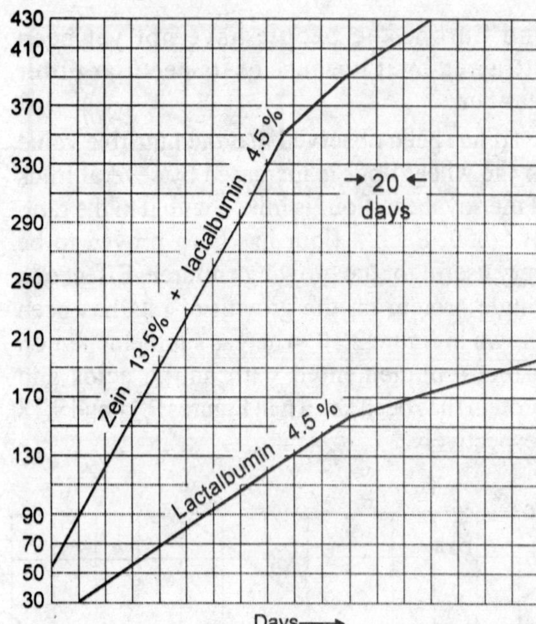

Fig. 9.12: Supplementation effect. Effect on rat growth after supplementing a zein diet with lactalbumin. Excellent growth is observed with the combination proteins.

Water

It constitutes nearly 70% of the total body weight and may be roughly compared to the ratio of water and land on the earth (Figures 9.13 and 9.14) where again water covers nearly 75% of the total area of the earth, thus emphasizing the contribution of water in the human body and on the earth.

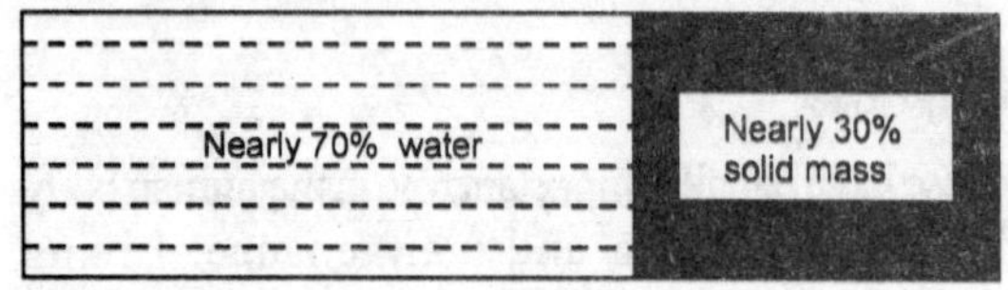

Fig. 9.13: Exhibiting ratio of water and solid mass in human body

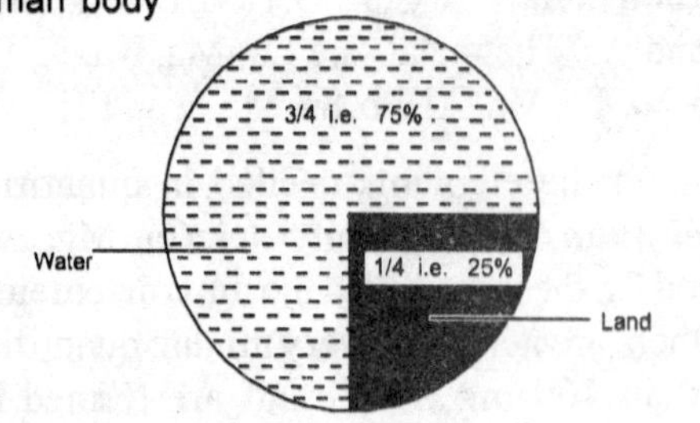

Fig. 9.14: Exhibiting the ratio of water and land on the earth

Loss of about 10% of body water causes illness and loss of about 20% may cause death. All the enzymatic reactions proceed in the human body in an aqueous phase of which water is the important component. Nearly 75% of the total diseases of the infants are caused due to giving them deficient and uncleaned water.

Diarrhoea and oral rehydration

Young children in our country suffer from various health problems. **Malnutrition and diarrhoeal diseases cause a large proportion of illness and death in young children.** Repeated attacks of diarrhoea often produce and worsen malnutrition.

What is diarrhoeal disease?

When a person passes liquid watery stools more than three times in 24 hours, he or she is said to have diarrhoea. It is very often accompanied by vomiting, fever and loss of appetite. This disease is caused by a variety of bacterial and viral agents which usually come from unclean surroundings. **Food, water, dirty hands and clothing carry these bacterial and viral agents.**

The immediate danger of diarrhoea is that it leads to dehydration (Fig 9.15) which may result in death if not corrected promptly. **Dehydration means loss of water.** When a person repeatedly vomits or passes watery stools, his body loses lot of water. Along with water, various important mineral salts, known as electrolytes are also lost. Mineral salts and water are vital for proper functioning of a body. When dehydration sets in, the following symptoms occur:

■ Increased thirst ■ Tongue and lips become dry ■ Weakness ■ Skin loses its elasticity ■ Eyes become sunken ■ In children below 18 months, the depression on their head - bone becomes more sunken ■ Urine output decreased

In diarrhoea in children, oral rehydration therapy (a mixture of pinch of sugar and salt in a cup of boiled and cooled water) should be started immediately (Fig 9.16) without any delay.

When liquid from the body is lost in large quantities and rapidly, particularly in very young children, dehydration can be very severe. This can lead to sudden death.

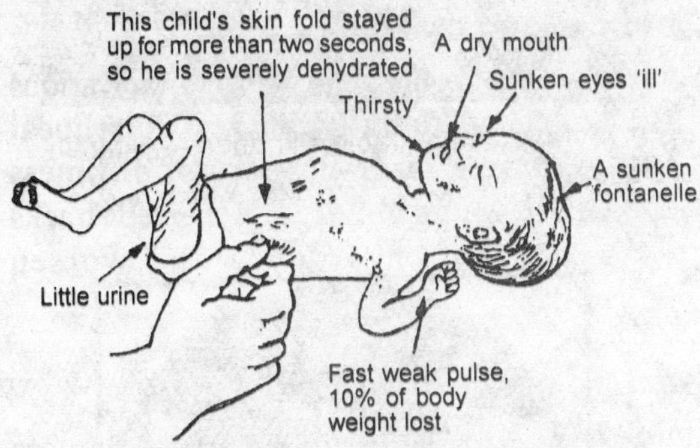

Fig. 9.15: Effect of dehydration

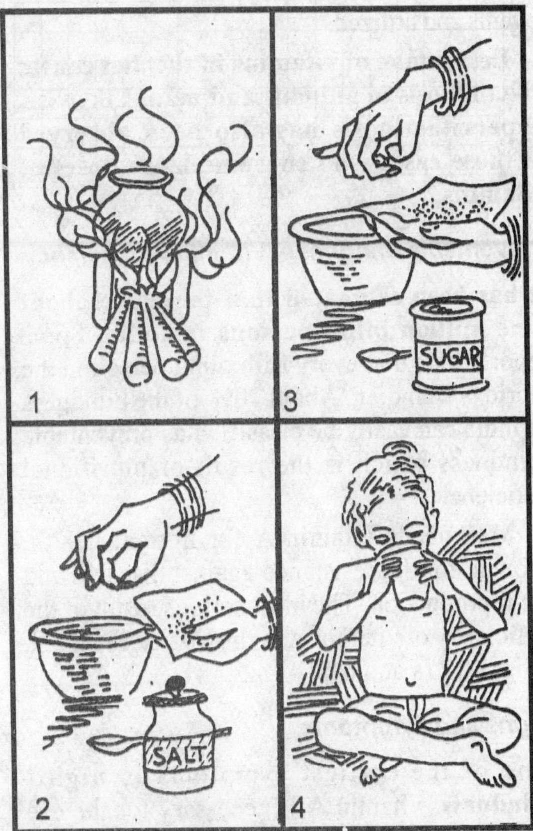

Fig. 9.16 : To show oral rehydration therapy

Vitamins

In addition to carbohydrates, lipids, proteins, inorganic salts and water, normal growth and good health in the mammals require the presence of additional compounds in the diet. These are organic in nature and are called vitamins. Not all living organisms require vitamins (some bacteria do not), nor do they necessarily need the same number or kind, since some vitamins can be synthesized by the organism. **For example, the guinea pig, man and other primates cannot synthesize vitamin C (ascorbic acid) due to the absence of enzyme L-gulono-oxidase and are therefore susceptible to scurvy,** whereas the rat can synthesize vitamin C and therefore does not require it in the diet. We do not know the biochemical functions of all the known vitamins, although many, especially those of the vitamin B group, are known to be precursors of coenzymes.

Vitamins are usually divided into two categories: those that are fat soluble and those that are water soluble. **Fat soluble vitamins are A, D, E and K; the water soluble vitamins are members of the B and C groups.** Nearly, all these vitamins are found in the consumable articles for instance vegetables, milk, meat, fish, pulses, corns(wheat, millet, gram, etc), fruits, cereals, etc.

Intestinal organisms play a role in the vitamin quota available to the animal or man. They may synthesize vitamins in significant amount. Vitamin K is an important example of a vitamin synthesized by intestinal organisms. Folic acid, nicotinic acid, pyridoxine, biotin, thiamine and riboflavin are other examples. These may be absorbed to varying extents and utilized.

Less intake of vitamins in the diet causes avitaminosis in animals and man. Likewise, hypervitaminosis has also been observed in those cases who consume large doses of vitamins.

Preventable Blindness- Vitamin A deficiency

It has been estimated that there are about nine million blind persons in India. Some reports state that every fifth blind person in the world is an Indian. About 20% of the blindness in India can easily be classified as preventable blindness which is the result of nutritional deficiencies.

Man needs vitamin A for normal health, growth, for the resistance against diseases and for reproduction. The most serious result of the deficiency of vitamin A is the loss of eye sight. {Fig. 9.17 (a and b)}.

Signs and Symptoms

One of the earliest symptoms is **night-blindness**. Vitamin A is necessary for the eye to respond or become sensitive to changes in light. If vitamin A is lacking, the person is unable to see clearly in dimlight or at night. Such children may be able to see perfectly well during day time. The condition is commonly known as night blindness. In addition, there are some visual changes in the eye. The white portion of the eye becomes dry and flaky. As a result, the thin membrane loses its lustre and appears rough and dry. This condition is known as **xerophthalmia** which means **'dry-eye'**. Wrinkled pearly grey spots, triangular or round in shape may appear on the white portion in chronic cases. These are known as **'Bitot spots'**.

These lesions by themselves do not affect vision. If the condition is not treated promptly, the black portion of the eye, that is the cornea also gets involved, resulting in keratomalacia and permanent blindness. This is a condition wherein the black portion of

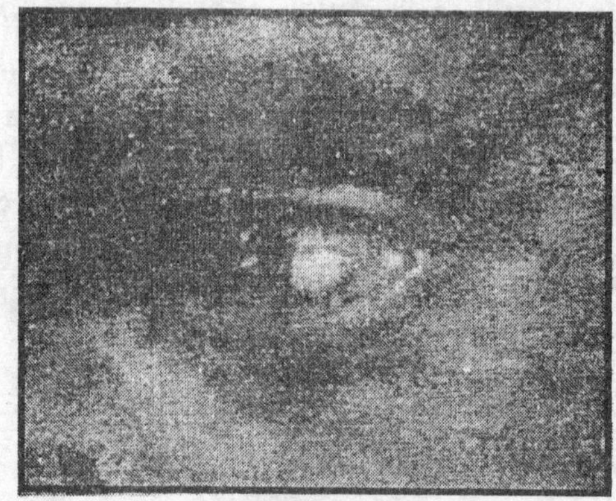

Fig. 9.17 (a) : Preventable Blindness - vitamin A deficiency

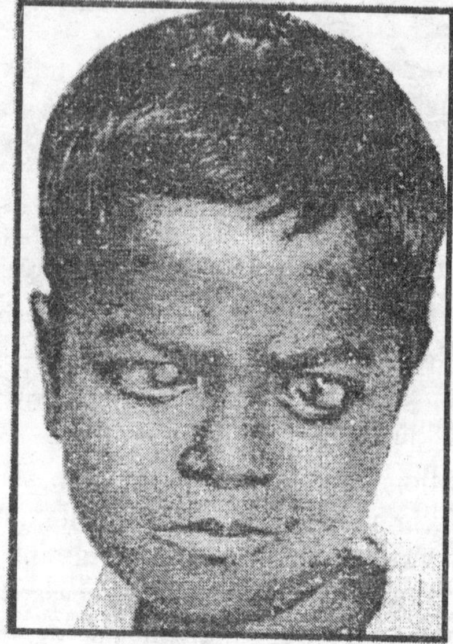

Fig. 9.17 (b) : To show the effect of vitamin A deficiency

the eye becomes softened into a cloudy, opaque mass.

In India, we have abundant sources of vitamin A that are easily and cheaply available. These include foods such as carrot, green leafy vegetables, namely drumstick leaves, amaranth, spinach and fruits like mango and papaya. Studies conducted by National Institute of Nutrition have shown that **if 40 g of green leafy vegetables**

are added to the existing diet, the child would get the required amount of vitamin A. This is because leafy vegetables are good sources of carotene which can be converted into vitamin A in the body.

Causes

However, intake of vitamin A by children as well as women is very low. In some areas, it is believed that children should not be given green leafy vegetables as it may cause diarrhoea. Others believe that pregnant women should not eat papaya; Thus, some of the rich sources of this vitamin are denied to those who need it most.

A well - nourished mother provides adequate vitamin A to her baby to be stored in its liver. After birth, the infant obtains vitamin A through the mother's milk. Therefore, a healthy mother provides enough vitamin A to her baby before birth as well as after birth.

Colostrum is the thick milky secretion of the breast in the first few days after child birth. This is a very rich source of vitamin A. Infants fed colostrum have better reserves of vitamin A. The practice of feeding colostrum should be encouraged.

During acute infections, vitamin A status of the child deteriorates. It has been shown that measles- common childhood infection is one of the important causes of keratomalacia. Acute respiratory and gastrointestinal infections also aggravate vitamin A deficiency. Intestinal parasites, especially round worms are common among children belonging to poor communities. **Incidence of vitamin A deficiency is higher among the children having round worms in their gastrointestinal tracts.**

Prevention and treatment

Even the most severe cases of vitamin A deficiency can be successfully treated. **The usual practice is to administer intramuscular injections of 30,000 μg of vitamin A for 2 or 3 consecutive days.** This is followed by oral doses for a few more days till the body reserves are built up. Conjunctival lesions and night blindness respond well to relatively small doses of vitamin A. **Oral administration of 1,000 μg daily for about a week usually reverses the changes.**

Corneal lesions should be treated as a medical emergency. **30,000 μg of water miscible vitamin A can be injected intramuscularly followed by 1000 μg of vitamin A orally for a period of 15 days. This helps in rapid clinical and biochemical improvement. Oil soluble vitamin A should not be injected as the absorption of this compound from the site of injection is poor.**

Diet improvement

The most logical method of prevention would be to improve the diet of the vulnerable groups.

Consumption of adequate amount of vitamin A is essential to keep the eyes bright. Drumstick leaves, spinach, amaranth, carrots and pumpkin contain large quantities of carotene. The substance is converted into vitamin A in our body. Even children suffering from mild forms of malnutrition are able to absorb carotene from amaranth. The presence of even small amount of fat helps in the absorption. Carotene is also present in large quantities in fruits like mango and papaya. **Consumption of such food [Fig. 9.18 (a & b)] should be encouraged.** Particularly pregnant and lactating women should eat sufficient quantities of foods rich in vitamin A. They can meet requirements easily if they eat atleast one medium sized bowl full of cooked greens every day.

As a short- term measure, periodical oral administration of vitamin A has been suggested for the prevention of vitamin A deficiency in children.

Based on the recommendations of the National Institute of Nutrition (NIN), Hyderabad,

the Government of India has launched a massive prophylaxis programme against vitamin A deficiency from 1970 in several states. In this programme children between 1-5 years are being given an oral dose of 2,00000 I.U. of vitamin A once in six months. The programme is implemented through the existing public health set up. Evaluation carried out in some states has shown a significant reduction in the incidence of xerophthalmia wherever the programme was well implemented.

A few paise spent on inexpensive foods rich in vitamin A can make all the difference between **good vision and no vision** (Fig. 9.19).

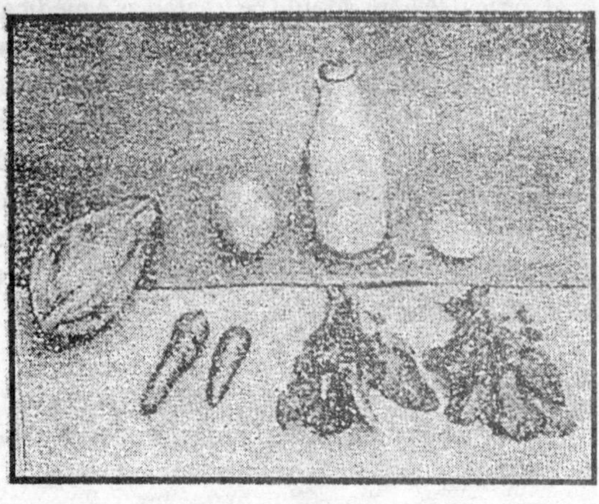

(a)

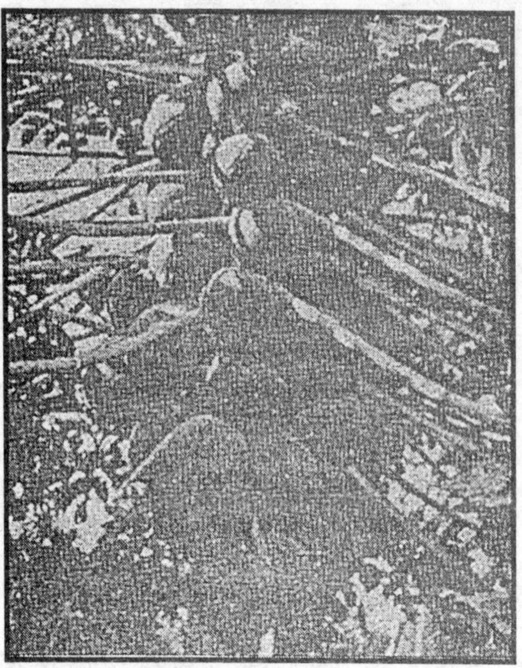

Fig. 9.18 (a & b) : Treatment part of vitamin `A' deficiency

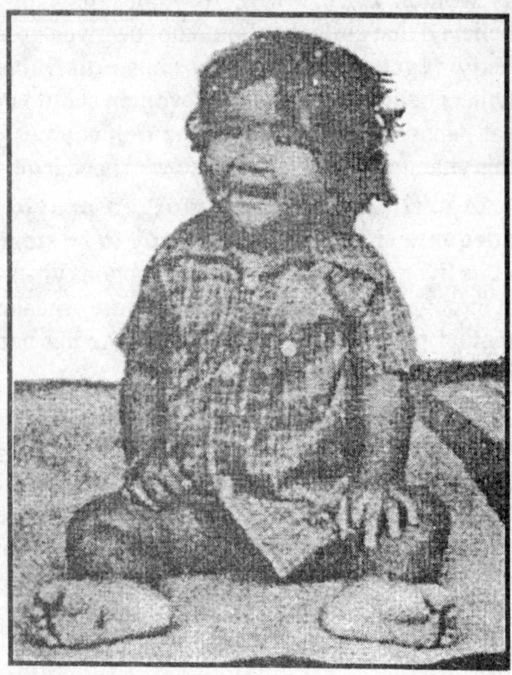

Fig. 9.19 : Normal child with good vision

TIPS FOR HEALTHY EATING

- **Eat whole grain cereals, millets and pulses.**
- Eat plenty of seasonal vegetables and one seasonal fruit daily.
- **Consume green leafy vegetables.**
- **Milk and milk products, fruits and vegetables are essential for healthy ageing.**
- Foods of animal origin, oil, fat and sugar are good for growing children, adolescents, pregnant and lactating women.

CHAPTER 10

METABOLISM OF CARBOHYDRATES

The major function of carbohydrate metabolism is to provide energy for various metabolic processes of the body. In this role, carbohydrates are utilised by the cells mainly in the form of glucose. Carbohydrates have the advantage of being cheap, easily digestible and rapidly metabolizable.

Carbohydrates' metabolism is basically the metabolism of glucose and substances related to it.

The sugar of the blood is glucose. The digestion of carbohydrates such as starch, sucrose and lactose produces glucose, fructose and galactose respectively which pass into the blood circulation. Conversion of fructose and galactose into glucose occurs in the liver.

Carbohydrates supply nearly 2/3 energy requirement of the body.

Glycolysis

The oxidation of glucose to pyruvate is termed as glycolysis (Fig 10.1).

Under aerobic condition pyruvic acid enters mitochondria and is completely oxidized to CO_2 and H_2O through TCA cycle, whereas under anaerobic condition, pyruvic acid is converted to lactic acid.

under aerobic conditions, i.e. in the presence of O_2 → acetyl CoA $\xrightarrow[\text{Cycle}]{\text{TCA}}$ CO_2 + H_2O

glucose $\xrightarrow{\text{glycolysis}}$ pyruvic acid

under anaerobic conditions i.e. in the absence of O_2 → lactic acid

The sequence of reactions from glucose to pyruvic acid is also called as **Embden-Meyerhof** pathway. **'Glycolysis is an extramitochondrial pathway which is carried out by a variety of enzymes (Figure 10.1).**

Salient features of Glycolysis

1. Successive phosphorylation of the glucose at C-1 and C-6 utilizes initially two molecules of ATP. These phosphorylations and an isomerization bring about the conversion of glucose to fructose 1,6-diphosphate.
2. After the split of the 6-carbon sugar to two 3- carbon molucules (by aldolase), there is immediate oxidation of the aldehyde to an acid with simultaneous formation of an anhydride bond between

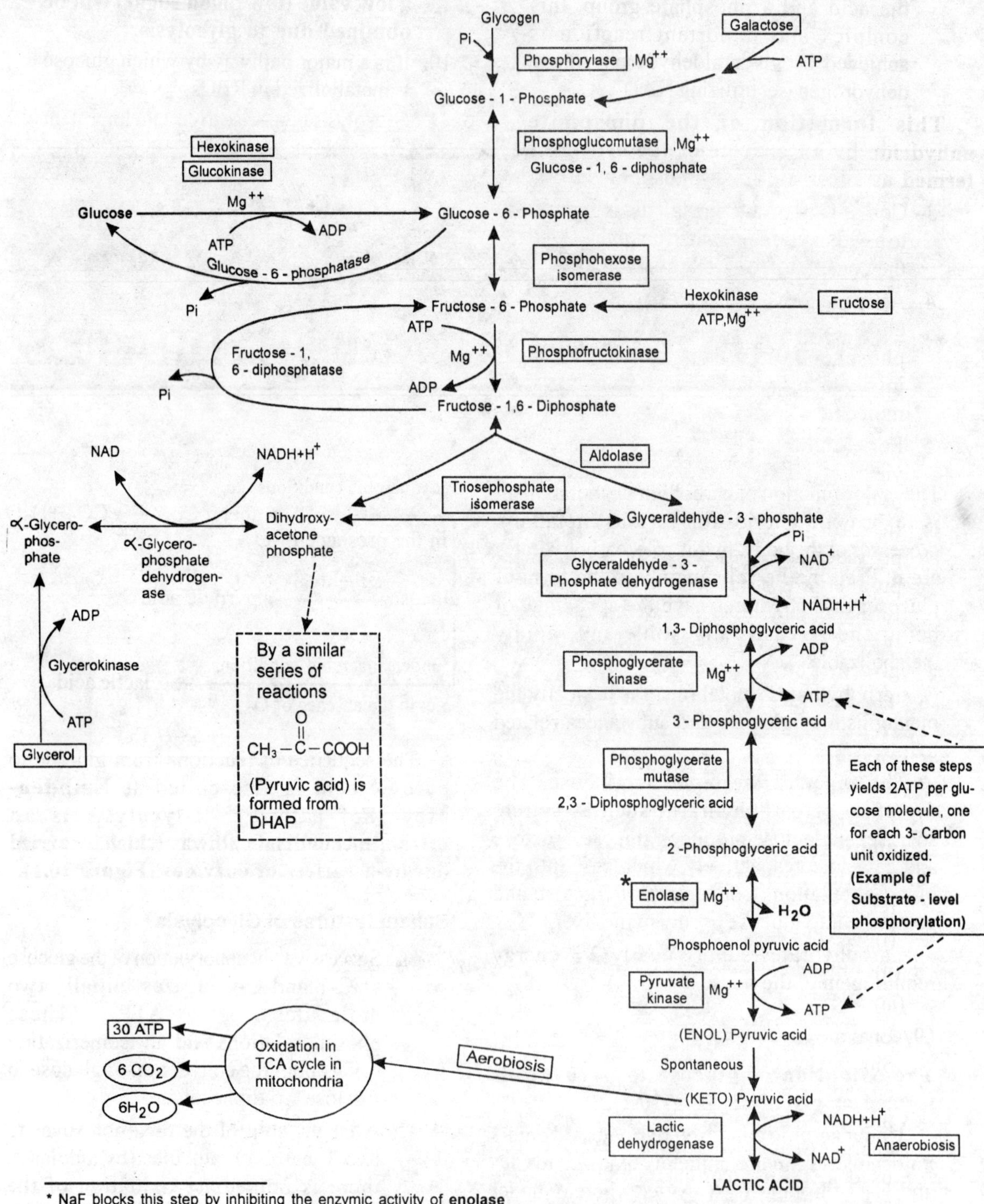

* NaF blocks this step by inhibiting the enzymic activity of **enolase**

Figure 10.1 : Glycolytic Pathway (Glycolysis)

the acid and a phosphate group, this complex and important reaction is achieved by glyceraldehyde phosphate dehydrogenase, utilizing NAD^+.

This formation of the phosphate anhydride by an enzyme of the cytosol is termed as substrate level phosphorylation.

3. Conversion of the phosphate anhydride to a carboxylic acid is then combined with the conversion of ADP to ATP.
4. After the move of the phosphate to C-2, enolase, by removing water, yields phosphoenolpyruvate, which is then involved in a reaction in which a further molecule of ATP is formed from ADP.
5. For each mole of glucose oxidized, the yield of ATP from glycolysis is two moles of ATP (4 ATP produced, 2 ATP utilized). In addition, 2 moles of NADH are produced (one for each of the 3- carbon products), each of which may yield a further two moles of ATP, if oxidized by the electron transport chain via the glycerol phosphate shuttle.
6. **The first rate limiting step (regulatory step) in glycolysis is catalysed by enzyme PFK. This enzyme is inhibited by citrate, ATP and NADH.**
7. **Pyruvate kinase is inhibited by ATP and NADH (second regulatory step).**
8. All the reactions of glycolysis are reversible except which are catalysed by
   (i) Hexokinase,
   (ii) PFK, and
   (iii) PK
9. Enzyme enolase is inhibited by fluoride. Since RBCs do not possess mitochondrial enzymes to oxidise glucose aerobically, they depend upon glycolysis only for their energy requirement, that is why, NaF is used in the collection of blood sugar samples because it prevents glycolysis by inhibiting the enzyme enolase, **otherwise a low value (low blood sugar) will be obtained due to glycolysis.**
10. It is a major pathway by which glucose is metabolized in RBCs.
11. Glycolysis gives rise to certain important compounds which are very important for other biochemical processes; those produced include:
    (i) Glyceraldehydade 3-PO_4: Required for the biosynthesis of triglycerides and phospholipids.
    (ii) Acetyl Co-A: Required for the biosynthesis of cholesterol.
    (iii) Pyruvate: Required for the biosynthesis of alanine by transamination.

Simplified schematic presentation of glycolysis is given in (Figure 10.2).

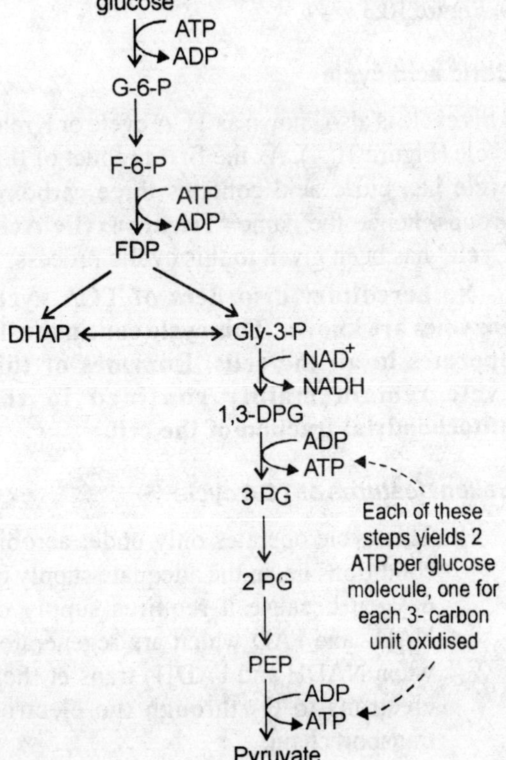

Figure 10.2 : Simplified schematic presentation of **'glycolysis'**.

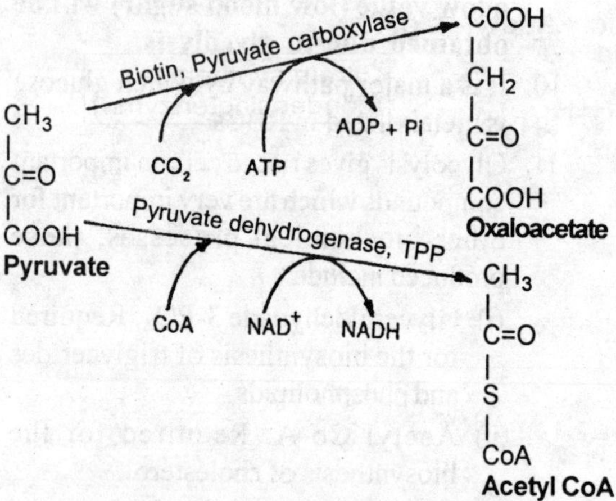

Figure 10.3 : Pyruvate metabolism

Further metabolism of Pyruvate

Pyruvate produced by glycolytic pathway and the other metabolic pathways can be converted either to oxaloacetate or acetyl CoA as shown in Figure 10.3.

Citric acid cycle

This cycle is also known as TCA cycle or Krebs cycle (Figure 10.4). As the first product of this cycle i.e., citric acid contains three carboxyl groups, hence the name **'Tricarboxylic Acid Cycle'** has been given to this cyclic process.

No hereditary disorders of TCA cycle enzymes are known. This cycle continuously operates in all the cells. Enzymes of this cycle remain mainly confined in the mitochondrial fraction of the cell.

Salient features of TCA cycle

1. This cycle operates only under aerobic conditions i.e. in the adequate supply of oxygen because it requires supply of NAD^+ and FAD which are regenerated when NADH and $FADH_2$ transfer their electrons to O_2 through the electron transport chain.
2. Before pyruvate gets entry into TCA cycle, it is oxidatively decarboxylated to acetyl CoA.
3. This cycle may be referred to as a mechanism whereby acetyl coenzyme A may be completely oxidized to CO_2 and H_2O.
4. The very first reaction of the cycle, which occurs in the presence of an enzyme called the **"condensing enzyme" (citrate synthetase)** is a condensation between acetyl CoA and oxaloacetic acid to form citric acid and coenzyme A. This reaction may be considered to be irreversible.
5. Aconitase and isocitric dehydrogenase play role as shown in the cycle.
6. α-ketoglutaric acid (α-keto acid) gets oxidatively decarboxylated forming succinyl CoA in the presence of TPP, NAD^+, FAD, CoA, lipoic acid and Mg^{++}.
7. The importance of this pathway lies in the fact that it is one of the pathways that generates the major part of the ATP and NADH in the cell.
8. NADP can be formed from $NADP^+$ and NADH by a mitochondrial transhydrogenase.
9. **ATP thus produced is utilized by the cell for its functions which are numerous and the NADPH for the biosynthesis of fatty acids, steroids and other important substances of the human body.**

Energetics of TCA cycle

(i) Pyruvic acid to acetyl CoA 2 x 3 = **6**
(ii) Isocitric acid to oxalosuccinic acid 2 x 3 = **6**
(iii) α-KGA to succinyl CoA 2 x 3 = **6**
(iv) Succinyl CoA to succinic acid 2 x 1 = **2** (substrate level phosphorylation)
(v) Succinic acid to fumaric acid 2 x 2 = **4**
(vi) Malic acid to oxaloacetic acid 2 x 3 = **6**

Total 30 ATP

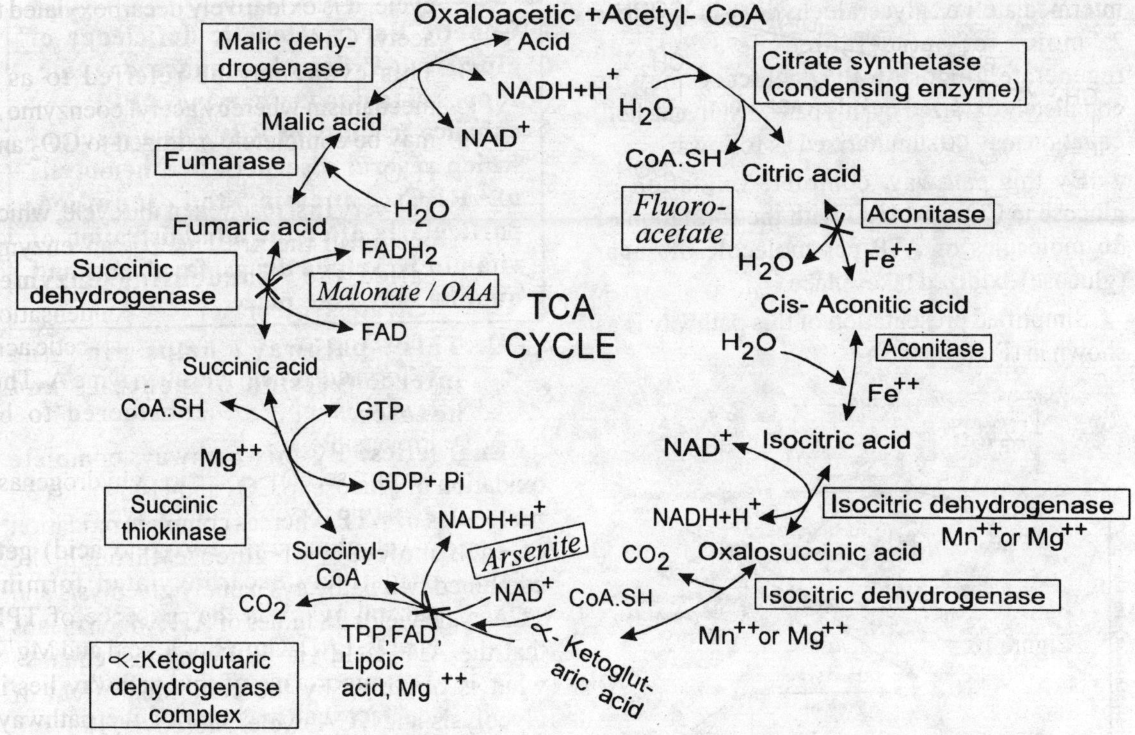

Figure 10.4 : TCA cycle (Krebs cycle)

Thus, total number of ATP molecules generated in TCA cycle under aerobic conditions is 30.

Hexose Monophosphate Shunt Pathway

This pathway is also known as **Warburg-Dickens Lipmann pathway or pentose phosphate pathway or phosphogluconate pathway or direct oxidative pathway or reductive pathway.**

Though, glycolysis is the principal pathway for the conversion of glucose into pyruvate in most of the tissues but still there exists an alternative pathway.

It is quantitatively insignificant in highly glycolytic tissues such as skeletal muscles and non-lactating mammary glands but is of considerable quantitative importance in tissues like adrenal cortex, testis, liver, adipose tissue and lactating mammary glands.

The enzymes of this pathway are found in the extra mitochondrial soluble fraction of the cell, the cytosol.

Besides the above tissues, it also operates in leucocytes and erythrocytes.

It is a multicyclic process in which 3 molecules of glucose-6-phosphate give rise to 3 molecules of CO_2 and three-5- carbon residues (namely: ribulose-5-PO_4). The latter are arranged to regenerate 2 molecules of glucose-6-phosphate and one molecule of the glycolytic

$$3 \text{ Glucose-6-phosphate} + 6 \text{ NADP}^+$$

$$\downarrow$$

$$3CO_2 + 2 \text{ glucose-6-} PO_4 + \text{glyceraldehyde-3-}PO_4 + 6 \text{ NADPH} + 6H^+$$

intermediate i.e. glyceraldehyde-3-PO_4. Since 2 moles of glyceraldehyde-3-PO_4,can regenerate glucose-6-PO_4, glucose may be completely oxidized by this pathway. In nutshell, equation may be summarized as follows:

By this pathway, complete oxidation of glucose to CO_2 and H_2O with the formation of 36 molecules of ATP per molecule of sugar (glucose) oxidized takes place.

Simplified presentation of this pathway is as shown in (Figure 10.5).

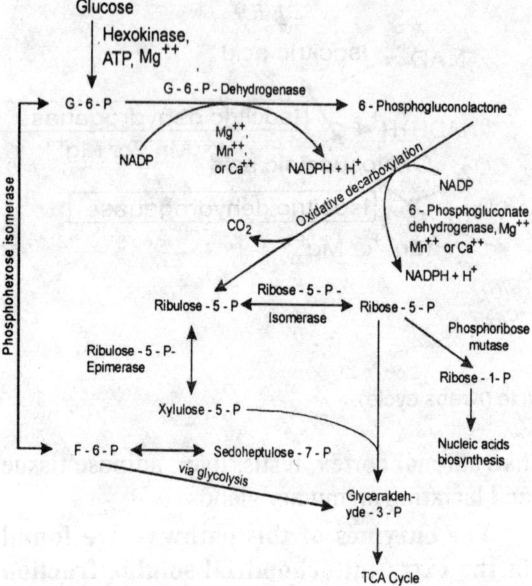

Figure 10.5: Pentose phosphate pathway (simplified presentation)

Importance of HMP shunt pathway

1. **One of the most important functions of this pathway is to provide NADPH which is required in the reductive synthesis of fatty acids, triglycerides, steroids and various other substances.**
2. **It gives rise to the formation of pentoses which are required in the synthesis of nucleic acids.**

> **Genetic Error: Genetic deficiency of glucose-6-P dehydrogenase enzyme, supposed to be a key enzyme of PPP may enhance fragility of RBCs as a result of which several disorders like hemolysis of RBCs, anemia and jaundice, particularly after the administration of vitamin K, sulpha drugs, favabeans and quinine may take place.**

3. **This pathway helps in the interconversion of pentoses and hexoses.**

Energetics: By this pathway, complete oxidation of glucose to CO_2 and H_2O yields 36 **molecules of ATP** whereas complete oxidation of each molecule of glucose through the combined two pathways namely glycolysis and TCA cycle yields 38 moles of ATP which means that the ATP yield via PPP is almost equal to what is obtained by the combined effect of glycolysis and TCA cycle. Moreover, PPP is a shorter route for the yield of ATP than the combined routes of glycolysis + TCA.

GLYCOGENESIS

This process may be referred to as the synthesis of glycogen from glucose or other sugars.

In the very first reaction glucose gets phosphorylated to form glucose-6-PO_4 in the presence of ATP; this reaction is catalysed by glucokinase. In the next step, mutation of the phosphate group of glucose-6-PO_4 from position 6 to the position 1 takes place in the presence of a cofactor glucose 1,6 diphosphate; this reaction is catalysed by the enzyme phosphoglucomutase. In the next reaction, glucose-1-PO_4 reacts with UTP to form active nucleotide i.e., uridine diphosphate glucose in the presence of enzyme UDPG pyrophosphorylase; in this process, two terminal phosphates are removed from UTP as inorganic pyrophosphate, while the remaining UMP portion gets joined by a pyrophosphate

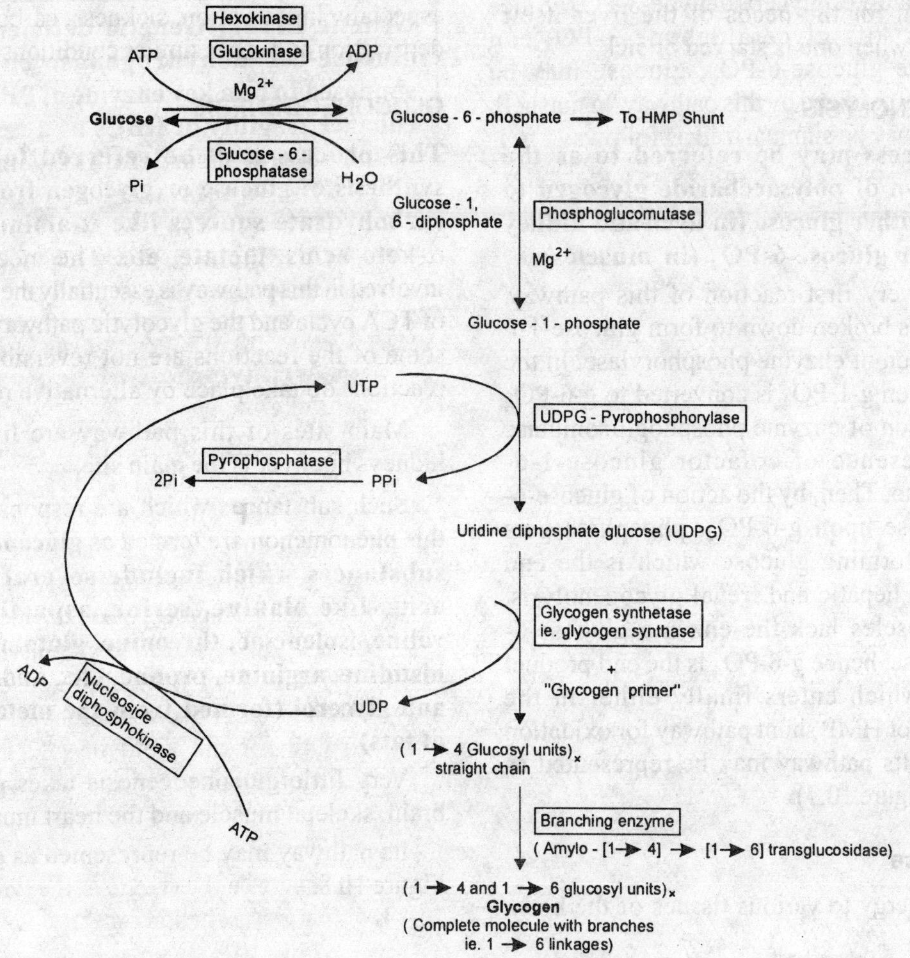

Figure 10.6 : Pathway of Glycogenesis

bridge to glucose-1-phosphate to form UDP-glucose.

The next reaction is catalysed by the enzyme glycogen synthetase, in this reaction, the C_1 of the activated glucose of UDPG forms a glycosidic bond with the C_4 of a terminal glucose residue of glycogen, liberating UDP with the formation of unnatural glycogen i.e., straight chain; a pre-existing glycogen or "primer" must be present to initiate this reaction. Afterwards, by the action of branching enzyme natural glycogen molecule bearing 1 → 4 and 1 → 6 linkages gets formed. Its pathway may be represented as in Figure 10.6.

Importance of Glycogenesis

Significance of this pathway lies in the fact that it acts as a source of energy (in the form of sugar), both for the blood that nourishes other

> ***Glycogen*** in fact, is a reservoir of energy. After a heavy intake of carbohydrates, as much as 1/10th of the liver mass may consist of this storage form of glucose, whereas in starvation or during illness when there is loss of appetite, the **glycogen reserve** may be almost depleted in order to meet out the energy requirements of the body.

tissues and for the needs of the liver itself especially when one is starved or sick.

GLYCOGENOLYSIS

This process may be referred to as the breakdown of polysaccharide glycogen to produce either glucose (in liver and kidney tissues) or glucose-6-PO_4 (in muscles).

In the very first reaction of this pathway, glycogen is broken down to form glucose-1-P by the action of enzyme phosphorylase. In the next reaction g-1-PO_4 is converted to g-6-PO_4 by the action of enzyme phosphoglucomutase in the presence of cofactor glucose-1-6-diphosphate. Then, by the action of glucose-6-phosphatase upon g-6-PO_4, phosphate gets liberated forming glucose which is the end product of hepatic and renal glycogenolysis. Since, muscles lack the enzyme glucose-6-phosphatase, hence g-6-PO_4 is the end product in them which enters finally either in the glycolysis or HMP shunt pathway for oxidation purposes. Its pathway may be represented as follows (Figure 10.7):

Importance

It gives energy to various tissues of the body, especially in starvation, sickness, carbohydrate deprivation and other similar conditions.

GLUCONEOGENESIS

This process may be referred to as the synthesis of glucose or glycogen from non-carbohydrate sources like α-amino acids, α-keto acids, lactate, etc. The mechanism involved in this pathway is essentially the reversal of TCA cycle and the glycolytic pathway. Since, some of the reactions are not reversible, such reactions do take place by alternative routes.

Main sites of this pathway are liver and kidneys but liver is the main site.

Such substances which are responsible for this phenomenon are termed as **gluconeogenic substances which include several amino acids like alanine, serine, aspartic acid, valine, isoleucine, threonine, glutamic acid, histidine, arginine, proline, etc., and lactate and glycerol (formed from the metabolism of fats).**

Very little gluconeogenesis takes place in brain, skeletal muscle and the heart muscle.

Its pathway may be represented as given in Figure 10.8.

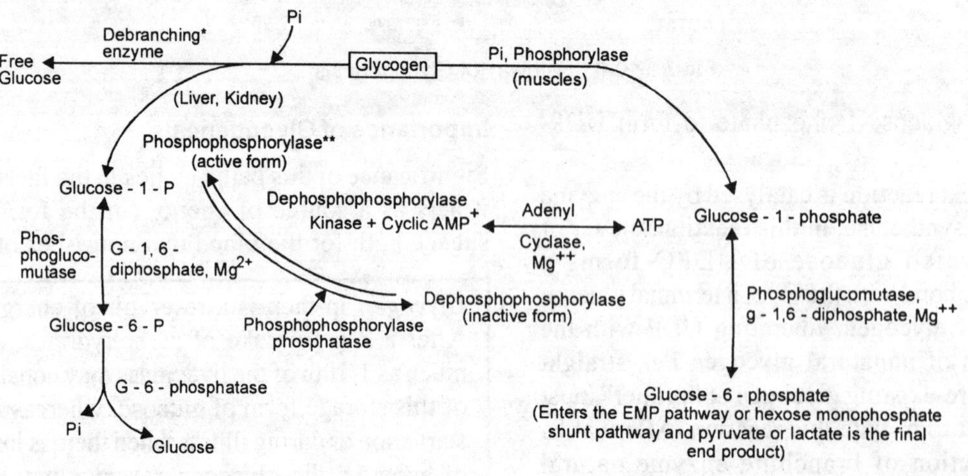

Figure 10.7 : Pathway of Glycogenolysis

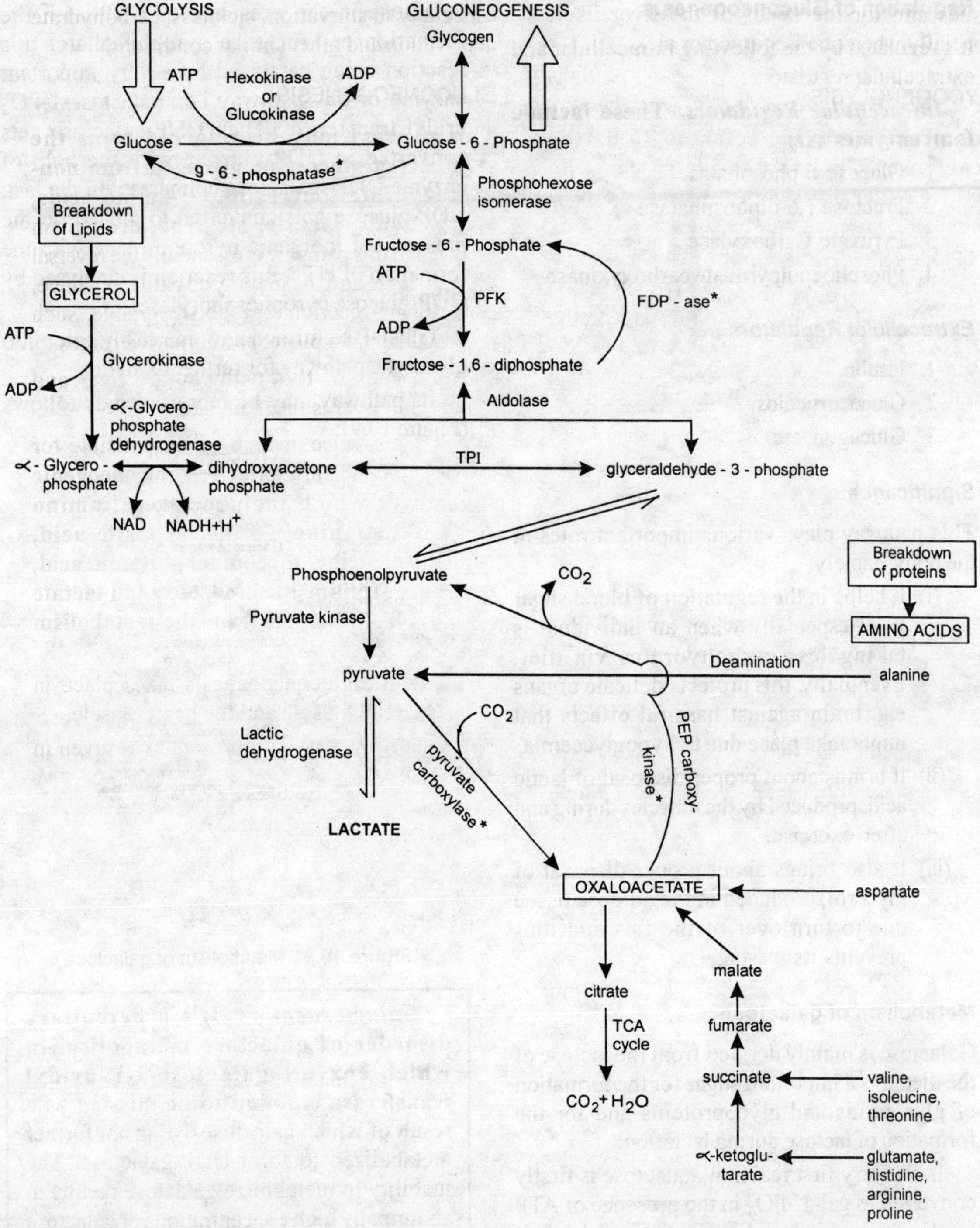

Fig. 10.8 : Pathway of gluconeogenesis showing the synthesis of glucose from (a) lactate (b) gluconeogenic amino acids and (c) glycerol

Regulation of Gluconeogenesis

It's regulated by the following intracellular and extracellular regulators :

***Intracellular Regulators:* These include four enzymes viz:**

1. Glucose-6-phosphatase
2. Fructose 1,6-diphosphatase
3. Pyruvate Carboxylase
4. Phosphoenolpyruvate carboxykinase

Extracellular Regulators

1. Insulin
2. Glucocorticoids
3. Glucagon, etc.

Significance

This pathway plays various important roles in the body, namely:

(i) It helps in the regulation of blood sugar level especially when an individual is taking less carbohydrates via diet. Eventually, this protects delicate organs e.g. brain against harmful effects that might take place due to hypoglycaemia.

(ii) It brings about proper disposal of lactic acid, produced by the muscles during and after exercise.

(iii) It also brings about proper disposal of glycerol, produced in the adipose tissue due to turn over of the fats and thus prevents its wastage.

Metabolism of galactose

Galactose is mainly derived from the lactose of the diet. It is a important sugar for the formation of glycolipids and glycoproteins and for the formation of lactose during lactation.

In the very first reaction, galactose is firstly converted to gal-1 -PO_4 in the presence of ATP by the enzyme galactokinase. Now, gal-1-P is metabolized to a nucleotide derivative i.e., UDP-galactose in the presence of UTP with the formation of inorganic pyrophosphate; this reaction being catalysed by a very important enzyme of this pathway i.e., galactose-1-PO_4 uridyl transferase. Then UDP-galactose gets converted to UDP-glucose with the help of enzyme UDP- galactose epimerase. In the last, UDP-glucose gets converted to glu-1-P in the presence of inorganic pyrophosphate with the formation of UTP, this reaction is catalysed by UDP-glucose pyrophosphorylase.

Glu-1-P so formed now can easily enter into glycolytic pathway for further oxidation.

Its pathway may be represented as follows (Figure 10.9):

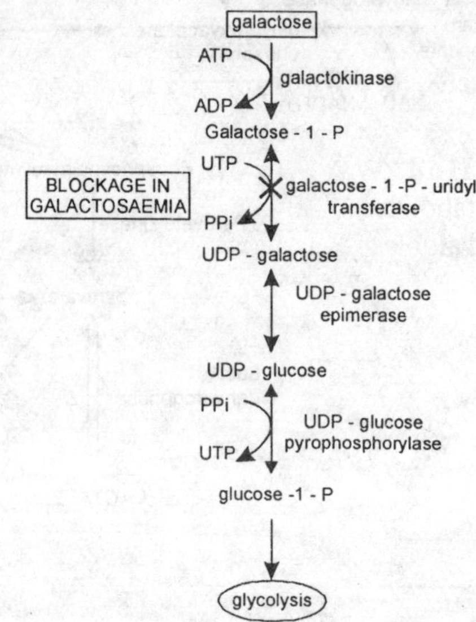

Figure 10.9 : Metabolism of galactose

> ***Galactosaemia* : It's a hereditary disorder of galactose metabolism in which enzyme galactose-1-P-uridyl transferase is found to be missing** as a result of which galactose-1-P is not further metabolized to form UDP-galactose. The inability to metabolize galactose results in abnormally high concentrations of galactose and gal-1-P in the blood and tissues.

Such infants are unable to digest milk. Treatment consists in giving them galactose (lactose) free diet i.e. milk should not be given to such infants.

Galactose-1-P accumulates in RBCs and other tissues causing damage particularly to the liver, brain and optic lens.

Fructose metabolism

There appear to be two ways by which fructose may be metabolized.

1st Way: Fructose may be phosphorylated by a hexokinase in the presence of ATP and Mg^{++} forming F-6-P which is an intermediate of glycolytic pathway.

$$\text{Fructose+ATP} \xrightarrow[Mg^{++}]{\text{hexokinase}} \text{fructose-6-P+ADP}$$

IInd Way: In this way, fructose is metabolized by two enzymes i.e. fructokinase and aldolase B as shown below (Figure 10.10) :

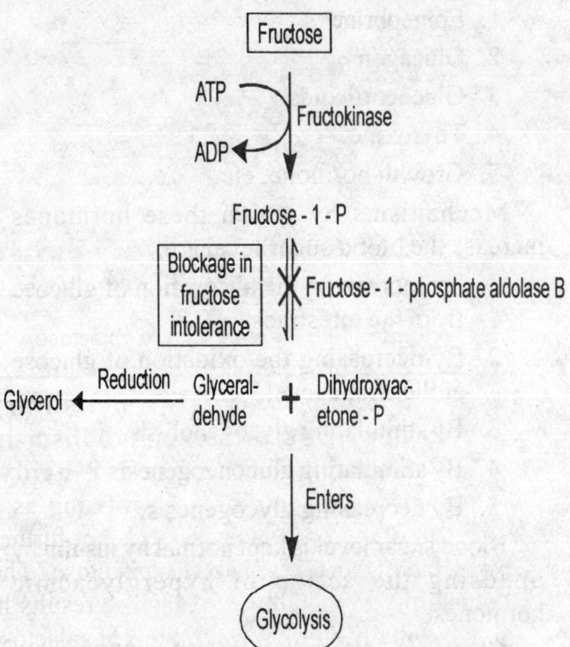

Figure 10.10 : Metabolism of fructose

> ***Hereditary disorder:*** There is a hereditary disorder of fructose metabolism which is known as ***fructose intolerance,*** the symptoms of which are lack of glucose in the blood stream and failure to gain weight which can result into *death.* In this disorder enzyme aldolase B is found to be missing. **Once diagnosed, the treatment is simple: replacement of the sucrose (cane sugar) in the diet by lactose or glucose.**

Regulation of blood sugar

Normal blood sugar level ranges between 80-120 mg%. Following a carbohydrate containing meal, concentration of sugar in blood may rise transiently to about 150 mg/dl (8 mM), which usually returns to normal within 2 hours.

The concentration of glucose in blood is the net resultant of the following two processes:

(a) Rate of glucose entrance into the blood stream.

(b) Rate of glucose removal from the blood stream.

Means by which sugar in added to the blood

1. By absorption from the intestines
2. By glycogenolysis (by breakdown of liver glycogen)
3. By gluconeogenesis

Means by which sugar is removed from the blood

1. Glycogenesis (conversion to liver glycogen and muscle glycogen)
2. In the synthesis of fats (i.e., triglycerides)
3. In the synthesis of glycoproteins, nucleic acids, lactose (during lactation), etc.
4. Loss in urine

A balance of above these two processes will keep the blood sugar within normal range.

Balance between the 'in' and 'out' of sugar may be summarised as follows:

Sources		Fate
Absorption →	Blood Sugar	→ Conversion in liver glycogen
Liver glycogen breakdown →		→ Conversion in muscle glycogen
		→ Synthesis of fats
Gluconeogenesis →		→ Synthesis of glycoproteins
		→ Synthesis of nucleic acids
		→ Synthesis of lactose(during lactation)
		→ Loss in urine

These two processes are influenced by a number of factors under physiological conditions.

The blood glucose level is most efficiently regulated by a mechanism in which liver, extrahepatic tissues and a battery of hormones play an important role.

1. ***Role of Liver:*** Liver, being the centre of all metabolic activities is mainly responsible for the regulation of blood glucose level. In liver, exist:

(i) the developed mechanism for uptake of glucose from the blood.

(ii) mechanism for the conversion of glucose to glycogen (glycogenesis).

(iii) mechanism for the release of glucose from glycogen (glycogenolysis), and

(iv) mechanism for the denovo synthesis of glucose from non-carbohydrate precursors (gluconeogenesis).

2. *Role of extrahepatic tissues*

(a) ***Role of muscles:*** Muscle glycogen does not contribute directly to the blood sugar due to the absence of the enzyme i.e. glucose-6-phosphatase. **Glycogenolysis in the muscles provides glucose to blood only through the formation of lactic acid which by Cori's cycle is converted to glucose in the liver.**

(b) ***Role of kidneys:*** These also exert a regulatory effect by reabsorbing glucose through the reabsorptive system of the renal tubules. When the blood glucose level rises above the renal threshold, **then the excess glucose is expelled through urine (glucosuria).**

3. ***Role of hormones:*** Several hormones play an important role in the homeostatic mechanism of blood sugar level. **Out of these, insulin is the only hypoglycaemic hormone whereas rest are hyperglycaemic** (tendency to raise blood sugar level) in nature.

Insulin: It plays an important role in the regulation of blood sugar level. It's secreted in the blood in response to hyperglycaemia. Insulin increases the transport of glucose across the cell membrances. It decreases the level of blood sugar by increasing the utilisation of glucose by glycolysis, by decreasing hepatic glycogenolysis and by increasing glycogenesis.

Hormones which raise the blood sugar level include:

1. Epinephrine
2. Glucagon
3. Glucocorticoids
4. Thyroxine
5. Growth hormone, etc.

Mechanisms by which these hormones increase the blood sugar level are:

1. By increasing the absorption of glucose from the intestines.
2. By decreasing the oxidation of glucose at the tissue level.
3. By stimulating glycogenolysis.
4. By stimulating gluconeogenesis
5. By decreasing glycogenesis.

Blood sugar level is kept normal by insulin by opposing the action of hyperglycaemic hormones.

Glucagon: It's a polypeptide of 29 amino acids. It's secreted by the α-cells of the pancreatic islets. It produces rapid hepatic glycogenolysis by activating hepatic phosphorylase. Glucagon has been regarded as part of a first line defence against hypoglycaemia.

Epinephrine (Adrenaline) : It stimulates the release of glucose from its store houses by activating the enzymes of the glycogenolytic pathway and it may be regarded as a hormone in the first line of defence against hypoglycaemia. Gluconeogenesis is also stimulated by the influence of adrenaline on the enzymes of this pathway.

Growth Hormone: It's hyperglycaemic character was observed for the first time by Houssay in Argentina and F. G. Young in London in 1924.

Adrenal Cortex hormones: Adrenal cortex secretes glucocorticoids which increase the rate of gluconeogenesis by increasing the rate of breakdown of proteins and also by increasing the activity of transaminases.

Glucocorticoids also inhibit glucose utilisation in extrahepatic tissues.

Thyroid hormones (T_3 and T_4) : These hormones are responsible for increasing gluconeogenesis, glycogenolysis and amino acids production from proteins and so tend to elevate blood sugar level. However, side by side, they also stimulate insulin secretion with resultant glucose uptake by peripheral tissues and promotion of lipid biosynthesis. Thus, overall, they have got little effect on blood sugar level.

Hypothyroidism has a tendency to elevate blood sugar level and is a cause of diabetes mellitus and aggravates it.

(Glycosuria) or carbohydrates in urine (melituria)

Appearance of unusually high amount of sugar in the urine is called glucosuria or glycosuria. Normally, 10-20 mg glucose may appear in urine per 100 ml. The most severe glucosuria is seen in severe diabetes mellitus, when the urine may contain as much as 10% or more glucose.

The excretion of detectable amounts of reducing sugar in the urine in called **Glucosuria. The general term for the presence of sugar of any kind in the urine is melituria or glycosuria whereas to be more precise and accurate, the presence of glucose alone is known as glucosuria.** Glucose is filtered by the glomeruli but is completely reabsorbed by the renal tubules. The reabsorption is effected by phosphorylation in the tubular cells. **The maximum rate of reabsorption of glucose by the tubules (TmG-Tubular maximum of glucose) is 350 mg/minute.** When the blood level of glucose is elevated, the filtrate contains more glucose that can be reabsorbed, whereas the excess passes into the urine and gives rise to glucosuria. **The renal threshold value for glucose is 160-180 mg%.**

There may be many reasons for the onset of glucosuria. Depending upon the cause, it has been classified into various groups:

1. Alimentary glucosuria
2. Diabetic glucosuria
3. Renal glucosuria
4. Adrenaline glucosuria

Except the diabetic glucosuria, rest others are temporary in nature in which the level of glucose in blood is found within normal range.

CHAPTER 11

METABOLISM OF LIPIDS

Blood lipids

The normal level of total serum cholesterol is from 150-200 mg/dl; normal level of HDL-cholesterol in serum is from 30-63 mg/dl (men) and 35-75 mg/dl (women); normal level of VLDL is upto 28 mg/dl, normal level of LDL-cholesterol in serum is upto 150 mg/dl; normal level of serum triglycerides is from 30-140 mg/dl; normal level of total lipids in serum is from 400 - 700 mg/dl; even then the intake of lipids via diet is very essential for various reasons. However, periodical checkup of various lipid fractions **(lipid profile)** in blood is also very essential and demand of the day especially in the society 40 plus in age because of the alarming rising trend in the incidence of cardiovascular disorders/ diseases.

In contrast to the blood glucose level, the normal fasting level of total blood lipids of about 500 mg/100 ml may be subject to much wide fluctuations (± 200 mg/100 ml) and will return much more slowly to baseline levels after a meal.

Since probably no absolute tissue demand for blood lipids exists, the consequences of lowered lipid levels are insignificant in comparison to the effects of hypoglycaemia. The pathology of the disorders in blood lipid metabolism tends to be related, rather, to excessive concentrations of lipids i.e., **hyperlipidaemia.**

Plasma lipoproteins

Virtually, all the phospholipids in liver or other

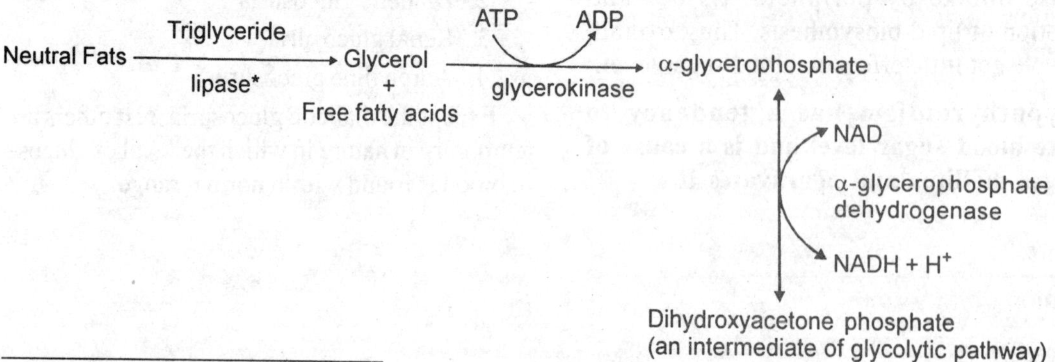

* *also known as lipoprotein lipase*

tissues exist in the membranes, with very few of them occurring in the form of solutions or micelles.

Lipids are water insoluble and are transported in the body in an aqueous medium in combination with various specific proteins. This results in lipid: protein complex called as lipoproteins, synthesis of which takes place in the liver.

Lipoproteins (phospholipid-carrier protein complex) are the important vehicles for the transfer of phospholipids.

Plasma lipoproteins occur in four major forms which are:

1. High or heavy density lipoproteins (HDL)
2. Low density lipoproteins (LDL)
3. Very low density lipoproteins (VLDL)
4. Chylomicrons.

Plasma lipoproteins always remain in dynamic state which are being continuously synthesized and degraded with rapid exchange of both lipid and protein among themselves. **Two enzymes namely, lecithin cholesterol acyl transferase (LCAT) and lipoprotein lipase (also called triglyceride lipase)** play a significant role in the catabolism of lipid fraction of lipoproteins.

Tangier Disease: An inability to carry normal amount of phospholipids and cholesterol in the blood is encountered in Tangier disease, which results from a congenital defect in the formation of a transport protein by the liver. A deficiency in the liver's capacity for the synthesis of albumin; which causes **analbuminemia**, leads to a decrease in the plasma's capacity to carry the fatty acids released from the fat depots.

Oxidation of fatty acids

The action of hormonally controlled lipase results in the hydrolysis of neutral fats to glycerol and free fatty acids. Glycerol enters the glycolytic pathway as shown below via the formation of glycerophosphate:

Fatty acids tightly bound with albumin are carried to various tissues for oxidation via blood.

Fatty acids oxidation takes place in mitochondria. Fatty acids are also oxidized to CO_2 and H_2O in the human body by the following three mechanisms:

(a) **β-oxidation**

(b) **α-oxidation,** and

(c) **ω-oxidation**

Out of the above, β-oxidation is the principal pathway, by which bulk of fatty acids gets oxidized liberating energy.

(a) β-*Oxidation Theory:* The term oxidation means that the oxidation takes place in the β-carbon of the fatty acid with the removal of two carbon atoms at a time from the carboxyl end of the molecule.

Fatty acids containing both the even number and the odd number of carbon atoms and as well as unsaturated fatty acids are oxidized by this theory. **Knoop** was the first who in 1904 invented this theory. In order to study the fate of fatty acids, he prepared a homologous series of phenyl fatty acid derivatives, which he fed to the animal; then he was able to isolate the phenyl labelled compounds in the urine. The simplest is benzoic acid, which is eliminated in the form of hippuric acid after combination with glycine.

C_6H_5-CO-OH (benzoic acid) + CH_2-COOH / H-N-H (glycine) ⟶ C_6H_5-CO-NH-CH_2-COOH (hippuric acid) (1)

C_6H_5-CH_2-CO-OH (phenylacetic acid) + CH_2-COOH / H-N-H (glycine) ⟶ C_6H_5-CH_2-CO-NH-CH_2-COOH (phenylaceturic acid) (2)

However, the next higher derivative i.e. phenylacetic acid is eliminated as the corresponding glycine derivative i.e., phenylaceturic acid.

With higher fatty acids, the products isolated were either hippuric acid (1) or phenylaceturic acid (2) for example,

$C_6H_5.CH_2\ CH_2\ COOH$ yields (1)
$C_6H_5.CH_2.\ CH_2.\ CH_2.\ COOH$ yields (2)
$C_6H_5.CH_2.\ CH_2.\ CH_2.\ CH_2.COOH$ yields (1)
$C_6H_5.CH_2.CH_2.CH_2.CH_2.CH_2.COOH$ yields (2)
etc.

From the results, he was able to draw the conclusion that oxidation of fatty acids occurred in such a way that at each stage in the degradation process there was a loss of two carbon atoms because of the oxidation at the β carbon atom, for example (Figure 11.1).

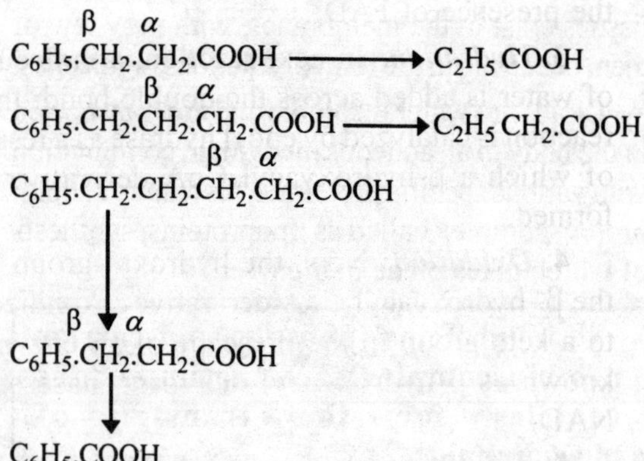

Mechanism of β-Oxidation of fatty acids

Five reactions are involved in the β-oxidation process as described below. All these reactions take place in the mitochondria of the cell.

1. ***Activation:*** The very first reaction consists in the formation of an acyl coenzyme-A derivative from the free fatty acid; this reaction is catalysed by a **thiokinase** which required the presence of ATP and CoA (Figure 11.1).

2. ***Desaturation*** : Once the fatty acid has been activated, it can now be dehydrogenated in the α, β position by acyl dehydrogenase in

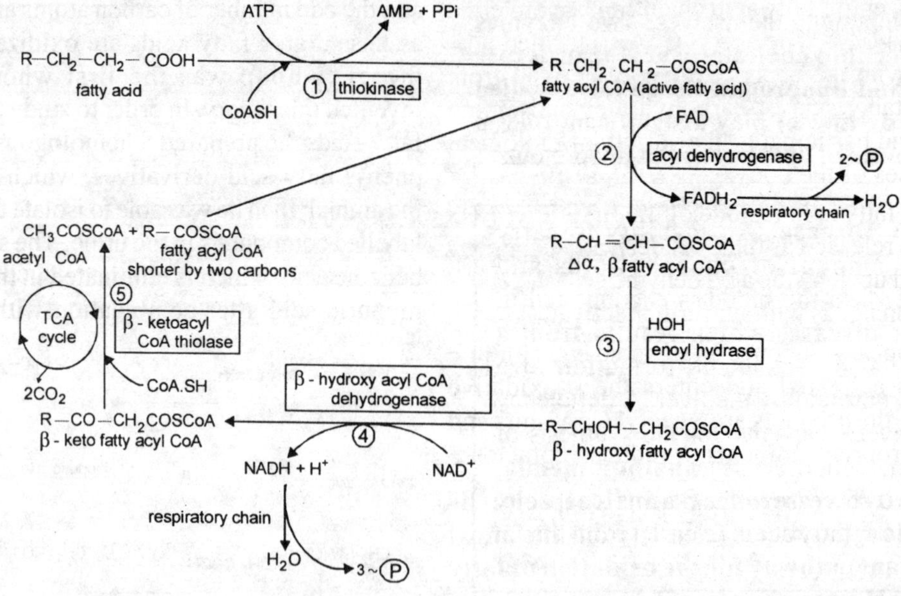

Figure 11.1 : Schematic diagram of β–oxidation of fatty acids (removal of one acetyl CoA unit from a fatty acid may be seen). Also known as ***Fatty Acid Cycle*** . [$FADH_2$ and $NADH_2$, when oxidized by the mitochondrial electron transport chain, generate two and three moles of ATP per mole of $FADH_2$ and $NADH_2$ respectively].

the presence of FAD.

3. *Hydration:* In next reaction, a molecule of water is added across the double bond; this reaction is catalyzed by enoyl hydrase as a result of which a β-hydroxyacyl CoA derivative is formed.

4. *Oxidation:* Now, the hydroxyl group of the β–hydroxyacyl CoA derivative is oxidized to a keto group in the presence of an enzyme known as β-hydroxyacyl dehydrogenase and NAD.

5. *Thiolytic cleavage:* The final step in the process of β-oxidation is the cleavage of the β-keto derivative by a molecule of coenzyme in the presence of enzyme β-ketoacyl CoA thiolase.

The products of the reactions are a molecule of acetyl CoA and a molecule of an activated fatty acid which is two carbon shorter than the fatty acid at the start. Now, the activated fatty acid can be further degraded by repetitions of the process, starting at the second reaction; reaction no. 1 i.e. activation step is not necessary at all. By the successive repetitions of the process, entire fatty acid chain can be converted to acetyl CoA. The acetyl CoA so formed now mixes with the acetyl CoA pool derived from the metabolisms of carbohydrates and amino acids and participates in a variety of biological processes of the body.

The fatty acid residue of the first turn of the cycle is released as the CoA derivative and may be acted upon by the acyl dehydrogenase system (reaction no. 2) without further activation.

It appears that once a fatty acid e.g. palmitic acid, is activated and enters the β-oxidative system, the products are 8 acetyl CoA units and the appropriate amounts of reduced cofactors.

(b) *α-Oxidation:* Quantitatively, β-oxidation has been found to be the most important pathway for the oxidation of fatty acids. However, α-oxidation, i.e. the removal of one carbon at a time from the carboxyl end of the molecule, has been found to occur in the brain tissue. It does not require CoA intermediates and does not generate high-energy phosphates.

(c) *Omega Oxidation (ω-Oxidation)* : It is normally a very minor pathway and takes place with the help of hydroxylase enzymes. The CH_3 group is converted to a CH_2OH group that subsequently is oxidized to-COOH, thus forming a dicarboxylic acid. This dicarboxylic acid is then β-oxidized usually to adipic (C_6) and suberic (C_8) acids, which are then excreted through urine.

Generation of ATP by the complete oxidation (β-oxidation +TCA cycle) of Stearic acid (18 carbon fatty acid)

The schematic diagram of fatty acid oxidation sequence in brief is as shown in Figure 11.2.

The net overall reaction involved in degrading a fatty acid by two carbons can be represented as follows:

By repetition of these reactions, the entire fatty acid molecule gets converted into acetyl CoA, which may enter the TCA cycle and be oxidized to CO_2 and H_2O liberating many molecules of ATP for energy purposes.

Steps	Moles of ATP
1. Stearate + ATP + CoASH ↓ Stearyl~SCoA	- 1
2. Stearyl~SCoA → 9 Acetyl-SCoA (a) 8 $FADH_2$ → 8 FAD (8 x 2=16) (b) 8 NADH → 8 NAD^+ (8 x 3=24)	+ 40
3. 9 Acetyl~SCoA + 18 O_2 (9 x 12=108) ↓ 18 CO_2 + 9 H_2O + 9 CoASH	+ 108
	147

Overall reaction

$$\underset{\text{Stearic acid}}{C_{17}H_{35}COOH} + 18O_2 + 147\ ADP + 147\ Pi \downarrow 18CO_2 + 18H_2O + 147\ ATP$$

Depending upon the needs of the organism for energy, **the remaining amounts of acetyl~SCoA may be diverted for the synthesis of important substances like cholesterol, acetylcholine, etc.**

As shown in figure 11.2 the pathway is used a total of 8 times to convert an 18-carbon fatty acid (e.g., stearic acid) to 9 moles of acetyl S~CoA. Upon oxidation of the acetyl groups, a total of 147 molecules of ATP can be generated in the mitochondria, which contain all enzymes required for the TCA cycle, oxidative phosphorylation and electron transfer system as well as for β–oxidation. The steps can be

$$CH_3(CH_2CH_2)_n - COOH + ATP + (n + 1)\ CoASH + nNAD^+ + nFAD + nH_2O$$

$$\downarrow$$

$$\left.\begin{matrix} (ADP + Pi) \\ (n + 1)\ CH_3\overset{\overset{O}{||}}{C} \sim SCoA + (AMP + PPi) \end{matrix}\right\} + n\,NADH + nH^+ + nFADH_2$$

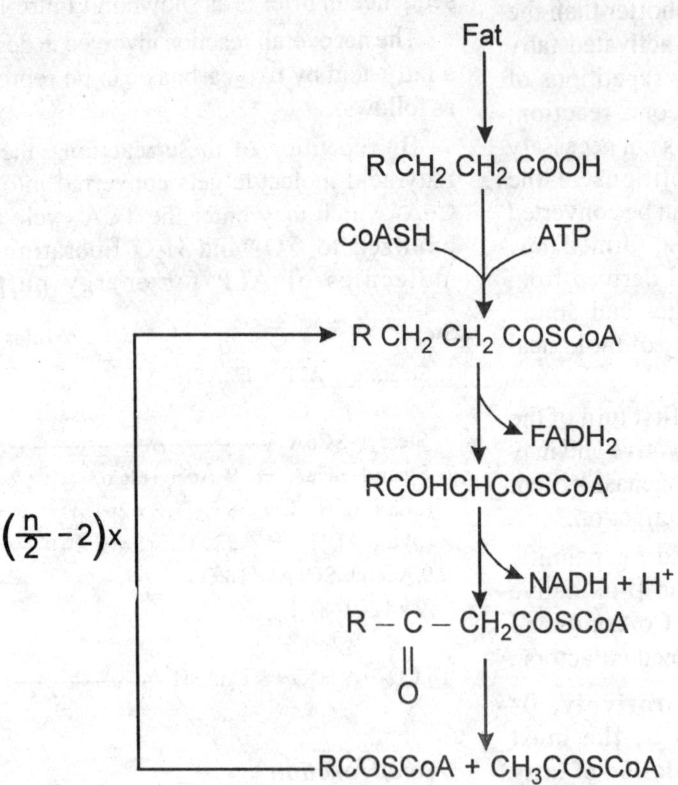

Fig. 11.2 : Fatty acid oxidation sequence. The pathway is used (n/2-1) times for each fatty acid. For instance, an 18 carbon chain would go through the cycle 8 times, i.e., once through and 7 repeats-to yield the nine two - carbon fragments as acetyl CoA.

summarised as follows:

Since the total free energy decrease is nearly 2600 kcal per mole, the "efficiency" of conversion of energy to ATP is :

$$\frac{147 \times 8}{2600} \times 100 = 45\%$$

Generation of ATP by the complete oxidation(β-Oxidation + TCA cycle) of palmitic acid (16-carbon fatty acid) :

If an even numbered fatty acid is taken into consideration e.g. palmitic acid (C_{16}), it gets split completely into 8 acetyl units in 7 rounds. On completion of each round, one mole of $FADH_2$ and mole of NADH are produced which are equivalent to 2+3=5 moles of ATP. In seven cycles (7 rounds), therefore, 35 moles of ATP are synthesized.

Each acetyl unit is oxidized by Krebs cycle to CO_2 and H_2O generating 12 moles of ATP. Thus, the total number of ATP generated during oxidation of 8 moles of acetyl coenzyme A would be 12x8=96. In total, 35+96=131 moles of ATP are generated per mole of palmitic acid oxidized. Since, the initial activation reaction requires the consumption of 2 moles of ATP {Fig 13.4 (a)}, therefore, the net gain of ATP per mole of palmitic acid oxidized would be 131-2 = 129. The steps of palmitic acid ($C_{15}H_{31}$ COOH) oxidation can be summarised as follows:

Energetics of palmitic acid oxidation :

Mechanism (steps)	ATP yield
I. β- oxidation 7 cycles	
7 $FADH_2$ (oxidized by electron transport chain (ETC), each $FADH_2$ yields 2 ATP	: 14
7 NADH (oxidized by ETC, each NADH liberates 3 ATP	: 21
II. From 8 acetyl CoA	
Oxidized by citric acid cycle, each acetyl CoA generates 12 ATP	: 96
Total energy from one molecule of palmitoyl CoA	: 131
Energy utilized for activation (formation of palmitoyl CoA)	: – 2
Net yield of oxidation of one molecule of palmitate	: 129

The ultimate aim of fatty acid oxidation is to generate energy. The energy obtained from the complete oxidation of palmitic acid (16 carbon) is as mentioned above.

The standard free energy of palmitate = 2,340 Cal. The energy yield by its oxidation is 129 ATP (129x7.3 Cal) = 940 Cal.

The efficiency of energy conservation by fatty acid oxidation

$$= \frac{940}{2,340} \times 100 = 40\%$$

Oxidation of fatty acids with an odd number of carbon atoms

In natural fats, the straight-chain, even-carbon

$$CH_3\,CH_2.COOH \xrightarrow[+CoA.SH]{ATP \quad AMP+PPi} CH_3.CH_2.CO.SCoA$$

propionic acid → propionyl CoA

$$CH_3CH_2.CO.SCoA \xrightarrow[+\,CO_2,\ biotin]{ATP \quad ADP+Pi} CH_3.CH\,(COOH).CO.SCoA$$

methyl malonyl CoA

$$CH_3.\,CH\,(COOH).\,CO.SCoA \xrightarrow{B_{12}\ Coenzyme} HOOC.\,CH_2.\,CH_2.CO.SCoA$$

succinyl CoA

fatty acids are found in abundance but they also contain odd carbon and branched chain fatty acids in minor quantity. The odd-carbon fatty acids e.g. propionic acid is oxidized as follows:

Succinyl CoA, so formed can now be oxidized via succinic acid and the TCA cycle to CO_2 and H_2O.

Heart mitochondria cannot oxidize propionyl CoA. The involvement of biotin in the CO_2 fixation reaction is a clear example of the function of this vitamin as a conenzyme.

Biosynthesis of cholesterol

Synthesis of cholesterol takes place in almost all the tissues of the body, liver being the most active site. Less important sites serially include skin, adrenal glands, gonads, adipose tissue, muscles, aorta, adult brain etc.

Acetate is the principal precursor of cholesterol biosynthesis. Its synthesis takes place as shown below (Fig. 11.3) :

1. *Activation of acetate to acetyl CoA* : This is brought about by a thiokinase in the presence of ATP and CoA with the formation of acetyl CoA.
2. *Condensation of two acetyl CoA to acetoacetyl CoA* : This is brought about by enzyme thiolase.
3. *Formation of β-hydroxy-β-methylglutaryl CoA* : Acetoacetyl CoA further condenses with another molecule of acetyl CoA in the presence of HMG CoA synthetase forming β-hydroxy-β-methylglutaryl CoA.
4. *Formation of mevalonic acid:* Now, β-hydroxy β-methylglutaryl CoA is reduced to mevalonic acid; the reaction is catalysed by the enzyme HMG-CoA reductase in the presence of reduced NADP.

Side-by-side, β-OH- β-methylglutaryl CoA (HMG—CoA) may also give rise to ketone bodies.

5. *Phosphorylation of mevalonic acid:* Mevalonic acid is phosphorylated to 5-phosphomevalonic acid in the presence of ATP and Mg^{++} ions. Reaction is catalysed by mevalonate kinase.

   5-phosphomevalonic acid is further phosphorylated to form 5-diphosphomevalonic acid in the presence of ATP and Mg^{2+}; the reaction is catalysed by the enzyme phosphomevalonate kinase.
6. Diphosphomevalonate loses CO_2 and H_2O to form isopentenyl pyrophosphate in the presence of an enzyme decarboxylase.
7. Isopentenyl pyrophosphate is now isomerized by a liver enzyme to form 3,3-dimethylallyl pyrophosphate which later on condenses with another molecule of isopentenyl-PP to form geranyl pyrophosphate.
8. Now, a molecule of isopentenyl-PP (C_5) reacts with geranyl-PP (C_{10}) to give rise to farnesyl pyrophosphate (C_{15}).
9. Now, in the presence of squalene synthetase reduced pyridine nucleotide and Mg^{++}, Mn^{++}, or Co^{++}, two moles of farnesyl-PP condense to form squalene.
10. Squalene in the presence of oxydocyclase I and a pyridine nucleotide undergoes cyclization process forming a steroid like structure called lanosterol (Figure 11.3).
11. Now, lanosterol is finally converted to cholesterol through a number of intermediates.

In this way, molecule of cholesterol is synthesized. Of the 27 carbon of cholesterol molecule, 15 arise from the methyl and 12 from the carboxyl of acetate. The first phases of synthesis involve activation of intermediates through union with CoASH, whereas the later stages of synthesis involve participation of phosphates.

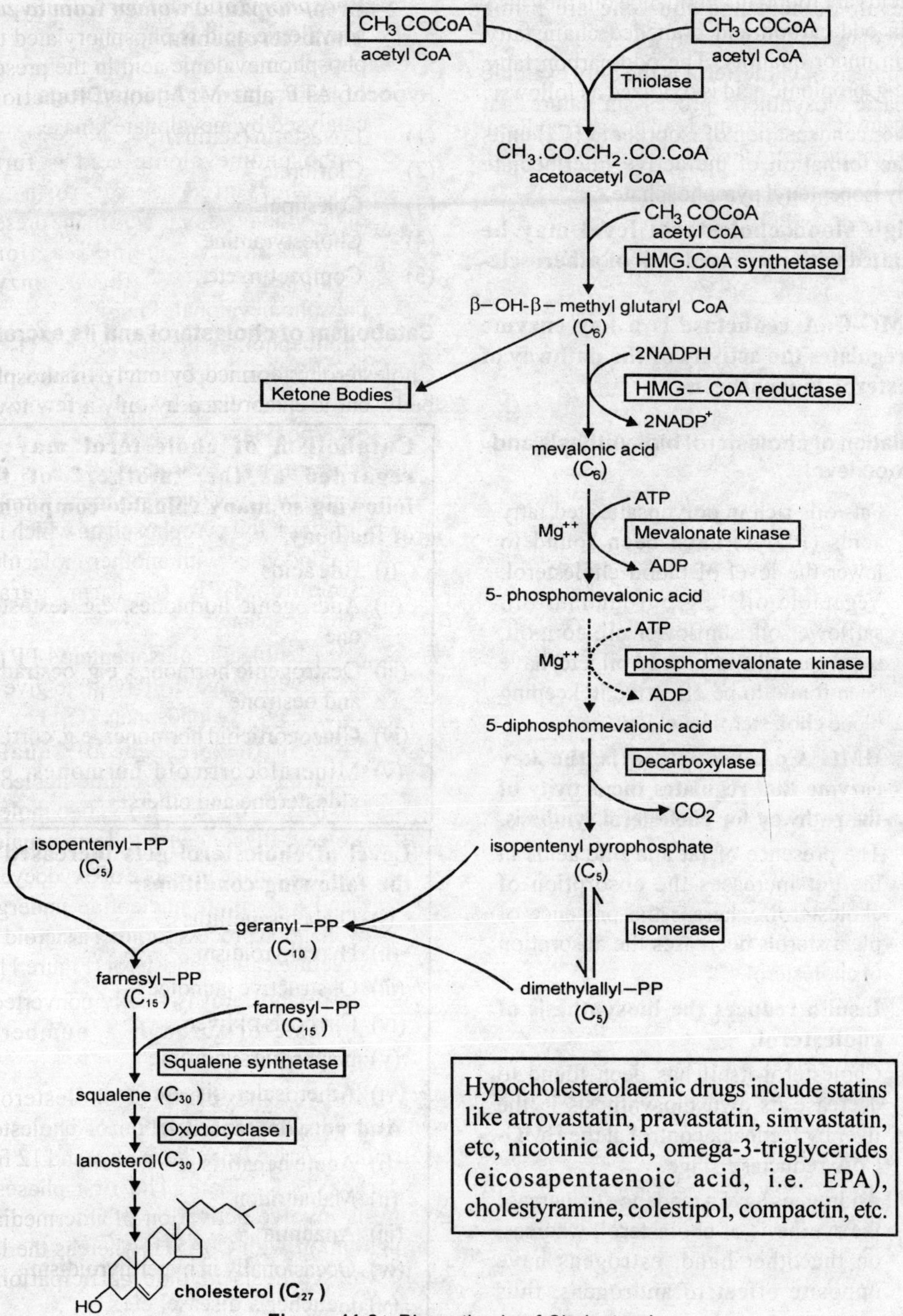

Figure 11.3 : Biosynthesis of Cholesterol

Mevalonic acid and squalene are prime intermediates in this pathway.

Synthesis of cholesterol is the only example of a basic biosynthetic process in nature that involves condensation of isoprenoid (C_5) units and the formation of the active intermediate namely isopentenyl pyrophosphate.

High blood cholesterol level may be associated with increased risk of atherosclerosis.

HMG-CoA reductase is a key enzyme that regulates the activity of the pathway of cholesterol biosynthesis.

Regulation of cholesterol biosynthesis and its blood level

1. Fats/oils rich in polyunsaturated fatty acids (PUFA) have been found to lower the level of blood cholesterol. Vegetable oils e.g., groundnut oil, safflower oil, sunflower oil, corn oil, soyabean oil and linseed oil, etc. have been found to be effective in keeping blood cholesterol level low.
2. **HMG CoA reductase is the key enzyme that regulates the activity of the pathway for cholesterol synthesis.**
3. The presence of fat and bile acids in the gut increases the absorption of cholesterol, whereas the presence of plant sterols decreases the absorption of cholesterol.
4. **Insulin reduces the biosynthesis of cholesterol.**
5. Cholesterol itself has been found to decrease its own biosynthesis in the liver by feedback control at the HMG-CoA reductase stage.
6. Androgens have a tendency to increase the synthesis of cholesterol, whereas, on the other hand, estrogens have opposite effect to androgens, thus **estrogens also protect the premenopausal women from hypercholesterolaemia.**

Hypocholesterolaemic Agents/Drugs

(1) Lovastatin (statins)
(2) Clofibrate
(3) Colestipol
(4) Cholestyramine
(5) Compactin, etc.

Catabolism of cholesterol and its excretion

Cholesterol is formed by many tissues of the body, but is catabolized by only a few tissues.

Catabolism of cholesterol may be regarded as the "mother" of the following so many valuable compounds of the body.

(i) Bile acids
(ii) Androgenic hormones, e.g. testosterone
(iii) Oestrogenic hormones, e.g. oestradiol and oestrone
(iv) Glucocorticoid hormones, e.g. cortisol
(v) Mineralocorticoid hormones, e.g. aldosterone and others.

Level of cholesterol gets increased in the following conditions:

(i) Diabetes mellitus
(ii) Hypothyroidism
(iii) Obstructive jaundice
(iv) Cirrhosis of liver
(v) Nephrotic syndrome
(vi) Atherosclerosis, etc.

And gets decreased in :

(i) Acute hepatitis
(ii) Malnutrition
(iii) Anaemia
(iv) Occasionally in hyperthyroidism
(v) Gaucher's disease, etc.

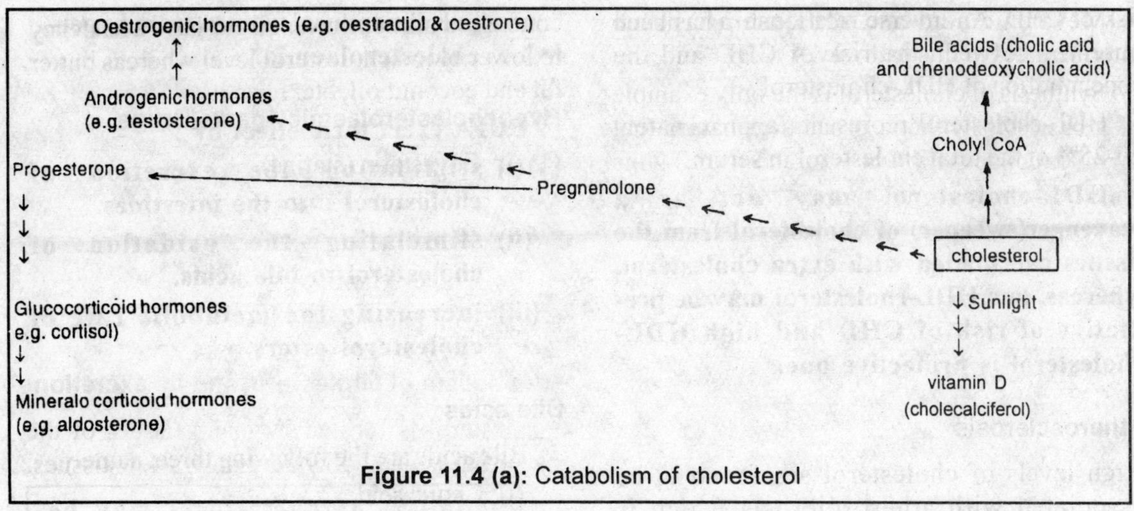

Figure 11.4 (a): Catabolism of cholesterol

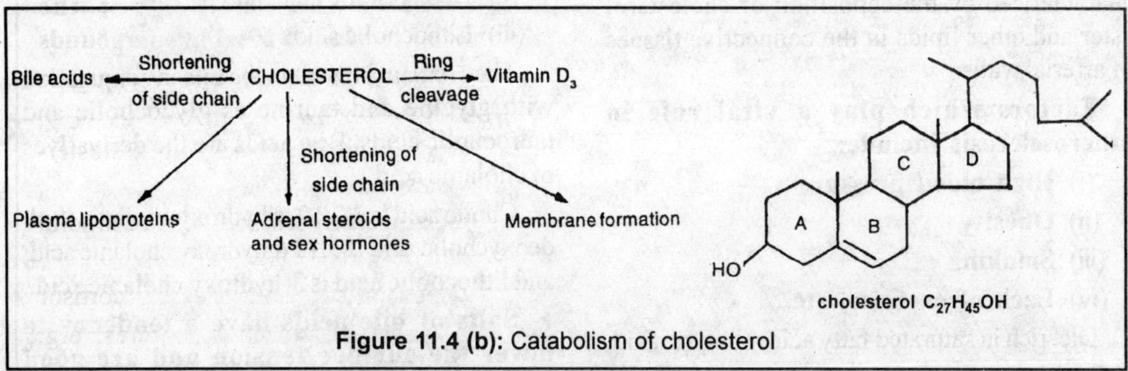

Figure 11.4 (b): Catabolism of cholesterol

The main catabolic fate of cholesterol is its oxidation to cholanic acids (cholic acids) and side by side, the main route of excretion is into the GI (gastrointestinal) tract via bile or through mucosal cells. Besides, gonads and the adrenals also utilize cholesterol for the biosynthesis of hormones (Figures 11.4 a & b).

The formation of bile acids from cholesterol in the liver represents the most important fate of cholesterol. Nearly, 80-90% of body's cholesterol is ultimately metabolized to bile acids for example cholic acid and chenodeoxycholic acid.

Cholesterol is transported in the blood as lipoproteins. The highest proportion of cholesterol is found in the low density lipoprotein fraction, **i.e. β-lipoprotein fraction (LDL).**

Cholesterol cannot be catabolised to straight chain molecule or to acetyl CoA, therefore, can't be used as a source of energy by the cells.

The combined risk factors of coronary heart disease (CHD) can be determined following the estimations of serum cholesterol and HDL-cholesterol. The ratio of cholesterol to HDL-cholesterol has predictive value in determining the risk of CHD more accurately. For normal males, the ratio of 5: 1 and for normal females, the ratio of 4.5: 1 are considered as average risk. Lower ratios significantly reduce the risk, whereas ratios 9.5: 1 and 7:1 for males and females respectively, are believed to double the risk of CHD. An inverse relationship has been observed between the risk of CHD and the concentration of HDL-cholesterol.

HDL-cholesterol represents approximately 20-25% of the total cholesterol in serum.

HDL-cholesterol may act as a scavenger(sweeper) of cholesterol from the tissues overloaded with extra cholesterol, whereas, low HDL-cholesterol may be predictive of risk of CHD and high HDL-cholesterol is protective one.

Atherosclerosis

High levels of cholesterol are found to be associated with atherosclerosis which is characterized by the deposition of cholesterol ester and other lipids in the connective tissues of arterial walls.

Factors which play a vital role in atherosclerosis include:

(i) **High blood pressure**
(ii) **Obesity**
(iii) **Smoking**
(iv) **Lack of exercise, etc.**

Diet rich in saturated fatty acids (butyric acid, caproic acid, caprylic acid, palmitic acid, stearic acid, etc.) increases the plasma cholesterol concentration, whereas diet rich in polyunsaturated fatty acids (PUFA) such as linoleic acid, linolenic acid and arachidonic acid decreases the plasma cholesterol concentration.

Corn oil, linseed oil, soyabean oil, peanut oil, cottonseed oil, sunflower oil etc. have a tendency to lower blood cholesterol level whereas butter fat and coconut oil, etc. raise it.

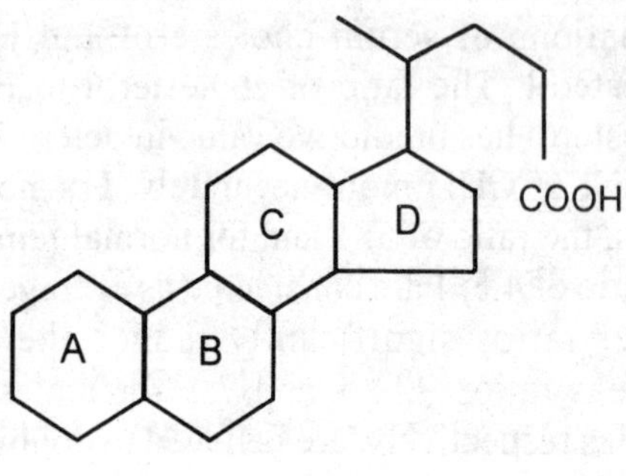

PUFA exert their effect by :

(i) **stimulating the excretion of cholesterol into the intestines.**
(ii) **stimulating the oxidation of cholesterol to bile acids.**
(iii) **increasing the metabolic rate of cholesterol esters.**

Bile acids

Bile acids are the following three, namely:

(i) Cholic acid
(ii) Deoxycholic acid, and
(iii) Lithocholic acid.

They remain present in the bile in conjugation with glycine and taurine as glycocholic and taurocholic acids. Bile acids are the derivatives of cholanic acid.

Cholic acid is 3,7,12 trihydroxy cholanic acid; deoxycholic acid is 3,12 dihydroxy cholanic acid; and lithocholic acid is 3-hydroxy cholanic acid.

Salts of bile acids have a tendency to lower the surface tension and are good emulsifying agents and hence play an important role in the absorption of fats from the intestines.

Ketone bodies (acetone bodies)

Ketone bodies are the three, namely:

(i) acetoacetic acid
(ii) β-hydroxybutyric acid, and
(iii) acetone

The principal ketone body is acetoacetic acid which gives rise to β-hydroxybutyric acid by reduction. and acetone by decarboxylation.

Ketone bodies are acidic in nature and when produced in excess over long period, as happens in diabetes mellitus, causes

$$CH_3COCH_2COOH \text{ (acetoacetic acid)} \xrightarrow[NAD^+]{\text{dehydrogenation}} CH_3-CH(OH)-CH_2COOH \text{ (β-hydroxybutyric acid)}$$

$$CH_3COCH_2COOH \text{ (acetoacetic acid)} \xrightarrow[-CO_2]{\text{decarboxylation}} CH_3COCH_3 \text{ (acetone)}$$

ketoacidosis which is ultimately fatal.

Ketone bodies are the intermediate breakdown products of fatty acid metabolism. Under normal conditions, fatty acids are oxidized to CO_2; these intermediates do not appear to any great extent either in the blood or urine.

Ketosis

Significant accumulation of ketone bodies in the blood (ketonaemia) and their excretion in urine (ketonuria) give rise to a condition known as **ketosis.**

Normal level of ketone bodies in blood is upto 3 mg per 100 ml and upto 50 mg in urine per day.

Under certain metabolic conditions such as starvation, high fat diet, severe diabetes mellitus, more fat is metabolized for energy purposes giving rise to increased formation of ketone bodies.

Increased fatty acid oxidation is a characteristic of starvation and diabetes mellitus, leading to the production of ketone bodies by the liver.

Under normal metabolic conditions, most of the acetyl CoA formed from the oxidation of fatty acids, pyruvate and other sources get condensed with oxaloacetic acid and oxidized through the TCA cycle. However, in circumstances when the metabolism of carbohydrate gets impaired or operating at a low level, such as in the diabetes mellitus, starvation, or prolonged living on a low carbohydrate diet, the fate of acetyl CoA gets altered for two reasons.

1. the oxaloacetate available to condense with acetyl CoA is in limited supply, and
2. a much greater proportion of the body's energy needs is being supplied by the oxidation of fatty acids, leading to the production of acetyl CoA in greater than normal amounts.

Because of this combination circumstances (large amount of acetyl CoA and small amounts of oxaloacetate), the metabolism of acetyl CoA instead of a normal route takes place through a different route in which the condensation of two molecules of acetyl CoA to form acetoacetyl CoA takes place; this reaction is catalysed by β-ketothiolase in which one molecule of coenzyme A gets liberated. Next reaction is catalysed by the enzyme HMG CoA synthetase forming β - hydroxy - β - methyl glutaryl CoA in which again one molecule of coenzyme A is liberated. Further reaction is catalysed by the enzyme HMG CoA lyase forming acetoacetic acid (figure 10.5) in which one molecule of acetyl coenzyme A is liberated. The final reaction takes place forming acetone and β-hydroxybutyric acid; first of all in a spontaneous reaction, acetoacetic acid gets decarboxylated forming **acetone** and side by side acetoacetic acid gets also dehydrogenated in the presence of $NADH_2$ and β-hydroxybutyrate dehydrogenase forming **β-hydroxybutyric acid (Figure 11.5).**

The three compounds, namely acetone, acetoacetic acid and β-hydroxybutyric acid are called as 'ketone bodies' or 'acetone bodies' and the process of their formation is known as 'ketogenesis'.

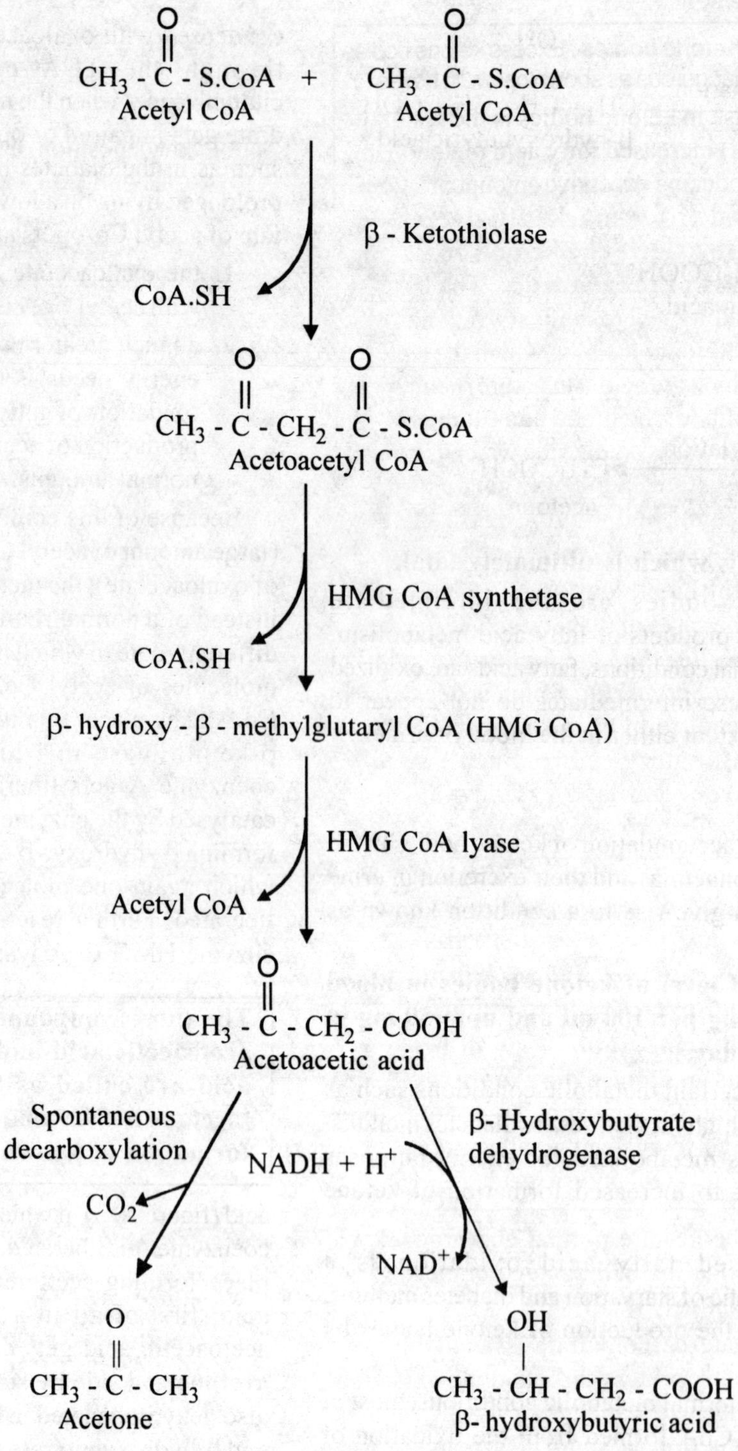

Figure 11.5 : Formation (synthesis) of Ketone bodies (Ketogenesis)

Danger of Ketone bodies : Excess ketone bodies are very dangerous as shown below 'in boxes':

An increase in ketone bodies is the result of both i.e. (i) increased fatty acid metabolism in liver producing excessive amount of ketone bodies and (ii) **a markedly decreased capacity to oxidize the ketone bodies by the muscles of the diabetics.** The ketone bodies lead to severe acidosis, a condition called as **'ketoacidosis'** in which the ketone bodies (which are acidic in nature) neutralize the alkalinity of the blood and tilt the pH of the blood towards acidic side which is a very dangerous state. **This dangerous state leads to coma and finally death ensues within 4-14 days.**

The typical breathing (smell of acetone) found in the cases of diabetic coma i.e. cases of ***uncontrolled diabetes mellitus*** is known as ***Kussmaul breathing*** which is due to the effect of enol form of the acetoacetic acid on the respiratory centre. Such patients exhibit hyperventilation i.e. air-hunger, meaning by they are always hungry of air.

Normal level of ketone bodies in blood is upto 3 mg per 100 ml. In diabetes mellitus as much as 300 to 400 mg per 100 ml and over has been reported.

In normal urine upto 50 mg of acetone bodies (as acetone) **may be excreted daily**, whereas in diabetics **10 to 50 g per litre** may be found, the greater proportion being that of β-OH butyric acid.

Ketone bodies are normal end products of fatty acid oxidation in the liver, but the amount formed is relatively small.

If adequate carbohydrate is available, the liver apparently prefers carbohydrate oxidation as a source of energy, as a result of which ketone bodies production is small. Carbohydrate is therefore treated to be an **'antiketogenic'** substance.

Fatty livers

Significant deposition of triglycerides in the liver leads to a condition known as **'fatty liver'. Normally, liver contains 5% of the lipids**, but under certain pathological conditions, the lipid content rises to 25-30%. The increased fat in the liver may result from:

(a) **Factors associated with increased free fatty acids (FFA) level are:**

(i) **Diabetes mellitus (severe uncontrolled)**

(ii) **Starvation**

(iii) **Ketosis**

(iv) **Toxaemia of pregnancy,** etc.

Here, the increased mobilization of FFA leads to the increased synthesis of triglycerides and then their accumulation.

(b) Due to the deficiency of **lipotropic factors such as choline, lecithin, methionine, vitamin E, vitamin B_6 i.e. pyridoxine, etc.**

(e) Other intoxicating agents like $CHCl_3$, CCl_4, phosphorus, arsenic, lead, alcohol, etc.

Biochemical basis of fatty liver

1. In one group, there is some primary factor which causes an increase in the FFA either due to increased mcbilisation from adipose tissue or increased hydrolysis of lipoproteins or chylomicrons by the enzyme **lipoprotein lipase.** This increased FFA level leads to the increased synthesis of triglycerides, vis-a-vis their accumulation later or in the liver. The production of lipoproteins (specifically the chylomicrons and VLDL) from triglycerides is unable to keep pace with the synthesis of triglycerides, which eventually leads to **'fatty liver'.** This is the mechanism in disorders like

uncontrolled diabetes mellitus, toxaemia of pregnancy, ketosis and starvation, etc.

2. In the other group, the defect lies in the production of plasma lipoproteins. Such a defect/blockade may be at one or more of the following sites:
   (i) **Synthesis of apoproteins**
   (ii) **Synthesis of lipoproteins from lipid and apoproteins**
   (iii) **Synthesis of lipids-specifically the phospholipids.**
   (iv) **Secretory mechanism of the lipoproteins.**

Substances which have got the capability to prevent or relieve such abnormal deposition of lipids in the liver are termed as **lipotropic factors** which are as mentioned just above.

Role of liver in the metabolism of lipids

Liver is the main site for the metabolism of lipids because it contains complete enzyme system to carry out the following major activities which are very important:

(i) **Synthesis of triglycerides**
(ii) **Synthesis of phospholipids**
(iii) **Synthesis of plasma lipoproteins such as VLDL, HDL, etc.**
(iv) **Synthesis of cholesterol and its derivatives such as bile acids, etc.**
(v) **Synthesis and degradation of fatty acids (β- oxidation)**
(vi) **Formation of ketone bodies**

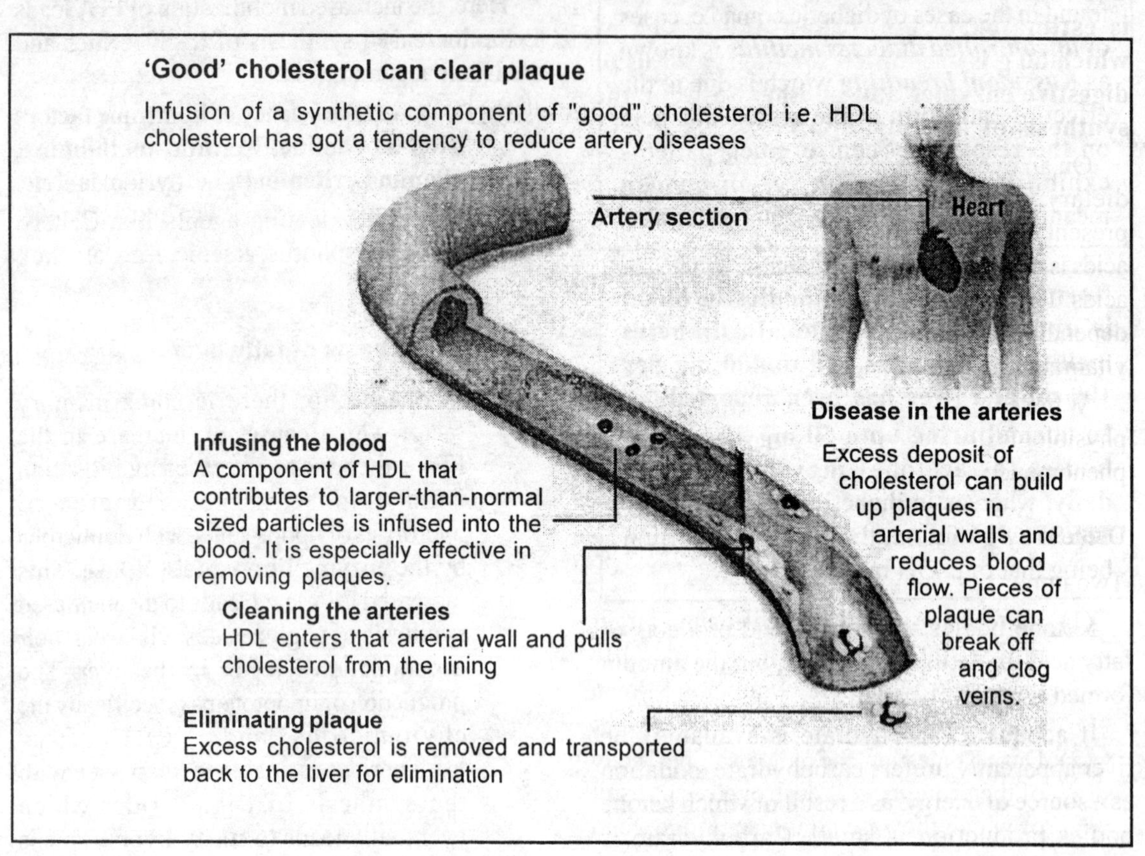

CHAPTER 12

METABOLISM OF PROTEINS

The total protein turnover of an adult male is estimated to be around 400 g/day, of which 50 g is accounted for the synthesis of digestive enzymes and another 15 g for the synthesis of haemoglobin.

On an overall, 20 amino acids are present in dietary proteins. These amino acids remain present in L-configuration. L-form of the amino acids is the physiological active form of the amino acids. The transport of such amino acids is energy dependent and requires ATP, Na^+, K^+,Mn^{++} and vitamin B_6.

Whereas D- form of amino acids is physiologically inactive and is transported by the phenomenon of diffusion.

DIGESTION AND ABSORPTION

Two important features of digestion are:

(1) It breaks down the non-diffusible larger molecules into smaller diffusible molecules which are commonly known as amino acids.

(2) During digestion, the biological specificity of the proteins gets destroyed as a result of which they are no longer antigenic in nature, thus avert allergic reactions to food.

Digestion of Proteins by various enzymes

Proteins are hydrolysed to their constituent amino acids by the action of a battery of enzymes found in the body, namely:

1. ***Pepsin:*** Responsible for the conversion of proteins to proteoses and peptones. It is secreted in the gastric juice as an inactive precursor i.e., pepsinogen. Pepsin is a very acidic protein and acts at pH between 1.5-2.5.
2. ***Trypsin:*** Responsible for cleaving peptide bonds involving carboxyl groups of arginine and lysine.
3. ***Chymotrypsin:*** Responsible for cleaving peptide bonds involving carboxyl groups of phenylalanine, tyrosine and tryptophan.
4. ***Carboxypeptidases:*** The two carboxypeptidases are secreted as precursor *procarboxypeptidases*. They cleave proteins and peptides from the carboxyl end.
5. ***Aminopeptidases:*** Responsible for cleaving proteins and peptides from the amino end.
6. ***Dipeptidases:*** Responsible for the cleavage of dipeptides.

Absorption

It is known that absorption is very rapid in man. The extent of hydrolysis of the food protein is low in the stomach which is nearly 10-15% but quickly reaches upto 50-60% in the duodenum. In the duodenal contents, the enzymes trypsin and chymotrypsin remain present at the concentrations of 200-800 μg per ml of fluid within a short time of stimulation. These high concentrations of enzymes are capable of rapidly hydrolyzing food proteins to small peptides. Absorption of protein fragments takes place in the duodenum and the jejunum, most of it is absorbed as di-and oligopeptides.

L- form of the amino acids is absorbed at much faster rate than the D-form. All amino acids are absorbed by active process which requires ATP, Na^+, K^+, Mn^{++} and pyridoxal phosphate.

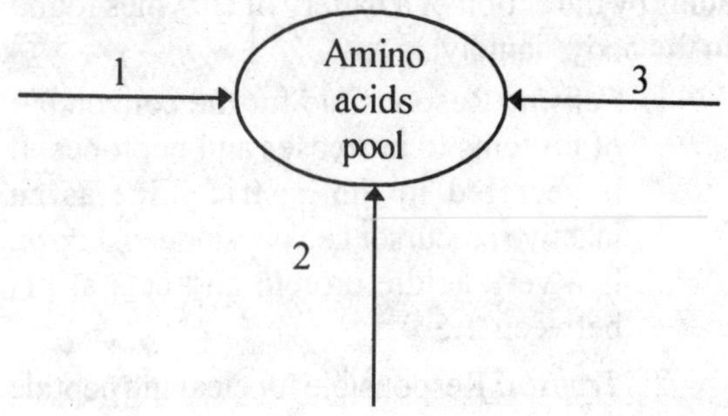

Sources of amino acids in the body pool include:

1. Dietary proteins
2. Intracellular synthesis } Metabolism
3. Tissue protein breakdown } (Table 12.1)

Transamination

It is a combined process of deamination and amination according to which the amino group of one amino acid may be reversibly transferred to the keto acid of another amino acid, thus effecting amino acid-keto acid interconversion. This phenomenon was for the first time discovered by two scientists namely ***Braunstein* and *Kritzmann.***

The process represents intermolecular transfer of amino groups without the splitting of ammonia. The reaction is reversible and is catalyzed by *transaminase enzymes,* which remain confined to almost every tissue or the animal but the major sites are heart, brain, kidney, testicle and liver.

The general process of transamination may be represented as follows:

It was earlier found that glutamic acid and its keto acid i.e., α - ketoglutaric acid participate in a large proportion of transamination reactions

Table 12.1 : Metabolism of amino acids within the cell

Anabolic phase	*Catabolic phase*
It is a synthetic process	**It is a breakdown process**
1. Biosynthesis of proteins which includes tissue proteins, blood proteins, enzymes and hormones.	1. Transamination
	2. Decarboxylation
	3. Oxidative deamination
2. Biosynthesis of non-protein nitrogen substances takes place for e.g., creatine, purines, pyrimidines, glutathione, choline, etc.	4. Utilization of nitrogen residue i.e., (i) Synthesis of glutamine (ii) Urea cycle

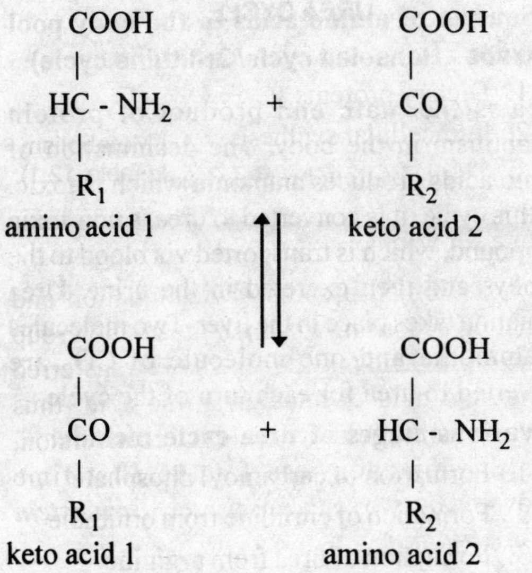

but now it has been concluded that all naturally occurring amino acids participate in transamination reactions.

There are two very important transaminases viz., glutamic-oxaloacetic transaminase i.e., GOT (AST) and glutamic-pyruvic transaminase i.e., GPT (ALT) which catalyze the following reactions:

L - glutamic acid + pyruvic acid

$\updownarrow$ transaminase

α - ketoglutaric acid + L - alanine

L - glutamic acid + oxaloacetic acid

$\updownarrow$ transaminase

α - ketoglutaric acid + L - aspartic acid

The transaminases require pyridoxal phosphate as cofactor. GOT is the most active and widely distributed of the transaminases. The most general type of transamination in animals and plants appears to be represented by the equation:

L - amino acid + α - ketoglutaric acid

$\rightleftharpoons$

α - keto acid + L - glutamic acid

In general, the transaminases of animal tissues and higher plants appear to be specific for L -amino acids, however, it has been noticed that certain bacteria, such as B. subtilis possess transaminases specific for both D and L - amino acids.

GOT activity of serum rises sharply following *myocardial infarction* and the rise appears to be proportional to the size of the infarcted area. Likewise, GPT activity of serum is of diagnostic value in liver disorders.

All available evidence indicates great importance of the transamination reaction in amino acid and protein metabolism. It represents a mechanism for the deamination of amino acids and also for the synthesis of amino acids from keto acids and glutamic acid. The key role of glutamic acid and α - ketoglutaric acid in amino acid and protein metabolism is obvious.

Decarboxylation

Amino acids are decarboxylated to produce amines. Such reactions are catalysed by enzymes known as decarboxylases which are found in liver, kidney and brain. These enzymes also require pyridoxal phosphate as a cofactor. Pyridoxamine phosphate is not required. The process is very important in the human body as it gives rise to important substances i.e., ***biologically active amines as follows:***

Tyrosine $\xrightarrow{\text{decarboxylation}}$ tyramine

Tryptophan $\xrightarrow{\text{decarboxylation}}$ tryptamine

Histidine $\xrightarrow{\text{decarboxylation}}$ histamine

$$\text{Glutamic acid} \xrightarrow{\text{decarboxylation}} \gamma - \text{aminobutyric acid (GABA)}$$

$$\text{5-Hydroxytryptophan} \xrightarrow{\text{decarboxylation}} \text{hydroxytryptamine (serotonin)}$$

Oxidative deamination

This process may be referred to as the liberation of ammonia oxidatively from amino acids, approximately two moles of NH_3 are formed for each molecule of O_2 taken up:

$$R-CH(NH_2)-COOH + 1/2O_2 \rightarrow R.CO\text{-}COOH + NH_3$$

Enzymes which bring about oxidative deamination are known as D- and L - amino acid oxidases; these act upon D - and L - amino acids respectively.

The D - amino acid oxidases are flavoproteins containing FAD, whereas L - amino acid oxidases are also flavoproteins but contain FMN (flavin mononucleotide).

The D - amino acids are not found in the tissues whereas L - amino acids are found which means that animal tissues are devoid of corresponding enzyme i.e., D - amino acid oxidases but contain L - amino acid oxidases. Both D - and L - amino acid oxidases are found in microorganisms. The function of D - oxidases is not yet known.

The mechanism of oxidative deamination may be represented by the following equations:

$$\underset{\text{amino acid}}{R-CH(NH_2)-COOH} + \underset{\text{flavoprotein enzyme}}{FP} \rightarrow \underset{\text{imino acid}}{R-C(=NH)-COOH} + \underset{\text{reduced enzyme}}{FP.H_2}$$

$$\underset{\text{imino acid}}{R-C(=NH)-COOH} + H_2O \rightleftharpoons \underset{\text{keto acid}}{R-C(=O)-COOH} + NH_3$$

UREA CYCLE

(Krebs - Henseleit cycle/Ornithine cycle)

Urea is the main end product of protein metabolism in the body. The deamination of amino acids produces ammonia which is toxic. By this cycle, it is converted to urea, a non-toxic compound, which is transported via blood to the kidneys and then excreted in the urine. Urea formation takes place in the liver. Two molecules of ammonia and one molecule of CO_2 are converted to urea for each turn of the cycle.

Various stages of urea cycle include:

1. Formation of carbamoyl phosphate
2. Formation of citrulline from ornithine
3. Formation of urea from arginine

1st stage: i.e. Formation of carbamoyl phosphate.

The first stage in the synthesis of urea in animals may be considered to be the formation of carbamoyl phosphate, the reaction is catalysed by the enzyme known as carbamoyl phosphate synthase (Fig. 12.1).

Carbamoyl phosphate is a reactive high energy compound. The enzyme requires an acyl glutamate such as N-acetylglutamate as a cofactor.

IInd stage i.e. Formation of citrulline from ornithine

Ornithine is converted to citrulline by the action of carbamoyl phosphate; this reaction is catalysed by the action of enzyme ornithine transcarbamoylase. **This reaction is not reversible.**

IIIrd stage i.e. Formation of arginine from citrulline

The syntheis of arginine from citrulline takes place in two stages. The first stage is the condensation of citrulline with aspartic acid to

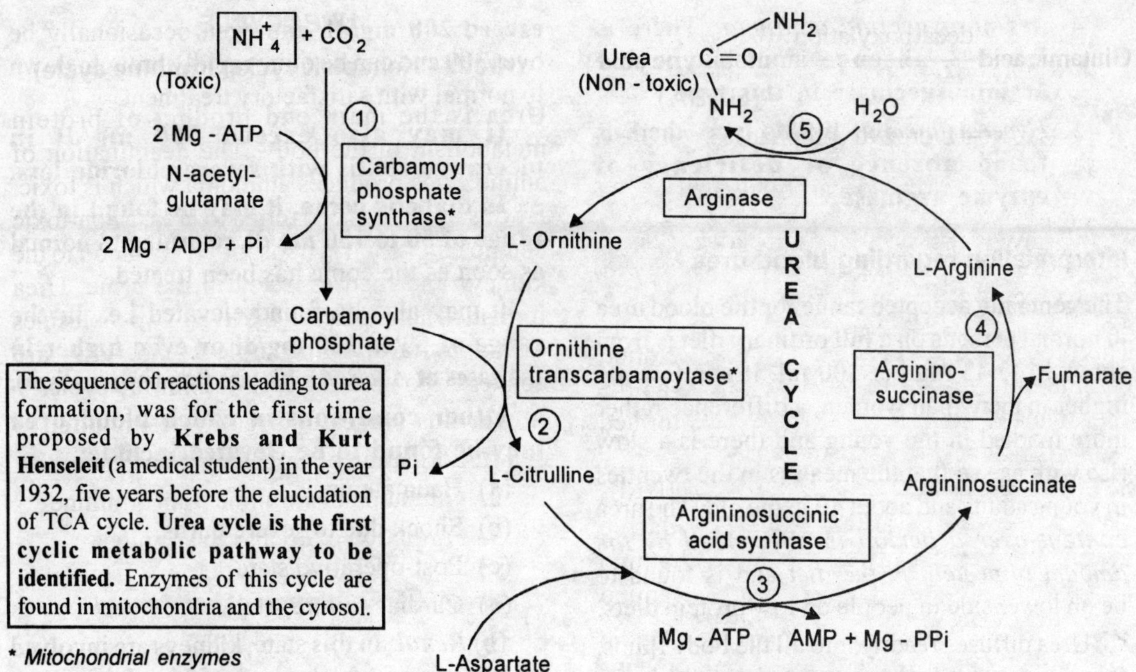

Fig. 12.1 : Reactions and intermediates of Urea Cycle

form argininosuccinic acid by the enzyme argininosuccinate synthetase. The arginino-succinate gets then split into arginine and fumarate by the cleavage enzyme known as argininosuccinase (Fig. 12.1).

IVth and last stage i.e. Formation of urea from arginine

Arginine is hydrolyzed to ornithine and urea by the enzyme arginase.

It has been observed that of the two N atoms in a molecule of urea, one is derived from *ammonia* through carbamoyl phosphate, and the other from *aspartic acid* through argininosuccinic acid.

$$
\begin{array}{c}
NH_2 \\
| \\
C=O \\
| \\
NH_2
\end{array}
$$

Urea
(non-toxic)

Metabolic disorders of the Urea Cycle (kerbs - Henseleit Cycle, Ornithine Cycle)

Hyperammonia or hyperammonaemic syndrome is caused due to the increased level of ammonia in the blood. Since, the formation of urea takes place from ammonia by urea cycle, therefore, any deficiency or defect of urea cycle enzyme (s) is responsible for elevated levels of ammonia. *Hyperammonaemia* gives rise to mental retardation.

There are five disorders:

1. *Hyperammonaemia type I:* In this type there is found **absence of enzyme carbamoyl phosphate synthetase.**
2. *Hyperammonaemia type II:* In this type there is found **absence of enzyme ornithine transcarbamoylase.**
3. *Citrullinaemia:* There is found **absence of enzyme argininosuccinate synthetase (synthase) in this type.**

4. *Argininosuccinic aciduria:* There is found **absence of enzyme argininosuccinase in this type.**
5. *Hyperarginemia:* In this type, there is found **absence or deficiency of enzyme arginase.**

Interpretation regarding blood urea

The generally accepted range for the blood urea in normal persons on a full ordinary diet is from about 14 to 43 mg per 100 ml. It is a few mg higher in men than women, a difference rather more marked in the young and there is a slow rise with age so that the mean is in the twenties in young adults and about 40 in the old. The urea *content over a period is influenced by the amount of protein in the diet* and is found to be on lower side in people on low protein diets.

Urea diffuses readily into all the body fluids. Its concentration in the water of plasma and cells is the same but as the water content of the cells is a little less per unit volume than that of plasma, the ratio of urea in plasma to cells is about 5:4.

Blood urea is found to be lower in pregnancy than in normal non-pregnant women.

Increases in the level of blood urea may occur in a number of diseases in addition to those in which the kidneys are primarily involved. For increases, three states may be responsible, namely:

(a) **Pre-renal**

(b) **Renal and**

(c) **Post- renal**

(a) *Pre-renal* : In this state, kidneys are not involved. In this state, blood urea level gets increased in cases of dehydration due to severe and protracted vomiting **as in pyloric and intestinal obstruction;** in chronic intestinal obstruction without vomiting; in diarrhoea; etc. *Very high values* of blood urea are encountered in these conditions if they are allowed to go untreated. **Thus, in *pyloric stenosis* with severe vomiting, the blood urea may exceed 200 mg/dl,** and even occasionally be over **300** and can be quite rapidly brought down to normal with satisfactory treatment.

It may also exceed 300 mg/dl in ulcerative colitis with severe chloride loss.

In diabetic coma, it may be found in the range of 50 to 150 *mg*/dl, returning to normal as soon as the coma has been treated.

It may also be found elevated **i.e., in the range of 50 to 100 mg/dl or even higher in the cases of *Addison's disease* (hypoadrenalism).**

Other conditions in which blood urea may be found to be elevated include:

(a) Haematemesis,

(b) Shock due to severe burns,

(c) Post-operative state,

(d) Cardiac failure, etc.

(b) *Renal:* In this state, kidneys are involved as a result of which level of blood urea gets increased **in all types of kidney diseases** which include:

(i) Acute glomerulonephritis

(ii) Ellis's Type II nephritis

(iii) Malignant hypertension

(iv) Chronic pyelonephritis

(v) Mercury poisoning

(vi) Hydronephrosis

(vii) Congenital cystic kidneys

(viii) Renal tuberculosis

(ix) Hyperparathyroidism

(x) Hpervitaminosis D

(c) *Post - renal:* Post renal diseases lead to increased blood urea level, are those in which there is obstruction to the flow of urine. **This causes retention of urine.** If prolonged, irreversible kidney damage results. **Most important among these is *enlargement of the prostate,*** in which estimation of blood urea is an essential part of the assessment of the condition. **Besides prostate, other conditions include:**

(i) **stones in the urinary tract**

(ii) **stricture of the urethra**
(iii) **tumour of the bladder affecting the ureters, etc.**

METABOLISM OF THE INDIVIDUAL AMINO ACIDS

According to the metabolic fate of their skeletons, amino acids have been classified in the following categories:

(a) Glycogenic or glucogenic amino acids
(b) Ketogenic amino acids

(a) Glycogenic (Glucogenic) amino acids:

These are those amino acids which may be responsible for the synthesis of glucose (see gluconeogenesis pathway). These include glycine, alanine, serine, threonine, valine, aspartic acid, glutamic acid, cysteine, cystine, methionine, proline, hydroxyproline, arginine and histidine.

(b) Ketogenic amino acids

Amino acids which have the capability to synthesize *acetate* or *acetoacetate* (the intermediates formed during fatty acid metabolism) are known as ketogenic amino acids. These include leucine, isoleucine, lysine, phenylalanine, tyrosine and tryptophan (see Table 12.2).

Table 12.2 : Classification of glycogenic and ketogenic amino acids

Glycogenic or glucogenic	*Ketogenic only*	*Glycogenic and ketogenic i.e., both*
glycine, alanine, serine, threonine, valine, aspartic acid, glutamic acid, cysteine, cystine, methionine, proline, hydroxyproline, arginine and histidine	leucine	isoleucine, lysine, phenylalanine, tyrosine and tryptophan

GLYCINE

It is one of the glycogenic (glucogenic) amino acids. It is a non-essential amino acid and is synthesized by the living cells. It contains no asymmetric carbon atom, hence does not exist in D or L form.

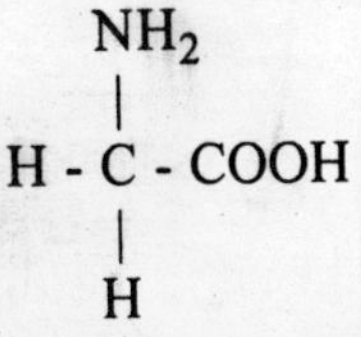

```
      NH2
       |
  H - C - COOH
       |
       H
    glycine
```

Glycine, {(Fig 12.2 (a) & (b)}, the simplest of

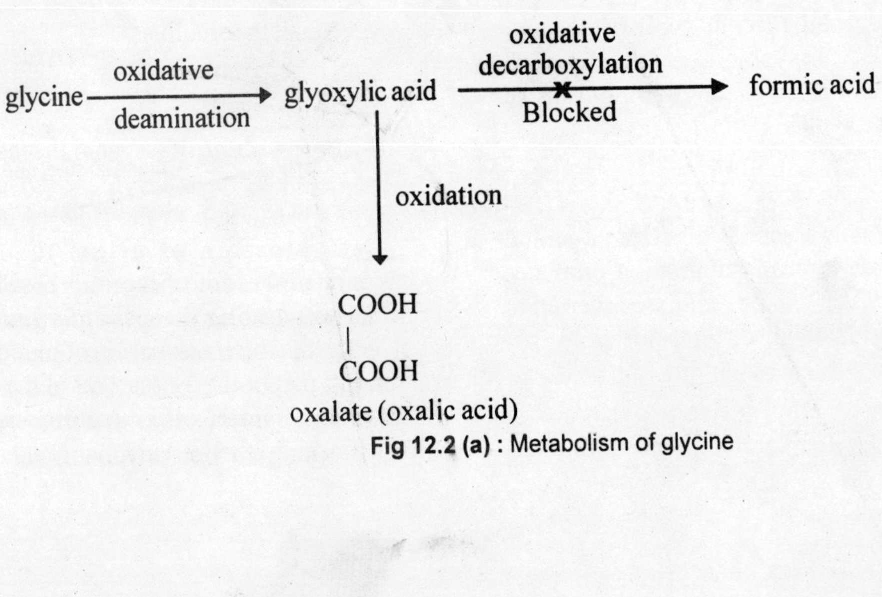

```
             oxidative                      oxidative
                                          decarboxylation
glycine ----------------> glyoxylic acid ------x------------> formic acid
            deamination         |              Blocked
                                |
                                | oxidation
                                v
                              COOH
                               |
                              COOH
                      oxalate (oxalic acid)
```

Fig 12.2 (a) : Metabolism of glycine

the amino acids, to date has been found to be utilized in more different ways in the animal body than practically any other amino acid. It is a very important and useful amino acid as its metabolism gives rise to several important substances as follows:

Formic acid
(one - carbon pool)
Protein

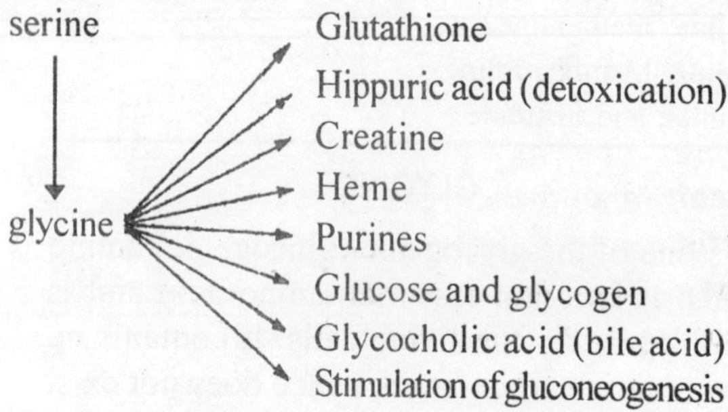

Fig. 12.2 (b): Metabolism of glycine

Abnormalities of glycine metabolism

1. Primary Hyperoxaluria

The metabolism defect in this disease in due to the disorder of glyoxylate metabolism where in glyoxylic acid is not oxidised to formic acid but is converted to oxalate, thus, giving rise to increased excretion of **oxalates** in urine.

2. Glycinuria

There is decreased tubular reabsorption of glycine in the kidneys as a result of which appreciable amount of glycine is found in the urine of such individuals.

ALANINE

This is also a non-essential glycogenic amino acid. Deamination or transamination produces pyruvic acid which can be readily converted to glucose or oxidized in citric acid cycle. β - alanine is a constituent of pantothenic acid.

Formation of alanine from pyruvate in muscles also helps in removing some of the NH_3 formed in that tissue during amino acid metabolism. The cycle of transport of glucose from liver to muscles and of alanine from muscles to liver is known as **glucose alanine cycle.**

The metabolism of alanine is as shown below:

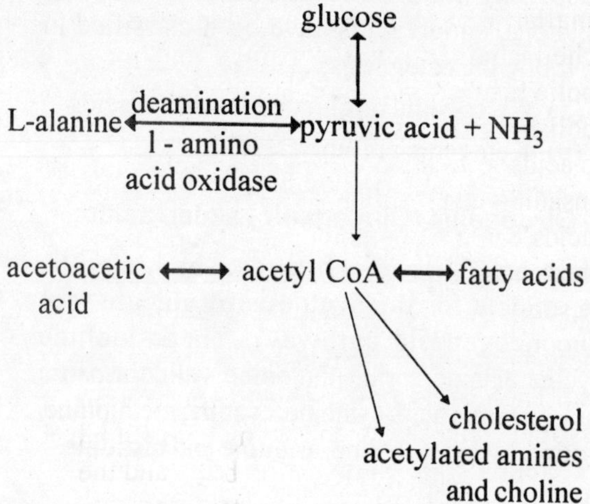

Serine

This is also a non-essential glycogenic amino acid. Serine and glycine are interconvertible in the body, as previously indicated. The metabolism of serine is as follows:

Glucose and glycogen
↑
Pyruvic acid + NH_3 ⟶ Other amino acids and urea
↑
Serine ⟶ Tissue proteins
Serine ⟶ Cysteine ↔ Cystine
Serine ⟶ Glycine
Serine ⟶ Ethanolamine and choline
Serine ⟶ Cephalins

It is of interest to note that certain moulds from serine derivatives like *azaserine* and *cycloserine* act as antibiotics. Azaserine is of great interest as it inhibits the growth of tumours and produces cell mutation. It interferes with purine synthesis through blocking reactions involving glutamine.

Branched chain amino acids

(A) Valine, (B) Leucine and (C) Isoleucine

These three amino acids are not **synthesized** by the mammals and all have been designated as essential amino acids **(EAA)** for the mammalian diet. Since all of them contain branched chain aliphatic groups and have metabolic features in common, therefore, their metabolisms are considered together. All these amino acids form the corresponding keto acids by transamination reactions. The corresponding keto acids can also be aminated to form these branched chain amino acids, hence the keto acids can be substituted for them in the diet.

These amino acids are taken up by brain and utilized. These are supplied by absorption from the gastrointestinal tract following a meal and are preferentially taken up by the brian and the muscles. In the post absorptive state, they are supplied by protein breakdown in the muscles.

(A) VALINE

It is glycogenic, on deamination, it forms α - keto isovaleric acid and later on succinyl Co-A. It's metabolism in brief is as follows:

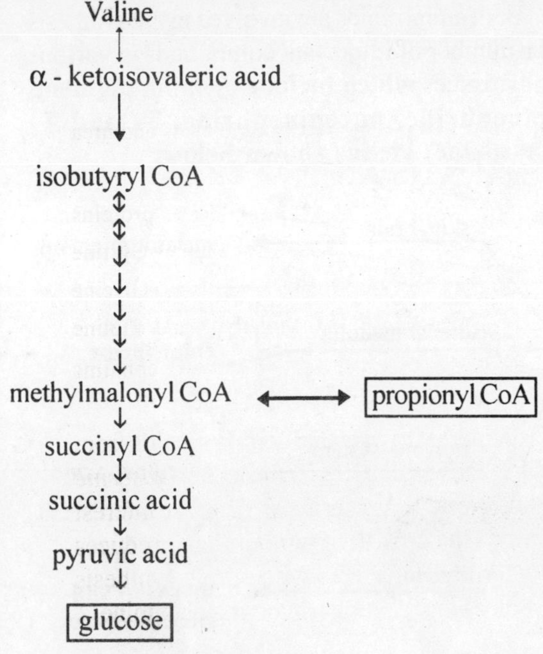

Hypervalinaemia

1. In this abnormal condition one finds raised level of valine in the blood and urine.
2. The infants suffer from stunted growth, muscle wasting and vomiting.
3. A diet containing protein hydrolysate low in valine prevents this condition effectively.

(B) Leucine

***Leucine,* on the other hand is most ketogenic of all the amino acids, i.e., it forms the ketone bodies.** Its metabolism in short may be represented as follows: Acetyl Co-A once formed may give rise to ketone bodies.

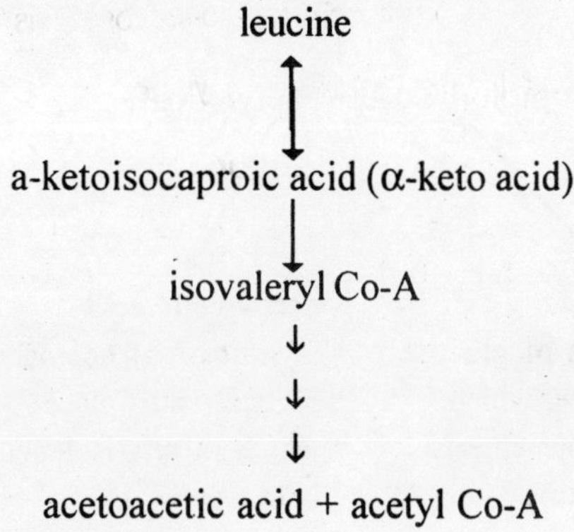

In step (2), the α - keto acid is converted by oxidative decarboxylation to the corresponding Co-A derivative (with one carbon less) i.e. isovaleryl Co-A. This reaction is catalysed by branched chain 2-keto acid dehydrogenase complex in the presence of TPP, lipoic acid, FAD, NAD and coenzyme - A as cofactors. The deficiency of this enzyme causes **maple syrup urine disease.** In this disease, there is metabolic defect involving the branched chain amino acids which results in the excretion of their keto acids in the urine. The defect is in step (2), the oxidative dearboxylation of the α- keto acids. **The urinc is said to have the odour of maple syrup. There is rapid deterioration in the**

first two months of life. If the child survives, he or she manifests serious mental retardation. It's a serious disease, the treatment of which is not available so far.

(C) Isoleucine

The metabolism of **isoleucine** may be represented in brief as follows:

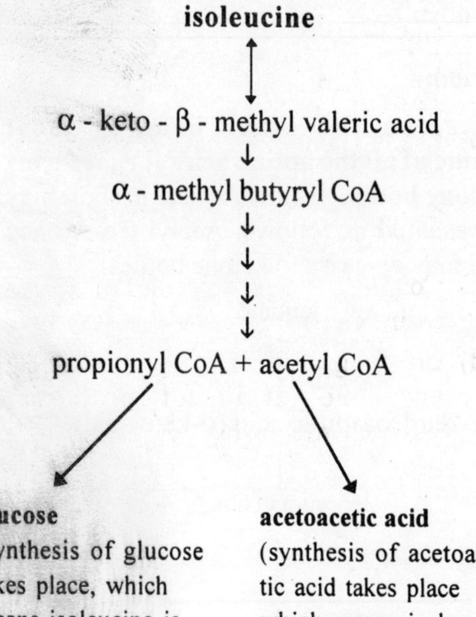

From the pathway of isoleucine metabolism, it is conclusive that two carbon atoms may lead to the formation of acetyl CoA and three carbon atoms to the formation of glucose.

Metabolism of Phenylalanine and Tyrosine

Both phenylalanine and tyrosine are aromatic amino acids. Tyrosine is hydroxylated phenylalanine. The structure of these are:

$C_6H_5-CH_2-CH(NH_2)-COOH$

Phenylalanine

$HO-C_6H_4-CH_2-CH(NH_2)-COOH$

Tyrosine (p - hydroxyphenylalanine)

Phenylalanine is an essential amino acid whereas tyrosine is a non-essential amino acid. Phenylalanine can be converted to tyrosine but the reverse is not possible, hence the requirement of tyrosine can be met by the intake of adequate amount of phenylalanine in the diet. Both are ***ketogenic amino acids.***

Both amino acids are involved in the synthesis of a number of important compounds in various body tissues **which include melanin pigment, epinephrine, norepinephrine, T_3 and T_4 (thyroxine) etc. as shown below:**

Phenylalanine —liver→ **Tyrosine**

Tyrosine —skin, brain→ **melanin pigment**

Tyrosine —adrenal medulla→ **epinephrine**

Tyrosine —nervous system→ **norepinephrine**

Tyrosine —thyroid→ **thyroxine and triiodothyronine**

Tyrosine —liver→ **glucose** + **ketone bodies**

(a) Formation of melanin

(a) Melanins represent the dark pigments of the skin, hair and retina of the eye and are formed from 3, 4 - dihydroxyphenylalanine (DOPA) through a complex series of reactions.

(b) Melanin forms a reversible oxidation-reduction system in which the reduced form is tan and the oxidized form is black.

(c) Melanins are produced in pigment - forming cells, the *melanocytes.*

(d) Melanins are very complex substances of high molecular weight and are insoluble in most solvents.

(e) The pathway of melanin formation is given below in Fig. 12.3.

(b) Formation of epinephrine (adrenaline) and norepinephrine (arterenol)

(a) Formation of catecholamines i.e., epinephrine and norepinephrine from tyrosine in the adrenal medulla proceeds through DOPA and hydroxytryptamine.

(b) Its pathway may be represented as shown in Fig. 12.4.

(c) Formation of triiodothyronine (T_3) and thyroxine i. e. tetraiodothyronine (T_4)

(a) Synthesis of important hormones like T_3 and T_4 takes place in the thyroid gland from phenylalanine and tyrosine (Fig. 12.4).

(b) Phenylalanine is converted to tyrosine which on iodination forms monoiodotyrosine; this on further iodination gives rise to diiodotyrosine.

(c) Coupling of two molecules of diiodotyrosine yields thyroxine (Fig. 12.5).

(d) Coupling of 1 mol. of monoiodotyrosine and 1 mol. of diiodotyrosine yields triiodothyronine (Fig. 12.5).

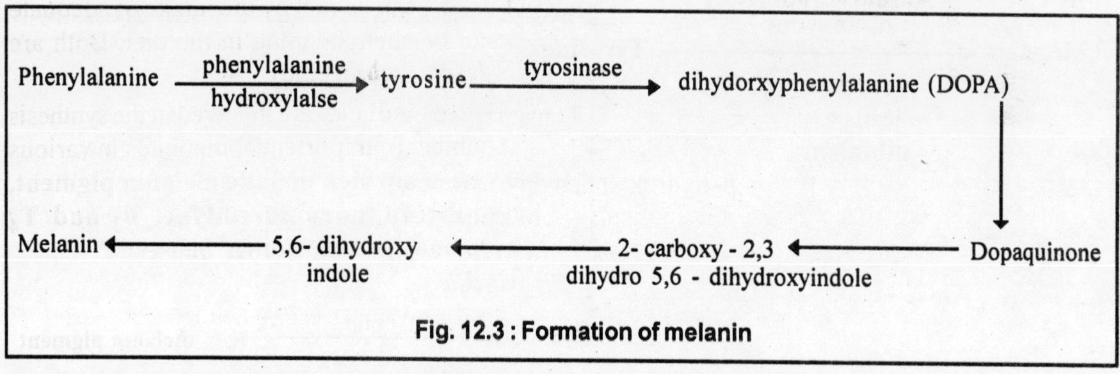

Fig. 12.3 : Formation of melanin

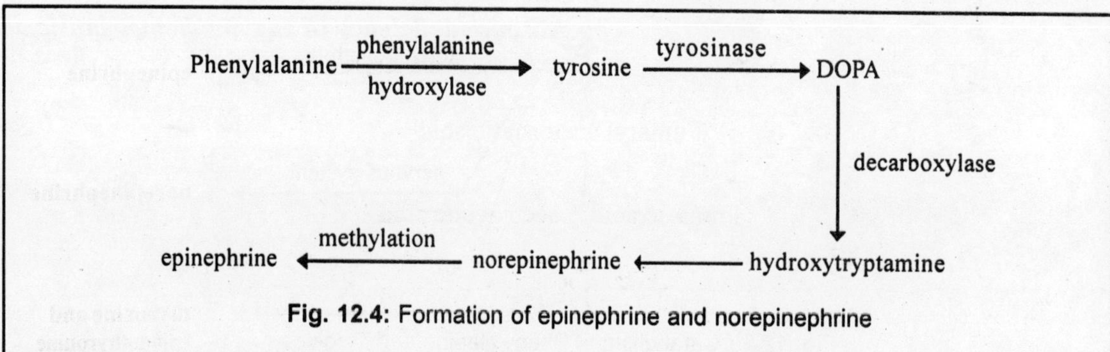

Fig. 12.4: Formation of epinephrine and norepinephrine

The steps are as shown below :

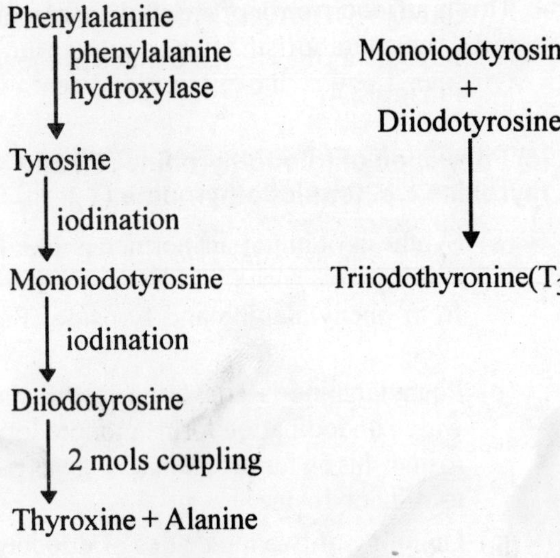

Fig 12.5 : Formation of T_4 and T_3

Inborn errors of the metabolism of phenylalanine and tyrosine (hereditary defects in phenylalanine and tyrosine metabolism).

There are number of metabolic abnormalities which are congenital and remain present throughout life. These disorders are hereditary (Fig. 12.6). Four well established hereditary defects in the metabolism of phenylalanine and tyrosine include **phenylketonuria (phenylpyruvic oligophrenia), tyrosinosis,**

Inborn error	*Enzyme defect*
(i) Phenylketonuria	Phenylalanine hydroxylase
(ii) Tyrosinosis	p- Hydroxy phenylpyuvate oxidase
(iii) Alkaptonuria	Homogentisic acid oxidase
(iv) Albinism	Tyrosinase

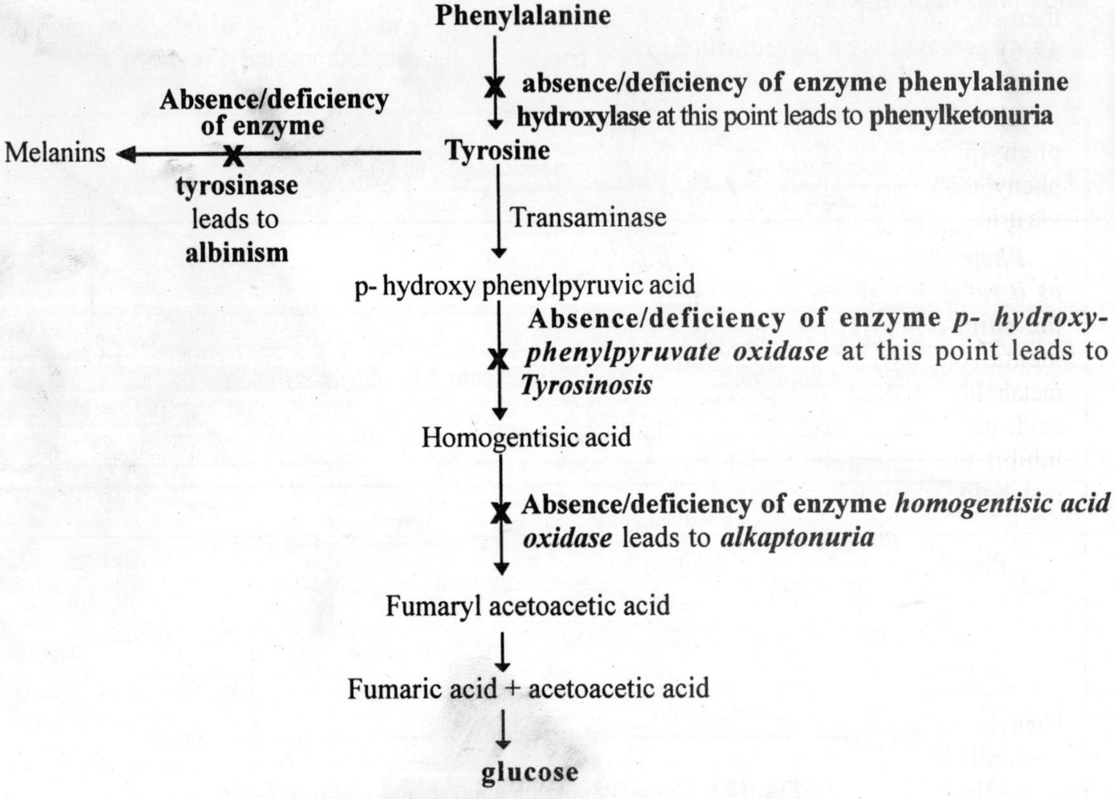

Phenylalanine

↓ ✗ **absence/deficiency of enzyme phenylalanine hydroxylase** at this point leads to **phenylketonuria**

Melanins ← ✗ **Absence/deficiency of enzyme tyrosinase** leads to **albinism** — **Tyrosine**

↓ Transaminase

p- hydroxy phenylpyruvic acid

↓ ✗ **Absence/deficiency of enzyme *p- hydroxyphenylpyruvate oxidase*** at this point leads to ***Tyrosinosis***

Homogentisic acid

↓ ✗ **Absence/deficiency of enzyme *homogentisic acid oxidase*** leads to ***alkaptonuria***

Fumaryl acetoacetic acid

↓

Fumaric acid + acetoacetic acid

↓

glucose

Fig. 12.6 : Catabolism of Phenylalanine and Tyrosine

alkaptonuria and albinism; in each case the defect is due to hereditary absence or deficit of a specific enzyme involved in a specific reaction. These conditions belong to what **scientist Garrod called 'inborn errors of metabolism'.**

Various blocks (checks) in the metabolism of phenylalanine and tyrosine give rise to different inborn errors of metabolism taking place either due to absence or deficiency of an enzyme which are as given in Fig. 12.6.

(i) Phenylketonuria

Phenylketonuria is an inborn error of metabolism associated with the metabolism of phenylalanine. The enzyme missing/deficient in this disease is known as ***phenylalanine hydroxylase*** which catalyses the conversion of phenylalanine to tyrosine. Due to the deficiency of the enzyme phenylalanine hydroxylase, the main pathway of the metabolism of phenylalanine via tyrosine (Fig. 12.6) gets blocked and the minor alternate pathway takes place as shown below. Various metabolites that accumulate in the blood are phenylpyruvic acid, phenyllactic acid and phenylacetic acid which later on are excreted via urine.

Phenylketonuria is a very serious disease as it results in severe mental deficiency and the children suffering from this disease are mentally retarded because of the fact that metabolites of phenylketonuria i.e. phenylpyruvic acid, phenyllactic acid and phenylacetic acid inhibit the formation of serotonin, a potent metabolite of brain.

Phenylalanine —(blocked ✗)→ Tyrosine

Phenylalanine ↕ (Transaminase) Phenylpyruvic acid

Phenylpyruvic acid —($-CO_2$)→ Phenylacetic acid

Phenylpyruvic acid ↕ (+2H / -2H) Phenyllactic acid

(ii) Tyrosinosis

This is an inborn error of metabolism associated with the metabolism of phenylalanine and tyrosine. The enzyme missing/deficient in this disorder is known as p - hydroxyphenyl pyruvate oxidase; due to the deficiency of this enzyme p - hydroxyphenylpyruvic acid is not converted to homogentisic acid resulting in the deposition of p-hydroxyphenylpyruvic acid in the blood. It's a very rare hereditary disorder in which p - hydroxyphenylpyruvic acid and tyrosine are excreted in the urine.

The first authentic case of ***tyrosinosis*** was described by the scientist *Medes* in the year 1932.

(iii) Alkaptonuria

It's an inborn error of metabolism associated with the metabolism of phenylalanine and tyrosine. The enzyme missing/deficient is known as **homogentisic acid oxidase**; as a result of the deficiency of this enzyme homogentisic acid is not catalysed to form fumarylacetoacetic acid. The net result is the accumulation of homogentisic acid in the blood and other body fluids which is later on excreted via urine.

Alkaptonuria is characterized by the excretion of urine which upon standing gradually **becomes darker in colour and finally turns black.** The urine is also strongly reducing and gives a *violet colour-with* $FeCl_3$. The substance responsible **for the formation of the black pigment has been identified as homogentisic acid.**

Deposition of *homogentisic acid* in the body fluids and the cartilages and other connective tissues gives rise to a condition known as *ochronosis.*

(iv) Albinism

This is also an inborn error of the metabolism of phenylalanine and tyrosine. The enzyme missing/deficient is known as ***tyrosinase,*** the deficiency of which does not catalyse the formation of melanins from tyrosine. **In this disorder, the natural melanin pigments of hair, skin and eyes are not formed.**

Total albinism is a hereditary condition in which there is complete absence of pigment in the skin, eyes and hair. It is due to absence of enzyme *tyrosinase* in the melanocytes and is transmitted as a simple recessive. **There are known various types of hereditary albinism in which pigment is only found to be lacking from certain parts of the body, such as the eye, areas of the skin and areas of the hair.**

Metabolism of Tryptophan

It's an aromatic amino acid and it is the only amino acid which contains indole ring in its structure. It is an essential amino acid. Omission of tryptophan from the diet of human beings is promptly followed by tissue wasting and negative nitrogen balance. Tryptophan has the metabolic distinction of giving rise to nicotinic acid, serotonin and indoles on the one hand and glucose and ketone bodies on the other hand as shown below:

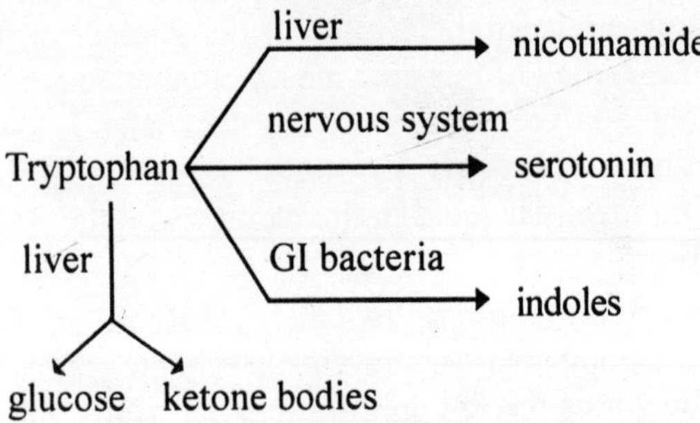

Tryptophan is metabolised in the following way:

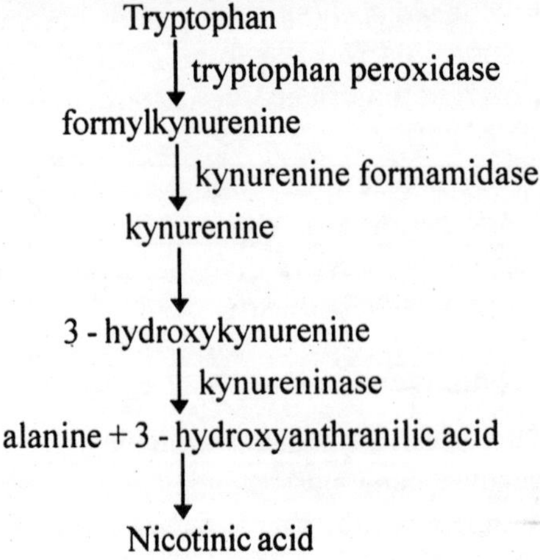

Salient features of this pathway are:

(i) **This pathway gives rise to the synthesis of niacin. 60 mgs of tryptophan gives rise to 1 mg of nicotinic acid in the human body.** In human diet, tryptophan is not in so much amount to meet the requirement of this vitamin.

(ii) **In the synthesis of serotonin: The vasoconstrictor substance 5 - hydroxy tryptamine** or **serotonin** is synthesized which remains present in the blood, particularly in the gastric mucosa, intestine, brain, mast cells and blood platelets. **It is an important substance in nerve impulse transmission (neurotransmitter). It regulates sleep, behaviour, blood pressure, etc.** This is synthesized, as mentioned below:

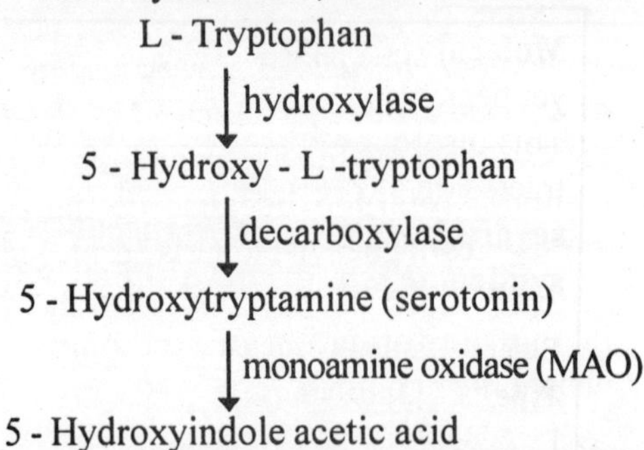

Carcinoid Syndrome : Patients with malignant carcinoid excrete large amounts of the serotonin metabolite i.e. 5- hydroxyindole acetic acid in the urine. Such patients have been estimated to utilize as much as 60 percent of the tryptophan metabolized in the formation of serotonin as compared with 1 per cent for the normal individual. **Serotonin is considered to function as a neurohumoral agent.**

(iii) In the synthesis of indole and skatole

This is the minor pathway by which tryptophan is metabolized as a result of which indole, indole acetic acid and skatole are formed in the large intestine due to action of certain bacteria. The foul smell of the faeces is due to these substances. These are excreted via urine or faeces.

Hartnup disease: This is an inborn error of metabolism associated with *tryptophan metabolism.* It has been named after the first detected family. **The enzyme deficient is *tryptophanperoxidase.*** This disease is characterized by the following three main symptoms:

(i) **Pellagra like dermatitis, the affected victims display skin lesions.**

(ii) **Sensitivity to sunlight**

(iii) **Motor ataxia characteristic of cerebellar dysfunction.**

Treatment: The treatment of patients with Hartnup disease consists in supplementing the diet with additional amount of niacin to alleviate the dermatological and neurological lesions together with protection from sunlight and the periodic sterilization of the gastrointestinal tract with antibiotics to reduce the formation of the bacterial breakdown products of tryptophan that may exert toxic effects.

The flow of information in all cells is from DNA to RNA to protein; this is known as **central dogma** of molecular biology; **it was formulated by scientist Francis Crick** shortly after the discovery of the structure of DNA. Information can also flow from DNA to DNA in both cells. Information also flows from RNA to RNA during the replication of RNA viruses such as polio virus. The final permitted information transfer is from RNA to DNA, which occurs only in the case of retroviruses such as **human immunodeficiency virus (HIV).** The only information transfer that is prohibited by the **central dogma is from protein to RNA or to DNA.** The permitted information transfers in cells (infected or uninfected) is summarized below:

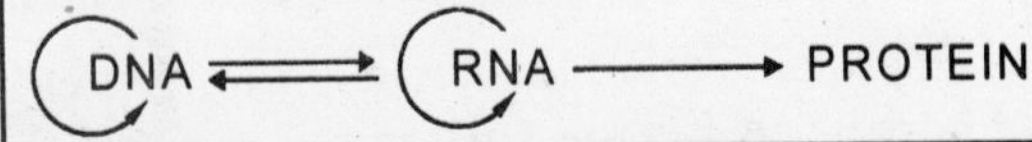

Molecular defects at the levels of transcription and translation of collagen polypeptides have not yet been clearly established but **may cause one type of Ehlers- Danlos syndrome (Type IV).** This disorder is characterized by decreased synthesis of type III collagen in the aorta, intestinal tract, skin and probably other tissues. Among the Ehlers- Danlos disorders, **Type IV is the most severe because of the threat of arterial rupture or gastrointestinal perforation. This syndrome is a group of inherited disorders as shown below:**

Ehlers- Danlos syndrome

Type	**Inheritance**	**Biochemical defect**	**Collagen fibril diameter**
I	AD	unknown	Increased
II	AD	"	"
III	AD	"	"
IV	AD or AR	Decreased type III collagen synthesis and its intracellular accumulation	Heterogeneous
V	XL	unknown	Heterogeneous
	XL	unknown	Increased
VI	AR	**Lysyl hydroxylase deficiency**	Decreased

AD = autosomal dominant, AR = autosomal recessive; XL = X- Linked.

CHAPTER 13

NUCLEIC ACIDS METABOLISM

Biosynthesis of the large complex molecules of the nucleic acids can be conveniently divided into synthesis of the monomers (mononucleotides) and the synthesis of the polymers (DNA and RNA).

Digestion and absorption of nucleoproteins

The protein part of the nucleoproteins is easily hydrolyzed by the following two types of enzymes viz:

(i) **gastric enzymes,**

(ii) **intestinal enzymes**

As a result of hydrolysis, the protein portion of nucleoproteins is broken down to its constituent amino acids; whereas the remaining part of nucleoproteins i.e., nucleic acids is not broken down in the stomach but is acted upon by pancreatic nucleases in the intestine. **Ribonuclease found in pancreatic juice hydrolyzes ribonucleic acid (RNA) splitting off particularly pyrimidine mononucleotides.**

Another enzyme which hydrolyzes deoxyribonucleic acid (DNA) to oligonucleotides (composed of a few mononucleotides) is a pancreatic deoxyribonuclease. Besides these two important enzymes, other enzymes found in intestinal mucosa are known as **nucleases** such as phosphodiesterase which hydrolyzes the nucleic acids completely to mononucleotides which are further hydrolyzed by intestinal phosphatases **(nucleotidases)** to inorganic phosphate and nucleosides. It appears that nucleosides are not further hydrolyzed in the intestine but are absorbed as such.

Corresponding enzymes which have got the capability to further hydrolyze nucleosides to form D-ribose, D-deoxyribose, purine and pyrimidine bases are known as **nucleosidases** which are found in the extracts of various tissues of the body like liver, kidney, bone marrow etc. Some examples of them are as given below:

$$\underset{\text{(uridine)}}{\text{uracil riboside}} + H_2O \xrightarrow{\text{nucleosidase}} \text{uracil + ribose}$$

$$\underset{\text{(guanosine)}}{\text{guanine riboside}} + \text{Pi} \xrightarrow[\text{phosphorylase}]{\text{nucleoside}} \text{guanine} + \alpha\text{-D-ribose-1-P}$$

Nucleoside phosphorylase found in liver and other tissues acts upon various nucleosides.

Biosynthesis of mononucleotides

Pyrimidine mononucleotides: The complete series of enzymic reaction giving rise to the parent pyrimidine mononucleotide (uridine 5'-monophosphate, UMP) is shown in Fig.13.1. **The**

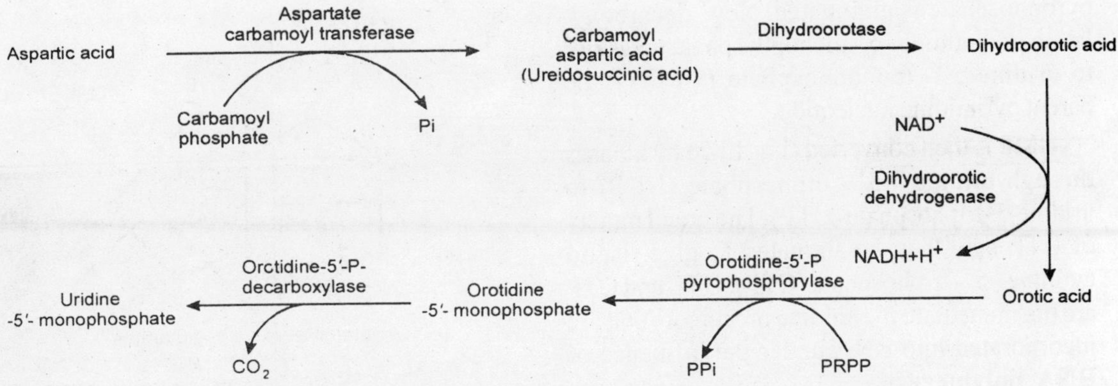

Fig. 13.1: Biosynthesis of UMP, the parent pyrimidine nucleotide

starting compounds are aspartic acid and carbamoyl phosphate (Fig.13.2) which combine to form carbamoyl - aspartate. Formation of the pyrimidine ring then takes place as a result of the action of **dihydro-orotase** forming dihydroorotic acid; dehydrogenation of which produces the important pyrimidine intermediate, orotic acid. A pyrophosphorylase reaction then follows in which orotic acid accepts a ribose - 5 - phosphate group from 5 - phosphoribosyl - 1 - pyrophosphate (PRPP). The resulting product is orotidine - 5′ - monophosphate; inorganic

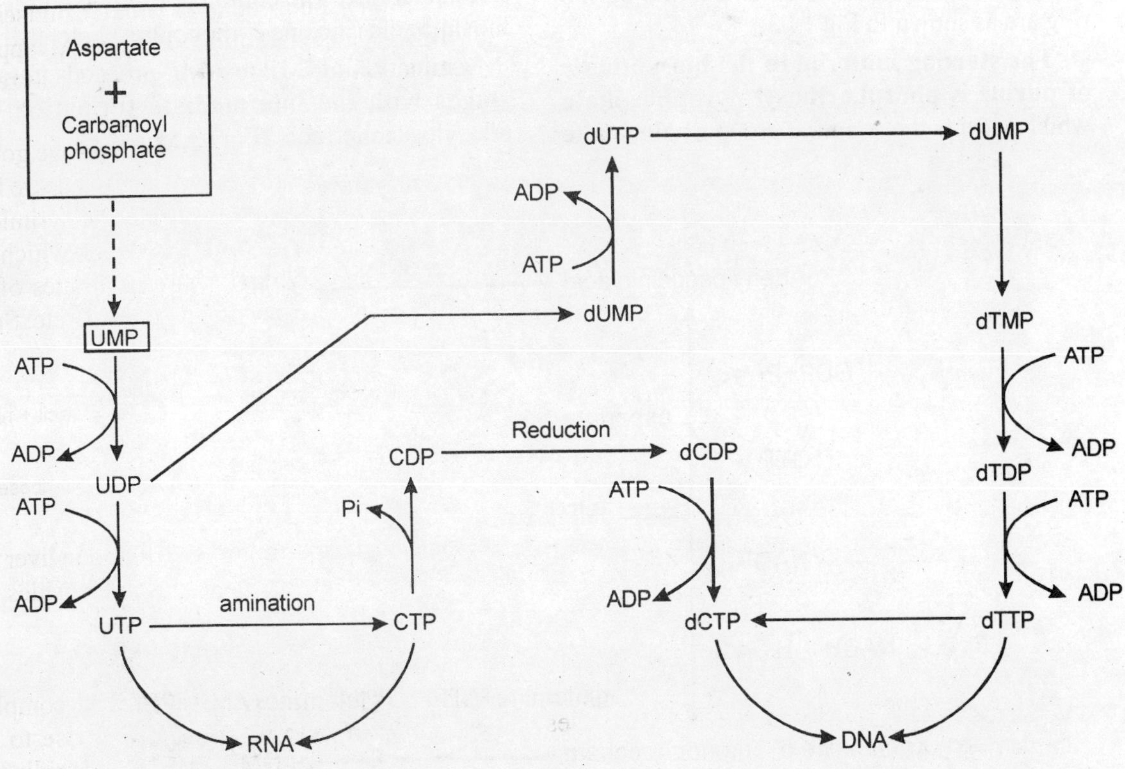

Fig13.2 : Biosynthetic pathways leading to the immediate pyrimidine precursors of DNA and RNA

pyrophosphate is eliminated. Now, decarboxylation of orotidine - 5′- monophosphate gives rise to uridine 5′ - monophosphate (UMP) - the parent pyrimidine nucleotide.

UMP is then converted (Fig 13.2) by kinases through uridine - 5′ - diphosphate (UDP) to uridine-5′-triphosphate (UTP). The uracil moiety of UTP may then be aminated to give rise to cytidine - 5′ - triphosphate (CTP). UTP and CTP are the immediate pyrimidine precursors that are incorporated into RNA under the influence of **RNA polymerase.**

Eventually dCTP and dTTP are the immediate pyrimidine precursors that are incorporated into DNA by the action of **DNA polymerase**.

Purine mononucleotides

It is known from experiments with isotope studies that the sources of various atoms in the purine ring are as shown in Fig 13.3.

The starting material in the biosynthesis of purine is phosphoribosyl pyrophosphate which accepts the α-amino group of glutamine

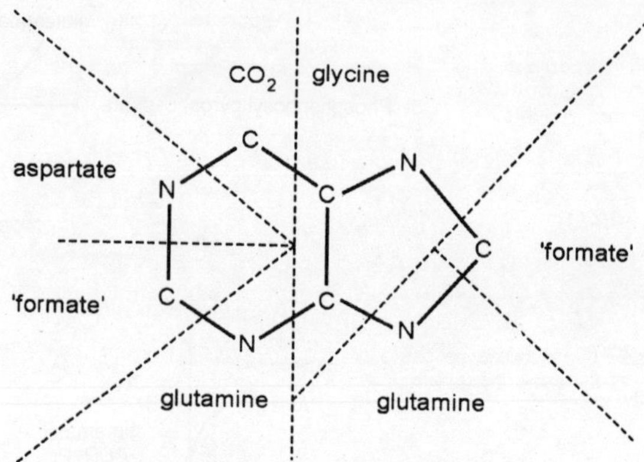

Fig 13.3 : Origin of the separate atoms in the purine ring. `Formate' stands for the formyl derivative of tetrahydrofolic acid.

to give 5- phosphoribosylamine (Fig 13.4).

The ring system is completed when N-formyl-tetrahydrofolic acid donates its formyl group to the 5-amino group of the imidazole carboxamide ribonucleotide. The complete ribonucleotide is inosinic acid (inosine 5'-monophosphate, IMP).

Amination of IMP to AMP proceeds in two stages with the intermediate formation of adenylosuccinic acid (Fig 13.5).

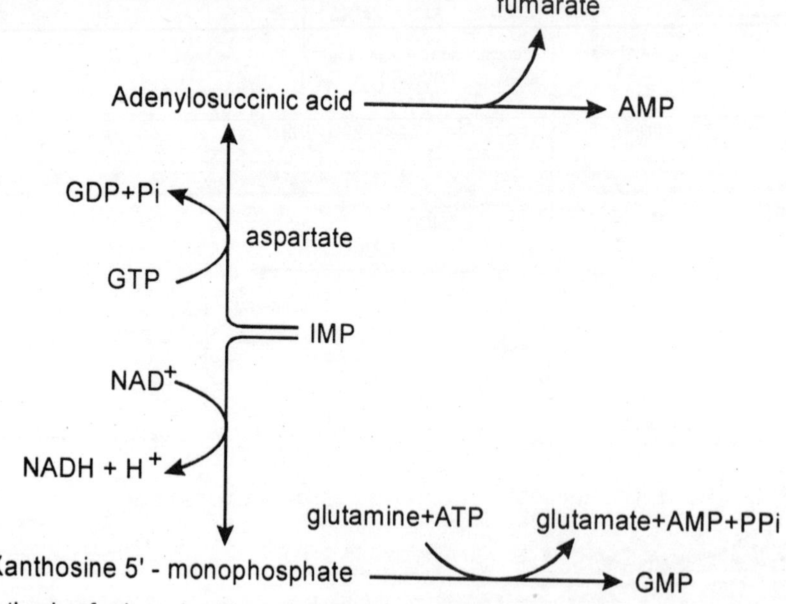

Fig13.5 : Biosynthesis of adenosine 5'-monophosphate (AMP) and guanosine 5'-monophosphate (GMP)

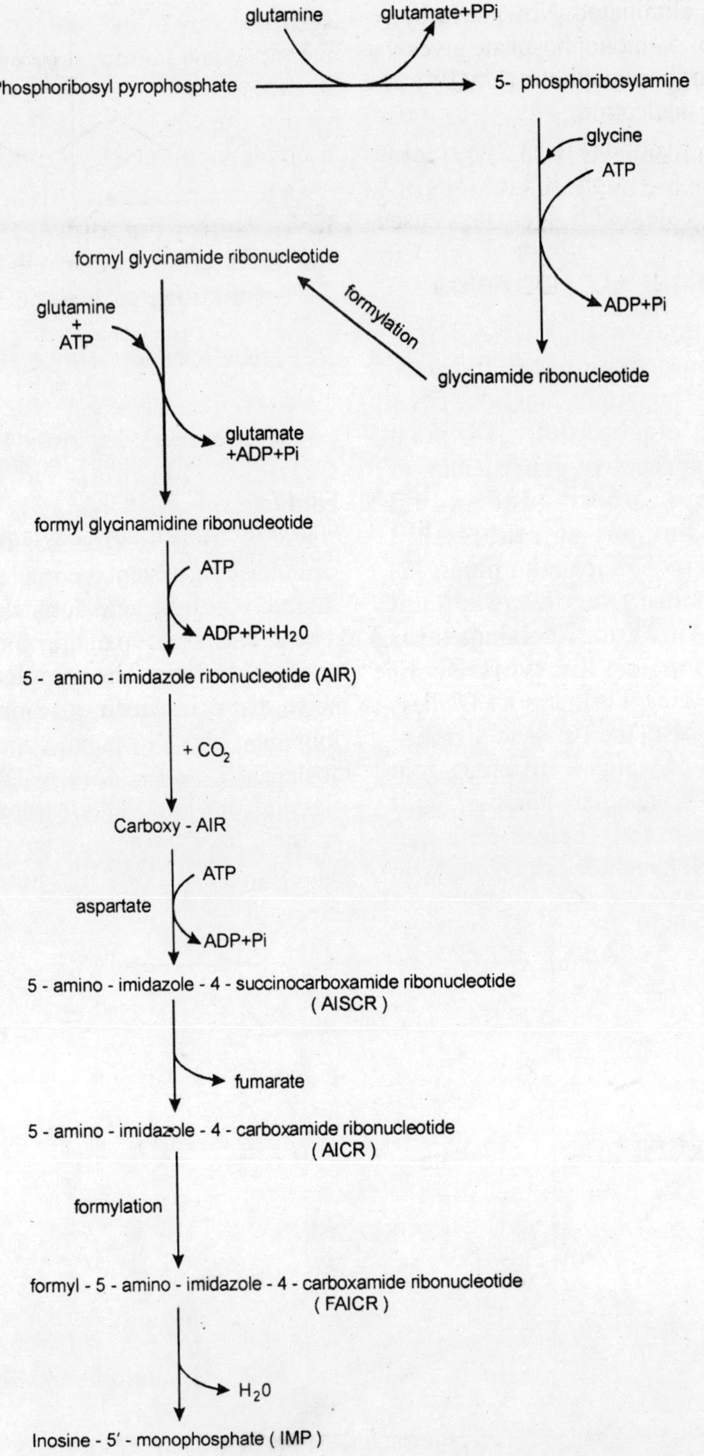

Fig13.4 : Biosynthesis of inosine 5′-monophosphate (IMP), the parent purine nucleotide

The formation of GMP from IMP is also a two stage reaction in which xanthosine 5'-monophosphate (XMP) is initially formed and then aminated to form GMP (Fig 13.5).

The two purine mononucleotides, AMP and GMP are phosphorylated by kinases through the diphosphate stage to give ATP and GTP.

BIOSYNTHESIS OF THE NUCLEIC ACIDS

It is now clearly known that DNA is the carrier of genetic information in living cells. To fulfil this vitally important function, DNA must have a number of properties. **(1) It must be stable so that successive generations of species maintain their individual characteristics, but not so stable that evolutionary changes cannot take place. (2) It must be able to store a very large amount of information. An animal cell contains genetic information for the synthesis of over a million proteins.** Furthermore DNA is the genetic material of all the 10^9 or so different living species, each of which is different from the others by at least one characteristic. (3) It must be duplicated exactly before each cell division, so that both daughter cells contain an accurate copy of the genetic information of the parent cells. (4) It must be expressed precisely in terms of protein synthesis as each cell grows so that the newly synthesized components are accurately produced.

An examination of the mechanism of DNA replication and protein synthesis at the molecular level reveals in detail how DNA functions as genetic material.

REPLICATION OF DNA i.e., DNA SYNTHESIS

The structure of DNA, with its two complementary strands led Watson and Crick to postulate a mechanism of replication which depends upon the base - pairing properties of the constituent nucleotides. Consider the small segment of double - stranded DNA as shown in Fig 13.6. The sequence of one strand is complementary to that in the other **that is adenine always pairs with thymine and guanine always with cytosine.** To allow such complementary base-pairing, the two strands of DNA must be anti-parallel, that is, if the orientation of one strand is in the 3' to 5' direction, then that of the other must be in the 5' to 3' direction (Fig13.6).

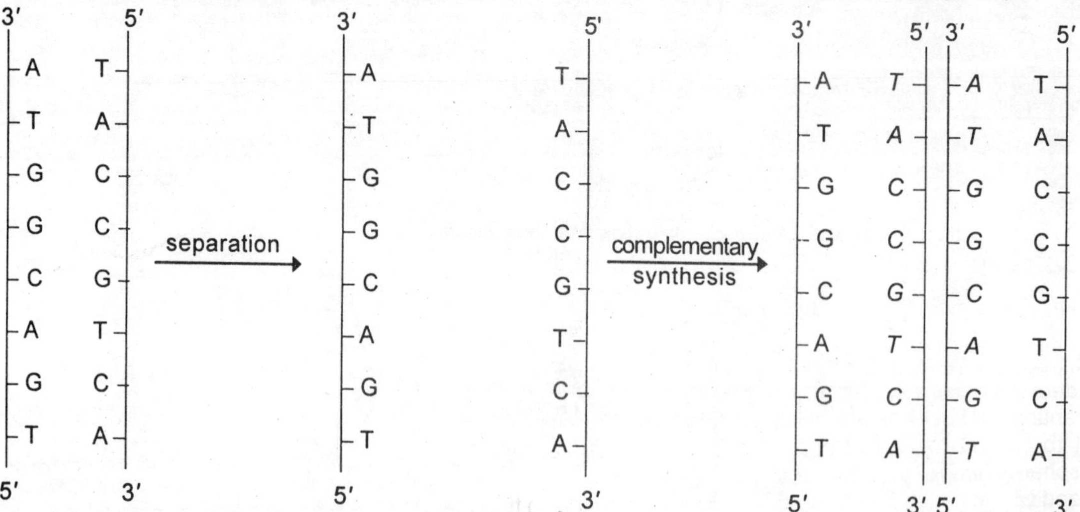

Fig. 13.6 : Schematic representation of DNA synthesis. The two strands separate and on each is built a new complementary strand (*italics*). The result is two indentical daughter DNA molecules, each of which is identical with the parental DNA molecule.

As a consequence of this complementary relationship, if the two strands are separated (Fig13.6); new complementary strands can be assembled on each, forming two identical double - stranded segment of DNA, each identical with the original.

Such replication is said to be semiconservative (one parental strand being conserved in each daughter molecule) and has been shown to be sequential, the two double stranded daughter molecules being synthesized progressively by a polymerizing enzyme which moves along the parental DNA molecule from one end to the other (Plates 13.1 and 13.2).

A more accurate representation of the process illustrated in Plates 13.1 and 13.2 is given in Fig 13.7 which takes into account the fact that native DNA is a double helix.

It is now known that this model of DNA replication is essentially correct but the nature of the polymerizing enzyme, probably part of a larger replicating complex, is unknown.

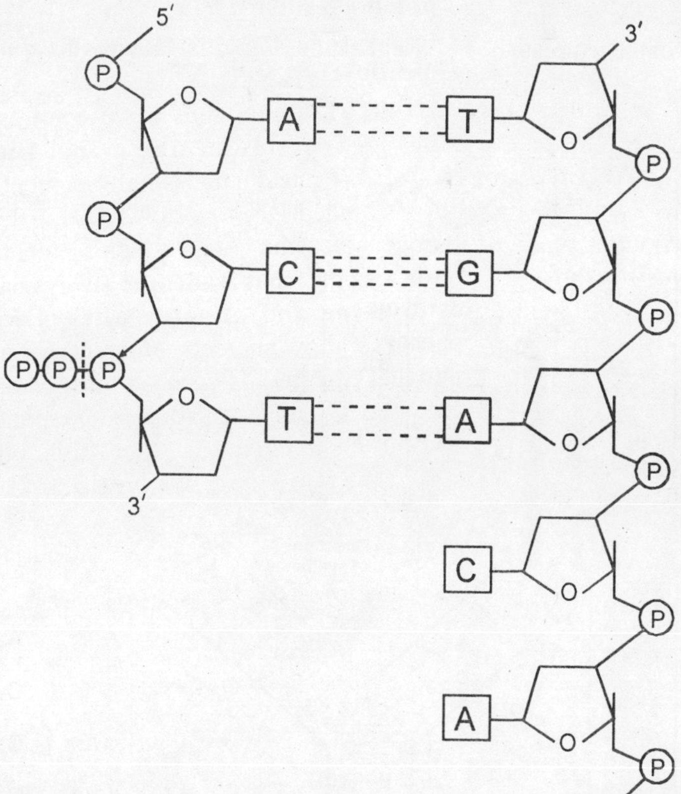

5′ 3′ P O A T O P P O C G O P P P P O T A O P 3′ C O P A O P 5′

Plate 13.1 Biosynthesis of DNA. A single- stranded template is shown on the right. Mononucleotides in the form of deoxyribonucleoside 5' triphosphates align themselves in appropriate sequence, and in keeping with the antiparallel orientation, along the template DNA. In the diagram, the nucleotide containing thymine is about to be linked to carbon-3' of the preceding nucleotide (containing cytosine), and inorganic pyrophosphate is about to be eliminated. In the same way, the next mononucleotide in the sequence to be synthesized will align itself opposite the cytosine nucleotide in the template; it will therefore be dGTP and the new chain is thus extended by one further unit. Dotted lines between the bases represent hydrogen bonds. A= adenine, C = cytosine, G = guanine, T = thymine and P = phosphate.

However, an enzyme discovered in 1957 by Arthur Kornberg and his colleagues, i.e. DNA polymerase (DNA nucleotidyltrans-ferase obviously closely related to the polymerizing enzyme of DNA replication. DNA polymerase catalyses the sequential polymerization of the deoxyribonucleotide **5'**-triphosphates (dATP, dCTP, dGTP and DTTP) in the presence of a template strand of DNA, to form a new complementary DNA strand (Plate 13.1). The 3′ hydroxyl of the growing strand reacts with the 5′-triphosphate group of the incoming deoxyribonucleotides are selected by complementarity with the base of the template strand.

The energy required during the formation of each 3′, 5′-phosphodiester bond of the polydeoxyribonucleotide is provided by the high energy bonds of the triphosphates as each monomer is incorporated into the new chain it loses its terminal pyrophosphate unit (PPi). The DNA template dictates the sequence of nucleotides in the newly synthesized strand, which is assembled in the 5′to 3′direction along the template, the template having an anti-parallel 3′to 5′orientation.

Replication (Fig 13.7) requires the coincident

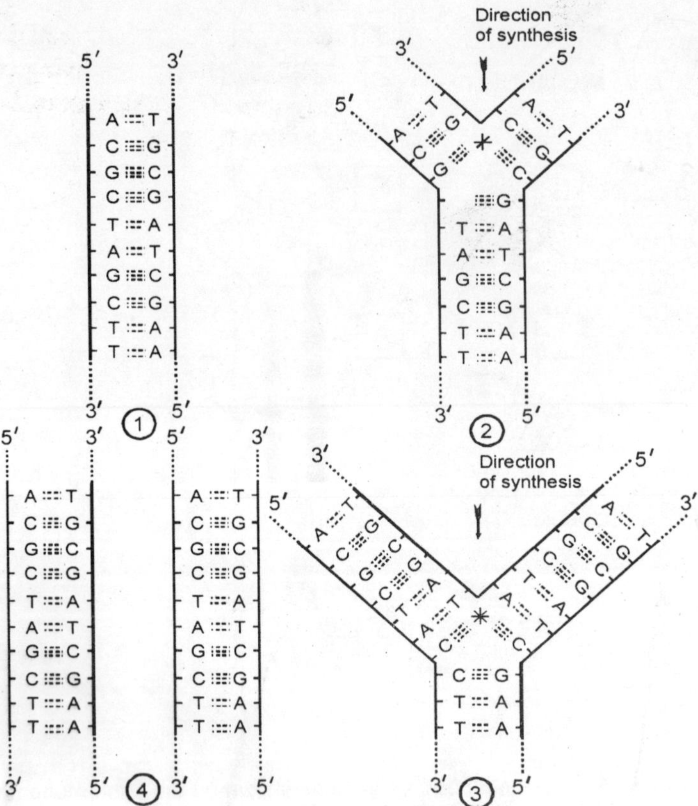

Plate13.2 : Replication of double- stranded DNA. 1. A small segment of double- stranded DNA showing the bases joined by hydrogen bonds. 2. An early phase of replication of the segment; newly synthesized DNA is shown in the diagram and the actual growing point is indicated by the asterisk. 3. A later stage of the replication process. 4. The two complete daughter segments are shown with the newly synthesized strands and appropriate complementary base- pairing. These double- stranded segments are identical with each other and with the parent segement as shown in 1.

synthesis of the two daughter strands, one in the 5′ to 3′ direction’ and the other in the 3′ to 5′ direction. **Kornberg’s DNA polymerase corresponds to the former, but no enzyme has been discovered which will synthesize a DNA strand in the 3' to 5' direction.**

DNA is very stable and is not synthesized in a non-dividing cell (that is there is no turnover). Furthermore, DNA replication is a very accurate process and consequently spontaneous mutations are very rare. If they occurred with anything more than an extremely low frequency, the daughter molecules of DNA would, after several generations, be quite different from the original parent molecule. In other words, there would be little resemblance between parent and offspring. **The frequency of mutation can be notably increased by means of certain agents such as ionizing radiation, ultraviolet radiation, alkylating agents and certain dyestuffs - all of which are known to alter the structure of DNA or interfere with normal replication.**

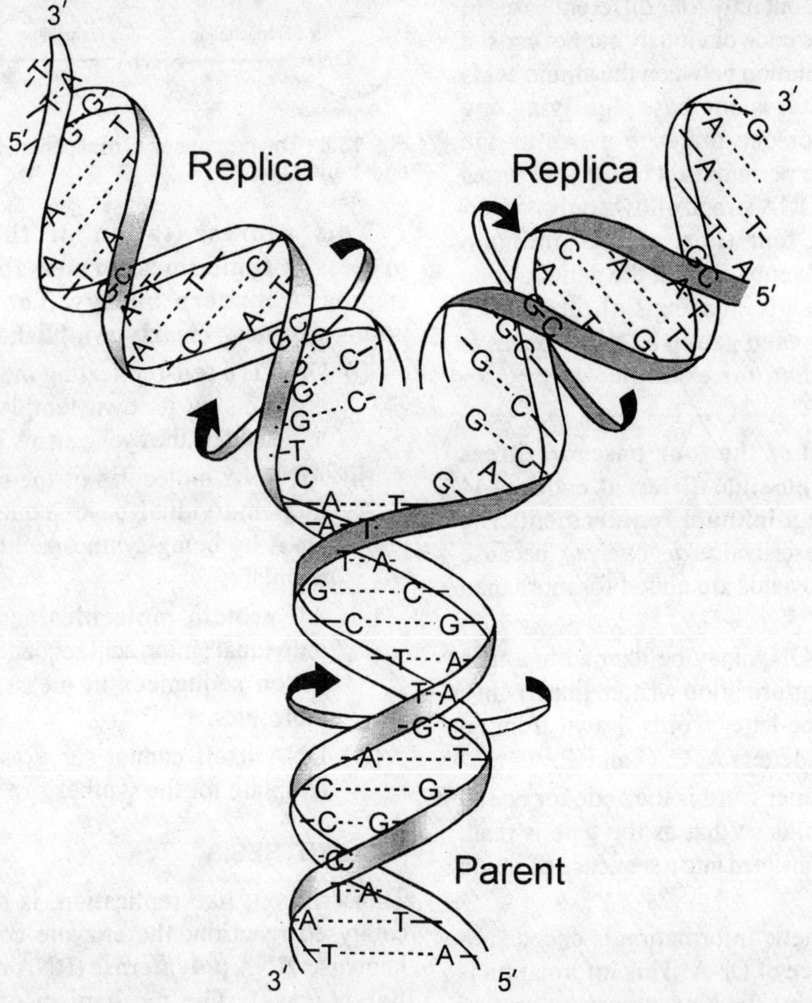

Fig.13.7 : A portion of native, double- helical DNA shown in the process of replication. The arrows indicate the directions of rotation that are necessary to allow unwinding of the parent helix with concomitant formation of the daughter helices. The two newly synthesized strands are growing in the downwards direction.

EXPRESSION OF GENETIC INFORMATION

The genetic information stored in DNA is known to reside in the linear sequence of bases in the molecule. Since genetic information in an organism is manifested mainly in the proteins synthesized by the organism, there must be some relationship between the base sequence in DNA and the amino acid sequence in proteins. In other words, the base sequence must constitute a code - **the genetic code** - that can be translated into protein. Since there are twenty different amino acids in proteins, but only four different bases in DNA, the genetic code obviously cannot consist of a one to one relation between the amino acids and the bases, **that is one base signifying one amino acid.** Nor can there be a two-to-one relation, because permutation of the four bases in twos along a DNA strand allows only $4^2 = 16$ different pairs, four short of the minimum requirement of twenty. In fact, the genetic code is translated linearly in groups of three bases along the DNA; **each group *of* three bases is known as a *codon,* for example:**

– C – T – A – | – A – C – T – | – A – G – C –

Permutation *of* the four bases in threes allows $4^3 = 64$ possible different codons, 44 in excess of the minimum requirement. The code has been described as *degenerate,* because almost all amino acids are coded for more than one codon.

The code in DNA may be likened to a tape which contains information written linearly in a language of three-letter words drawn from an alphabet of four letters A, C, G and T.

Each three-letter word is the code for one of the 20 amino acids so that as the tape is read, information is translated into a sequence of amino acids.

Thus the genetic information is encoded in the base sequence of DNA. This information is used to programme the biosynthesis of protein in two stages. In the first, the information is transcribed from DNA on to a large intermediate molecule of messenger RNA(mRNA). In the second stage, the messenger RNA- intermediary transports the information to the protein-synthesizing centres of the cell where the information is translated from the linear sequence of codons in the RNA into a linear sequence of amino acids which are concurrently polymerized into protein.

At this point, it is convenient to integrate these concepts with the replication of DNA in the form of Fig13.8.

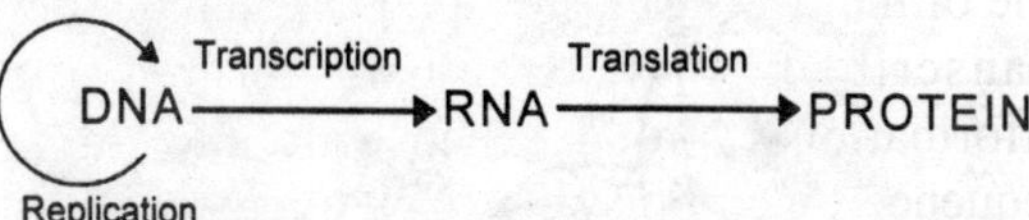

Fig. 13.8 : The processes of replication, transcription and translation

This representation of the overall process is sometimes termed the Central Dogma of modern biology. The following points are now clearly established.

(i) DNA is a self-replicating molecule, that is it acts as its own template. This is indicated by the cyclic arrow in Fig. 13.8.

(ii) All RNA molecules of the cell acquire their individual base sequences from DNA by being synthesized on DNA as template.

(iii) All protein molecules acquire their individual amino acid sequences from the codon sequences in messenger RNA molecules.

(iv) DNA itself cannot serve as the direct template for the synthesis of protein .

RNA SYNTHESIS

Transcription, like replication, is an enzyme-catalysed reaction; the enzyme concerned is known as **RNA polymerase (RNA nucleotidyl polymerase).** The mechanism of action of RNA polymerase is closely similar to that of DNA polymerase; in both, a DNA template and four nucleoside triphosphates are required.

Transcription differs from DNA replication in that (a) the triphosphates are ribonucleoside 5'triphosphates, (b) the product of the reaction is a single strand of RNA, and (c) the double stranded DNA template remains unaltered.

3′5′- phosphodiester bonds are synthesized and inorganic pyrophosphate is eliminated during the incorporation of the monomer units into the RNA product. An important feature of transcription by **RNA polymerase** is that only one of the two strands of the DNA template is transcribed; this strand is termed the informational strand because its nucleotide sequence determines the nucleotide sequence in the transcribed RNA. The DNA strand complementary to the coding strand has merely a supporting function which ensures that DNA is replicated accurately before cell division. The mechanism of transcription is illustrated in Plate 13.3 which shows that the enzyme RNA polymerase is engaged in transcribing the informational strand of a segment of DNA. It is clear that the RNA product has a nucleotide sequence complementary to that of the informational strand of the DNA template. The complementary arises because the process follows the usual rules of hydrogen bonding and antiparallelism. The RNA contains uracil (U) in place of thymine (T), but each of these pyrimidine bases forms the same specific hydrogen-bonding arrangement with adenine (A).

The detailed molecular mechanism of transcription (Fig 13.9) shows that the RNA polymerase starts transcribing at a specific point on the DNA template, and that the linear 5' triphosphate unit of the first nucleotide incorporated remains on the newly synthesized RNA product. The direction of transcription is therefore 5′→3′, that is, the 5′-end is synthesized first and the 3′-end last.

All of the RNA of the cell, the rRNA, the tRNA and the mRNA, is transcribed from DNA. Although the bulk of the RNA of anyone cell consists of ribosomal RNA (rRNA) and transfer RNA (tRNA) only a very small proportion of

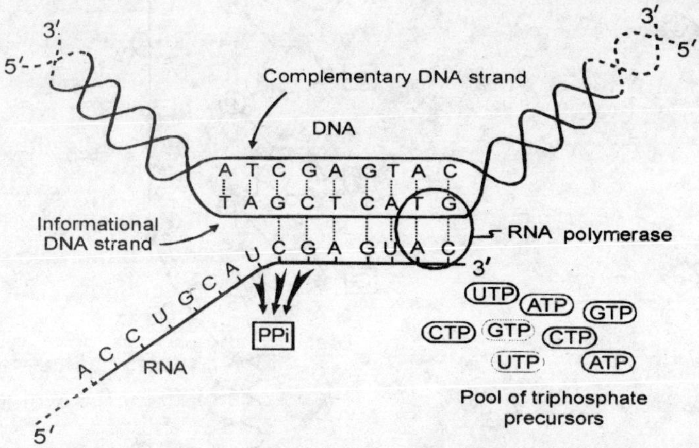

Plate 13.3 : Biosynthesis of RNA by transcription from a DNA template. The double- helical configuration of the DNA has become 'loosened' at the point of active transcription catalysed by the RNA polymerase. Transient base- pairing (A with U, C with G, G with C and T with A) is thus permitted between the coding strand of the DNA and the incoming ribonucleoside 5'- triphosphates. Polymerization of the monomers ensure by formation of 3', 5'-phosphodiester bonds. The polymerase advances to the right along the double-helix, opening new transcription sites. Concurrently, the section of 'loosened' DNA at the left resumes its original 'tight', double- helical configuration, and the product RNA peels off the template. Note that the nucleotide sequence of the RNA product is complementary to that of the coding strand. PPi = Inorganic pyrophosphate.

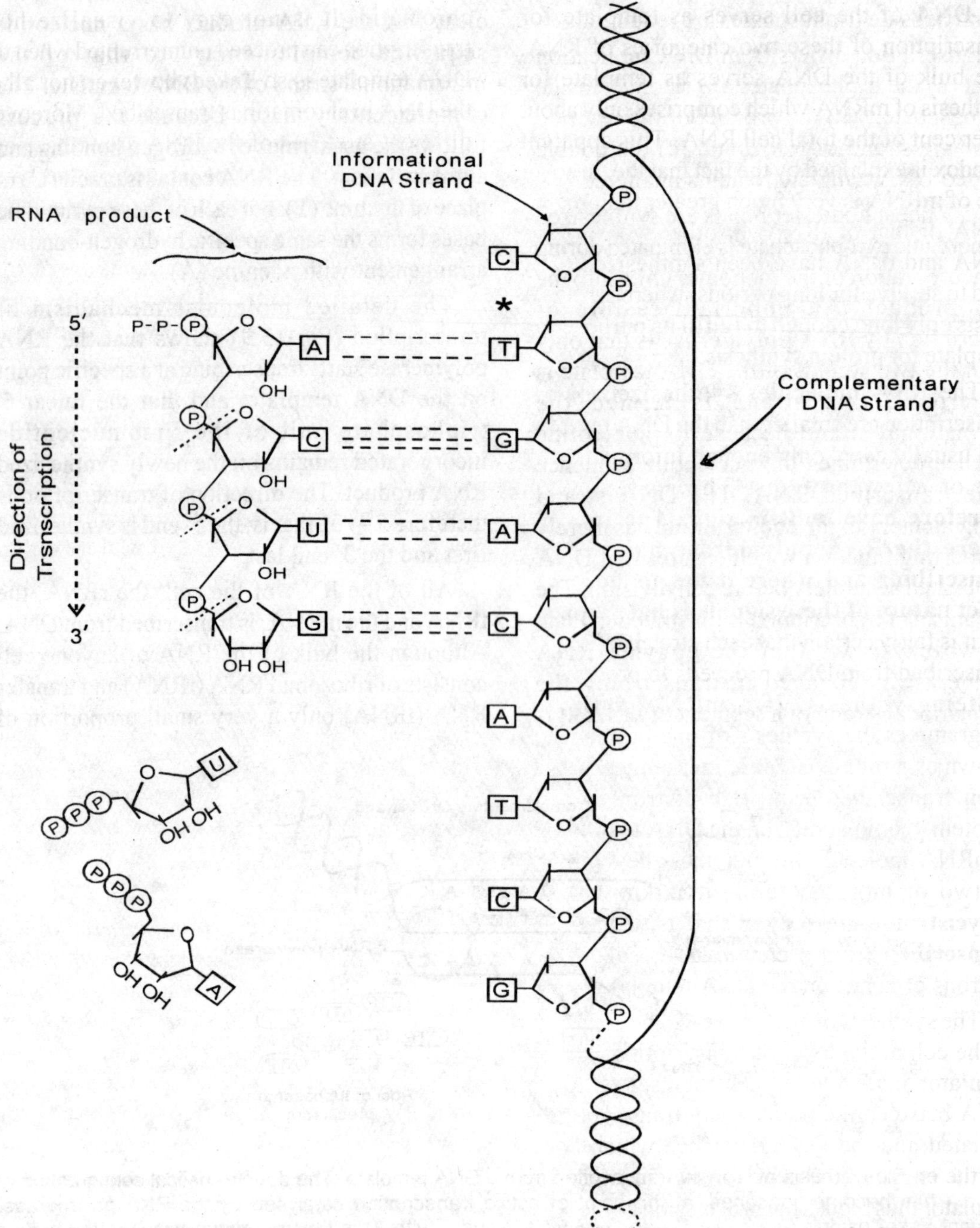

Fig 13.9 : Mechanism of biosynthesis of RNA on a DNA template. For the sake of clarity only one of the two strands (the coding strand) of the DNA is drawn out in detail in the region of transcription. This diagram should be compared with **Plate 13.3.** The initiation point for transcription is indicated by the asterisk. Note that the biosynthesis is proceeding in the 5′→3′ direction and in accordance with the rule of complementarity and antiparallelism. Ⓟ represents phosphate.

the DNA of the cell serves as template for transcription of these two categories of RNA. The bulk of the DNA serves as template for synthesis of mRNA which comprises only about 1 per cent of the total cell RNA. This apparent paradox is explained by the fact that the turnover rate of mRNA is very much greater than that of rRNA or that of tRNA. In other words, once rRNA and tRNA have been synthesized, they tend to survive for long periods, whereas mRNA exists only long enough to fulfill its purpose as a template for protein synthesis.

The RNA molecules synthesized during transcription are smaller than the DNA template and usually carry only enough information for one or a few proteins. **The system must therefore have built-in signals to indicate where the RNA polymerase has to start transcribing and where it has to stop. The exact nature of these signals is not yet clear,** but it is fairly certain that each stretch of mRNA transcribed from DNA proceeds to programme protein synthesis. If a mRNA molecule programmes the synthesis of one protein, it is known as a **monocistronic messenger,** having been transcribed from one cistron or gene (protein - coding unit), on the DNA template. If a mRNA molecule programmes the synthesis of two or more proteins, it is known as a **polycistronic messenger,** that is, it has been **transcribed** from a consecutive sequence of cistrons or genes on the DNA template.

The synthesis of an enzyme can be controlled in the cell at the level of transcription. Protein regulator molecules attach themselves to the DNA between the point where transcription is initiated and the DNA sequence which codes for the enzyme (the gene for the enzyme). The regulator thus blocks the progression of the RNA polymerase along the DNA and prevents the synthesis of mRNA from the gene.

In the cells of higher organisms the DNA is associated with histones and other proteins in a deoxyribonucleoprotein complex called chromatin. It is not easy to visualize how transcription can proceed uninterrupted when the DNA template is so linked; however, not all of the DNA in chromatin is transcribed. Moreover, different stretches of the DNA are transcribed in the cells of different tissues of the same animal. This implies that different species of mRNA are elaborated and go on to programme the synthesis of different proteins in various tissues, and in conformity with this, it is found that different cell types do indeed synthesize different sets of protein. For example, muscle cells (but no other cells) produce vast amounts of actin and myosin, and cells of the pancreas produce certain digestive enzymes not synthesized by the cells of other tissues. It is possible that the proteins in the chromatin mark certain regions of the DNA (different regions of the DNA in different tissues); thereby preventing transcription from these regions.

Since all cellular synthesis of RNA occurs on a DNA template, the process has been described as DNA-dependent synthesis of RNA and the. enzyme has been termed **DNA dependent RNA polymerase.** Events are quite different when a RNA-virus invades a cell. In these circumstances, the viral RNA serves as mRNA for the synthesis of virus-specific proteins and also as template for its own replication. Among the virus-specific proteins synthesized is a RNA polymerase which uses the parental viral RNA as template in a replicative reaction which synthesizes many daughter copies of the parent molecule. **This process is termed RNA-dependent synthesis of RNA and the virus-induced polymerase is called a RNA dependent RNA polymerase.**

NUCLEASES

Nucleases catalyse the hydrolysis of internucleotide bonds. Some are specific for DNA, and others for RNA, while some are capable of hydrolysing both types of nucleic acid. Nucleases specific for DNA are termed **deoxyribo-**

nucleases, and those specific for RNA are termed **ribonucleases.**

Some nucleases hydrolyse only the internucleotide bonds located at the ends of the nucleic acids, and thus release **mononucleotides,** one at a time, from the end. These enzymes are known as **exonucleases.** Some of these attack the internucleotide bonds consecutively from the 5′ - end of the nucleic acid, others from the 3' end. In contrast, other enzymes hydrolyse internucleotide bonds located at points throughout the length of the nucleic acid chains. These enzymes are termed **endonucleases.**

A well-known ribonuclease from bovine pancreas (pancreatic RNase) hydrolyses internucleotide bonds within RNA chains to give mono- and oligonucleotide products bearing 3′-phosphoryl groups. The specificity of this enzyme is such that bonds between purine nucleotides are not hydrolysed, bonds between adjacent pyrimidine nucleotides are hydrolysed; bonds between purine (Pu) nucleotides adjacent to pyrimidine (Py) nucleotides are hydrolysed only if the sequence in the RNA chain is 5′-Py-Pu-3′ and not 5′-Pu - Py-3′.

Endonucleases may hydrolyse internal internucleotide bonds in nucleic acids to produce oligonucleotides bearing either 3′- phosphoryl-terminal or 5′ phosphoryl-terminal groups. For example, a DNA-endonuclease from bovine pancreas (pancreatic DNase) has a **pH optimum of 7 to 8,** and hydrolyses **internucleotide** bonds in double-helical DNA (single-chain scission) to yield oligodeoxyribonucleotides terminated by 5′ - phosphoryl and 3′ - hydroxyl groups. **This enzyme has been termed deoxyribonuclease I. A DNA-endonuclease from bovine spleen has a pH optimum of 4.5 and hydrolyses both chains in double helical DNA at the same point (double chain scission)** to yield oligodeoxyribonucleotides terminated by 3′- phosphoryl and 5′ - hydroxyl groups. This enzyme has been termed **deoxyribonuclease II.**

Exonucleases may hydrolyse the terminal internucleotide bonds in nucleic acids to produce either nucleoside 3′ - monophosphates or nucleoside 5′ - monophosphates. **Well-known examples of exonucleases are the DNA exonucleases, (a) from bovine spleen, which starts at the 5′ - end of DNA chains and consecutively releases deoxyribonucleoside 3′ - monophosphates, and (b) from snake venom, which starts at the 3′ - end of DNA chains and consecutively releases deoxyribonucleoside 5′ - monophosphates** (these two enzymes have also been referred to as **phosphodiesterases).**

Some deoxyribonucleases show a preference for, or in some cases an absolute specificity for double - helical DNA, others show the reverse type of specificity, that is they prefer single stranded, or denatured DNA as substrate.

In summary, the nucleases show specificity in action that relates to one or more of the following:

(i) DNA and/or RNA as substrate;

(ii) exo- or endo-nucleolytic action;

(iii) 3' - or 5' - phosphoryl-terminal groups produced;

single-stranded and/or double-helical condition of the substrate.

Important functions of Nucleases

Nucleases are involved in many of the important reactions of DNA. They are required for the repair of damaged DNA, for genetic recombination, where sections of the double-stranded DNA of homologous chromosomes are interchanged, and also probably for the complex process of DNA replication. Endo - and exonucleascs with lower specificity also catalyse the hydrolysis of nucleic acids to nucleotides, in the living cell (for example, degradation of mRNA) and in the course of degradation of dead cells. Foodstuff derived from cellular material also contains nucleic acids which are degraded by pancreatic nucleases in the duodenum.

REPAIR OF DAMAGED DNA

Single-strand scissions in double-stranded DNA which have a 3′ - hydroxyl group on one side and a 5′ - phosphate group on the other (like those formed by pancreatic DNase can be repaired by the enzyme **polynucleotide ligase** (Fig 13.10).

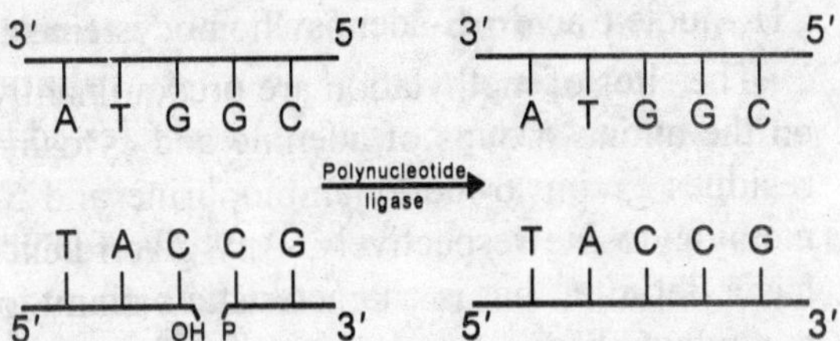

Fig 13.10: The mode of action of polynucleotide ligase.

Similar breaks are produced in DNA in vivo by X-irradiation and many of them are repaired by a polynucleotide ligase.

Ultraviolet radiation, on the other hand, gives rise to thymine dimers in DNA. Absorption of energy at 260 rim causes the 5, 6 double bonds of adjacent thymine bases in one strand of the DNA to rearrange and form dimers (Fig 13.11).

Thymine dimers locally distort the regular form of the DNA double helix and block replication. The reaction is enzymically reversible in the presence of light, but in the dark such thymine dimers are removed by a complicated series of reactions (Fig 13.12).

An endonuclease recognizes the distortion in the double helix and forms a single strand scission (3′ - hydroxyl, 5′ - phosphate) on the 5′ side of the thymine dimer. An exonuclease, working from the scission in the 5′ to 3′ direction, removes nucleotides and the thymine dimer. Concurrently, a DNA polymerase (with the properties of Kornberg's DNA polymerase, adds nucleotides sequentially (using the deoxyribonucleoside triphosphates, dATP, dCTP, dGTP and dTTP) starting at the free 3′ - hydroxyl of the original scission, and using the other strand of the double helix as template. Eventually, polynucleotide ligase joins the gap left by the joint action of the exonuclease and the DNA polymerase. The product has the same structure as the DNA prior to ultraviolet irradiation. This process, which is probably carried out by a complex of enzymes, is summarized in Fig 13.12.

Repair can be envisaged as the continual monitoring of the DNA by the repair complex, which cuts out and replaces irregularities in the double helix. **A heritable disease in man,**

Fig. 13.11: The formation of a thymine dimer under the influence of ultraviolet light. Two adjacent thymine residues (left) in DNA become linked together as shown on the right.

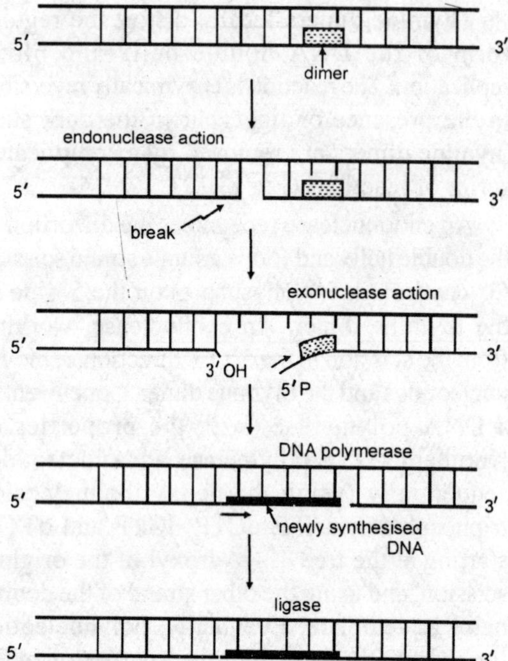

Fig. 13.12 : The repair of damaged DNA. An endonuclease cuts the affected strand on the 5' side of the dimer. An exonuclease then excises a length of the affected strand including the dimer leaving a gap which is filled in by the polymerase. The final join between the newly synthesized DNA filling the gap, and the remainder of the original strand is brought about by the ligase.

xeroderma pigmentosum, which in homozygous individuals is characterized by an extreme sensitivity to sunlight and the eventual development of multiple carcinomas on the exposed parts of the body, is caused by a defect in DNA repair. The lesion has been identified with the absence of the specific endonuclease which forms single-strand scissions as the first step in the repair process.

ENZYMIC MODIFICATION OF NUCLEIC ACIDS

Some enzymes can modify the nucleic acids at the polynucleotide level. **Thus, after synthesis of nucleic acids, methylation, glucosylation, phosphorylation, acylation, thiolation and other alterations of the macromolecule may take place. Of these reactions, methylation is quantitatively the most important.**

Methylation of DNA and RNA is affected by specific enzymes **(methyltransferases)** which recognize not only the ribo- or deoxyribo-type of nucleic acid but also specific nucleotides at specific sites within the nucleic acid chain. Only a small proportion of the bases is methylated. The general reaction is:

nucleic acid + S-adenosylmethionine ⟶
CH_3-nucleic acid + S-adenosylhomocysteine

The sites of methylation are predominantly on the amino groups of adenine and cytosine residues giving 6-methylaminopurine and 5-methylcytosine respectively. Any given DNA has a definite, that is characteristic amount of methylated bases.

tRNA contains a number of methylated bases and also contains methyl groups at the 2' hydroxyl position of the ribose moiety at certain specific sites in the polynucleotide chain.

CATABOLISM OF NUCLEOTIDES

Nucleotidases and nucleosidases

Some of these enzymes have very low specificities and hydrolyse both 5' - monophosphates and 3′ - monophosphates, while others display a much higher degree of specificity, degrading only the 5′- or the 3′-monophosphates. **Nucleotidases are known which hydrolyse the phosphate from one specific nucleotide only.**

The collective action of these enzymes gives rise to pentose, pentose phosphate, and to the free purine and pyrimidine bases.

Catabolism of pyrimidines. The pyrimidine bases are catabolized in mammalian tissues by preliminary reduction of uracil and thymine to the corresponding dihydro-derivatives, followed by ring opening to give the appropriate ureido-acid, and removal of ammonia and carbon

uracil ⟶ dihydro uracil ⟶ β–ureido propionic acid ⟶ $NH_2CH_2CH_2COOH$ (β- alanine)

thymine ⟶ dihydro thymine ⟶ β - ureido isobutyric acid ⟶ $NH_2CH_2CH(CH_3)COOH$ β - amino isobutyric acid

Fig 13.13 The catabolism of pyrimidine bases

dioxide to give β-alanine or its methylated derivative β-aminoisobutyric acid (Fig. 13.13).

Catabolism of purines. The purine bases arising from degradation of the nucleic acids are conveyed in the blood to the liver where they are catabolized still further through a well-known series of changes resulting in the formation of uric acid (Fig.13.14). Adenine is deaminated by **adenine deaminase** (adenase) to yield hypoxanthine.Guanine is deaminated by **guanine deaminase (guanase)** to give xanthine. Further oxidation is brought about by **xanthine oxidase** in the liver. This enzyme oxidizes hypoxanthine to xanthine, and xanthine to uric acid which, in primates, is excreted by the kidney. **The amount of uric acid excreted per day in human urine varies widely from 0.1 to 2.0 g.**

Uric acid is excreted in large amounts by birds and reptiles, but in them it is the end product not only of purine catabolism but also of protein catabolism. **Instead of excreting urea, they excrete uric acid as a semisolid paste.** They can thus conserve water by avoiding the necessity of producing urine in the form of a dilute aqueous solution.

Human blood normally contains 3.0 to 6.0 mg of uric acid per 100 ml. This value tends to rise whenever cells are being destroyed and nucleoprotein liberated. **Raised levels are therefore encountered in such conditions as leukaemia, polycythaemia, and in pneumonia during the process of resolution. In chronic renal disease, the excretion of uric acid, like that of other nitrogenous compounds, is impaired and retention of uric acid occurs. Probably the highest values for uric acid in plasma are found in gout immediately before an acute attack.** In this disease, salts of uric acid are actually deposited in the tissues, causing the typical chalky swellings **(tophi)** but it is not clear why such large amounts of uric acid should be formed in gouty persons; there may be a defect in the feed-back control of the enzyme that forms 5′-phosphoribosylamine (PRA), a precursor of purine nucleotides. The disorder is found mainly in males and appears to be genetically determined. **Gout may be controlled effectively by the substance allopurinol which inhibits xanthine oxidase and so**

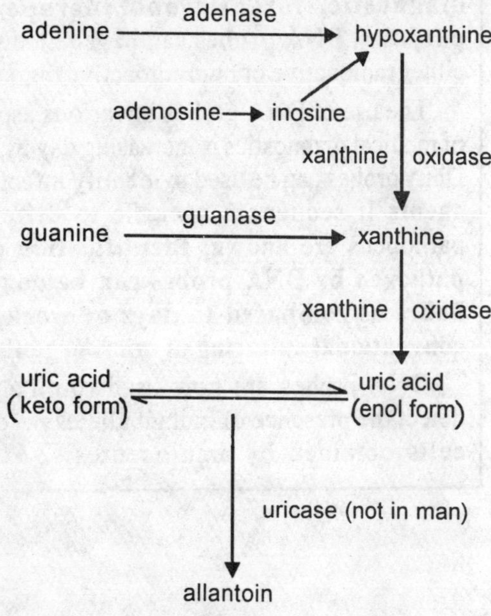

Fig. 13.14 The catabolism of purine bases

prevents the formation uric acid. The end products of purine metabolism excreted in the urine of patients treated with allopurinol are the much less insoluble compounds i.e., hypoxanthine and xanthine.

Most mammals, apart from man and other primates, oxidize uric acid further by the action of uricase to give allantoin. **Hydrolysis of allantoin by the enzyme allantoinase yields allantoic acid, the end-product of purine catabolism in certain teleost fishes.** In most fishes and in amphibians, however, allantoic acid is hydrolysed to glyoxylic and urea and in these species purine catabolism does not proceed further. Some marine invertebrates degrade urea to ammonia and carbon dioxide and in these species, the original purine- nitrogen is excreted as ammonia. The relationship of allantoin to these other metabolites is as shown below.

Allantoin

Allantoic acid

Urea

Glyoxylic acid

Diagnostic and Clinical applications of DNA

DNA probes: The ability to isolate specific fragments of DNA containing known sequences of genes gives rise to **DNA probes which can be used for a variety of diagnostic, forensic and therapeutic purposes. DNA probes** can be labelled with either radioactive or nonradioactive markers.

The use of DNA probes in various aspects of medical diagnostics is increasing day by day. DNA probes can be used to identify infectious agents if sequences specific to different pathogens are known. **Identification of a pathogen by DNA probes can be done in hours as compared to days or weeks by conventional culturing of microorganisms.**

DNA probes are now used routinely to detect the presence of mutant alleles in foetal cells obtained by amniocentesis. **Many inherited disorders, such as sickle cell anaemia, cystic fibrosis, Huntington's disease, Duchenne's muscular dystrophy and dozens of other mendelian (single-gene) disorders, can** now be diagnosed in foetus and adults.

In addition to inherited disorders, DNA probes are used to detect the presence of active oncogenes or inactive tumor suppressor genes in cancerous tissues removed from patients.

Southern Blot Analysis :

The **southern blot (named after the inventor, E.M. Southern)** is a method for hybridizing one or more labelled DNA probes to a large number of DNA fragments and discriminating them. The procedure depends upon the ability of denatured DNA single strands to bind tightly to nitrocellulose under certain conditions.

CHAPTER 14

METABOLISM OF INORGANIC ELEMENTS (MINERALS) AND WATER METABOLISM

MINERALS

The main minerals that are required by the human body are listed below in the Table 14.1 along with the daily requirement and the deficiency symptoms. Main minerals are sodium, potassium, magnesium, calcium, iron, copper, chloride, phosphate, iodine and fluoride. Requirement for Na^+ and Cl^- reflects the fact that these are the main ions excreted in urine and sweat; whereas requirement for iron is determined largely by the rate of its excretion in the faeces. The ions are digested in a number of ways. The bulk of Na^+ and Cl^- is eaten in the form of salt. The other ions are present either as free salts in food and water, examples K^+, Mg^{2+}, Ca^{2+} and F^- or bound to other molecules, examples Fe^{2+} Zn^{2+}, PO^-_4 and I^-.

Each ion performs a number of functions in

Table14.1: Mineral requirements and deficiency symptoms

Sl. No.	Ion	Approximate daily requirement	Deficiency symptoms
1.	Na^+ (Sodium)	5g; 200 m mol	Dehydration, acidosis
2.	K^+(Potassium)	3g; 75 m mol	Acidosis, renal damage, cardiac arrest
3.	Mg^{2+} (Magnesium)	0.3g; 15 m mol	Muscular tremor,mental depression
4.	Ca^{2+} (Calcium)	0.8g; 20 m mol	Rickets in children and osteomalacia in adults
5.	Fe^{2+} (Iron)	10 mg; 200 μmol	Anaemia
6.	Zn^{2+} (Zinc)	15mg; 200 μmol	Anaemia, stunted growth
7.	Cu^{2+} (Copper)	3mg; 50 μmol	Anaemia (hypochromic), various nervous lesions
8.	Cr (Chloride)	7g; 200 mmol	Alkalosis
9.	Phosphate	0.8g; 30mmol	Renal rickets
10.	Iodine	0.1 mg; 1 μmol	Endemic goitre (hypothyroidism)
11.	F (Fluoride)	2mg; 100 μmol	Dental caries

the body.

A requirement for chromium has been reported, **and in animals selenium is required for satisfactory reproduction but is toxic if taken in excess.**

The most important inorganic requirements for the human beings are Na, K, Ca, Mg, Fe, Cu, Zn, Mo, Cl, I, and P. (Table 14.1). Sulphur as sulphate is essential for the formation of certain body constituents, but it is always organic sulphur, in the form of sulphur-containing amino acids, which is oxdized to sulphate *in vivo.* Co, as far as known at present, is only necessary in the form of vitamin B_{12}. Se is a constituent of glutathione peroxidase. The involvement of Cr and V in normal human physiology is not yet proven. **Fluoride does not form part of the normal body requirements, but it should be added regularly in traces to drinking water as a preventive factor of dental caries.**

Potassium is the main inorganic cation present in the intracellular fluid, as distinct from plasma and extracellular water. Its concentration is about 3.2 g (80 meq) per kg (muscle). It also occurs to the extent of about 4 meq per litre in plasma. Since it is universally abundant in foodstuffs, whether of plant or animal origin, there is usually no difficulty in supplying the daily requirements, probably in the order of 1 g per day (20-30 meq). Disturbances of potassium metabolism may occur, particularly in derangements of the adrenal cortical gland.

Besides the main minerals as mentioned above, our body also requires large number of elements called as **'trace elements'** in minor quantity for proper functioning. **These include sulphur, zinc, manganese, cobalt, molybdenum, selenium, chromium, copper, iodine, iron, etc.**

SODIUM

It is the main ion of the plasma and other extracellular fluids. Under normal dietary conditions, human beings are not subject to the deficiency of sodium. However, excessive diarrhoea, pernicious vomiting or extreme sweating over a long period may bring about the deficiency of sodium and chloride. Now a days, it is a common practice to supply extra amount of sodium chloride either in the form of salt water or salt tablets to those, who are subjected/ exposed to excessive heat like **labourers, workers, rikshaw pullers etc.** Normal sodium chloride consumption of an individual is nearly 10g per day (about 4g of sodium) which is supplied easily by the dietary ingredients. This is many times the actual requirement. In health, excess salt consumed is excreted by the kidneys.

Main functions of sodium are:

(a) It maintains the osmotic pressure i.e. osmolarity throughout the body. Osmolarity is maintained at approximately 0.3 mol/l (it is approximately made up of 0.15 mol/l of Na^+ and 0.15 mol/l of Cl^-).

(b) It maintains the normal state of acid-base balance.

(c) It maintains the normal state of water balance.

(d) It plays a role in gaseous transport.

> An average adult requires about 4 g Na^+ per day (150-200 meq), of which about 1g (50 meq) is in foodstuffs before flavouring is added. Intakes lower than 50 meq may be tolerated with difficulty, but the requirement may be greatly increased in many circumstances, particularly when a hot climate or prolonged exercise have caused a considerable loss of Na^+ in perspiration. Insufficient Na^+ intake can give rise to heat exhaustion or heat stroke, characterized by muscular weakness, nausea and fever. The excretion of sodium is carefully regulated by renal mechanisms under the control chiefly of aldosterone, and may be abnormal in the diseases of the adrenal gland.

(e) It maintains the muscle and nerve irritability at the proper level.

(f) In blood plasma sodium chloride has got an outstanding function of keeping the globulins in physical solution. It also regulates the degree of hydration of the plasma proteins, vis-a-vis the viscosity of blood.

(g) Gastric HCl is derived from the sodium chloride of the blood.

Saline depletion causes cramps, weakness and faintness and clinical features of 'dehydration', diminished tissue turgor, hypotension and peripheral circulatory failure.

Saline overloading is most often the result of a primary disturbance of the function of the heart, kidneys, or liver which leads to complex causes like oedema and raised central venous pressure. Occasionally, it is caused by the excess intravenous infusion of saline.

POTASSIUM

It is a very important mineral for various functions of the human body. Under normal dietary conditions, human beings do not suffer from potassium deficiency. The human potassium intake is around 2 to 4 g per day which is supplied easily by the dietary items that we eat daily. Again this is far more than our requirement, and the excess is excreted in the urine. It is the principal cation of intracellular fluid. Its metabolism is regulated by the hormone named as ***aldosterone.***

Important functions of potassium in human body are as given below:

(a) It maintains the osmotic pressure (osmolarity) in its normal range throughout the body.

(b) It helps in maintaining the normal state of acid base balance.

(c) It maintains water balance.

(d) It plays an important role in gaseous transport.

(e) It helps in maintaining muscle and nerve irritability at the proper level.

(f) Like sodium chloride, potassium chloride has also an outstanding function of keeping the globulins in physical solution and also helps in the regulation of the degree of hydration of the plasma proteins which is eventually very important for proper viscosity of the blood:

(g) Potassium is required by several enzymes of glycolysis and other pathways. It may be required for nuclear activity and also for protein synthesis.

***Hypokalaemia* causes tiredness, muscle weakness, paralysis, mental confusion and polyuria. It is commonly noticed after the prolonged administration of powerful diuretic drugs.** Such drugs provoke an increased flow of urine by inhibiting the activity of enzymes in the renal tubules that are responsible for the absorption of Na^+ and Cl^-. When, however, there is low dietary intake of Na^+ and high level of circulating aldosterone, these diuretics promote the exchange of Na^+ for K^+ in the distal tubule and thus lead to an increased excretion of K^+. Chronic diarrhoea and repeated vomiting also are responsible for **hypokalaemia.**

Potassium is toxic in high amounts (hyperkalaemia) by virtue of the fact that it stops the heart beat and thus leads to death. Besides, hyperkalaemia also causes small bowel ulcers.

MAGNESIUM

Adult human body contains nearly 20-25 g magnesium. It is an indispensable constituent of all living cells. About 60 percent of the magnesium of the body remains present in the bones. In muscles magnesium exceeds calcium as regards amount, whereas in blood, the reverse is true. In blood it remains very constant.

Biological functions: Magnesium ions act as activator for number of enzymes such as hexokinases, phosphorylases enolase, alkaline phosphatase, DNA polymerase, phosphoglucomutase, etc.

Absorption and excretion: About one-third or less of the magnesium in the diet is absorbed. In a state of balance, the amount of magnesium in the urine equals that absorbed, which in normal men has been found to average 162 ± 45 mg per day. Faecal magnesium represents that which remains unabsorbed. High dietary intake of fat, calcium and phosphorus reduces its absorption and so is the condition with alkaline food.

It is excreted both in urine and faeces. Nearly 70% of it is excreted via faeces. Intake of alkaline food reduces its excretion via urine.

Urine is the principal route of its excretion; most magnesium filtered by the glomeruli is reabsorbed by the renal tubules.

Requirement:

Its daily requirement is 250 - 300 mg.

Sources:

It is found in such amount in plant foods and meat that there is little possibility of the diet being inadequate in it. However, the main sources include meat, eggs, green leafy vegetables, potato, cereals, fruits, etc.

Deficiency symptoms: These may be observed in chronic alcoholics, uraemics, tetany, children suffering from kwashiorkor, pregnancy (particularly toxaemia of pregnancy), rickets, diabetic acidosis, diarrhoea and vomiting. Its deficiency causes depression, hyperirritability (muscle spasm or convulsions), cardiac arrhythmias, muscular weakness and convulsions. Its normal level in blood is from 1-3 mg/dl.

Hypermagnesaemia: Excess magnesium in the body can occur when absorption from the gut exceeds excretion by the kidneys, as happens in renal insufficiency. Its pharmacological effects are characterized by:

(i) Depression of the central nervous system
(ii) Depression of the cardiovascular system
(iii) Depression of the blood pressure

IRON

Introduction and Storage:

Our body contains nearly 4 g iron; nearly 70% of which remains present in blood in the form of **haemoglobin** or similar structures such as **myoglobin. Small amount of iron acts as cofactors in many enzyme reactions, notably those of oxidation. The remaining, about 25% is stored in the following:**

(i) Liver
(ii) Reticuloendothelial system
(iii) Spleen, and
(iv) Bone marrow, bound to protein

Nearly 3 mg of iron is found in transit in blood plasma which remains bound largely to a β-globulin called as **transferrin.** Iron is found in the body in two forms, i.e., the essential iron and the storage iron.

Absorption: Its absorption occurs mainly in the stomach and the duodenum. Normally nearly 6.5% of the dietary iron is absorbed. The absorption may be increased by 20 percent in mensurating and pregnant women. Its absorption from the food depends upon several factors such as the form of iron and other constituents present in the diet. **Alcohol, hydrochloric acid, Vitamin C, etc. promote its absorption while tea decreases it.** The amount absorbed depends upon the individual's need for iron.

The well known mechanism for absorption of iron in the mucosal cells is known as **mucosal block theory.** After digestion, iron present in the diet gets converted into the ferrous form (Fe^{2+}) by the H^+ and the reducing substances, such as vitamin C present in the intestinal lumen.

It is the only form in which iron is absorbed. Transfer of iron from the intestinal lumen into mucosa is an energy dependent process. After absorption Fe^{2+} is oxidised to Fe^{3+} and combines with apoferritin which is converted to ferritin. Apoferritin has got a very rapid turnover which is degraded and reformed when the absorption of iron takes place. The high concentration of ferritin in the mucosal cell further blocks the absorption of iron.

Iron from ferritin (Fe^{3+}) is reduced to Fe^{2+} and passes into the blood capillaries which is again oxidised to Fe^{3+} and combines with apotransferrin for its conversion to transferrin, the form in which iron is transported in plasma. The excess of iron which cannot be stored as ferritin is then stored in liver as **haemosiderin.** When excessive haemoglobin iron is given repeatedly to an individual by transfusion then it results into excess storage **(haemosiderosis).** In iron- deficiency anaemia, utilization of iron is increased considerably; under this condition average absorption of dietary iron increases to 20% as compared to nearly 6.5% under normal conditions.

The oxidation of Fe^{2+} to Fe^{3+} is catalysed by ferroxidase I (ceruloplasmin) and ferroxidase II. Ferro-reductases reduce Fe^{3+} iron to Fe^{2+} form. This oxidation and reduction of iron is essential as it remains present in the Fe^{2+} form in haemoglobin whereas in the Fe^{3+} form in ferritin and transferrin.

Iron is used with great economy in the body. Daily destruction of the red blood cells (RBCs) contributes nearly 25 mg of iron to the iron pool which is stored as ferritin and reused whenever required for the synthesis of haemoglobin.

Excretion of iron gets increased particularly in the hot moist climate which causes **iron deficiency anaemia.** Normally, its excretion takes place through the following routes:

a) Faecal: (The unabsorbed iron is excreted via faeces which is nearly 90% of the food iron).
b) Renal: (Nearly 0.05 mg/day through urine).
c) Dermal : (0.5 - 1.8 mg/day through sweat)
d) Menstrual : (35-70 ml per period, average daily loss would amount to 0.5 to 1.0 mg/ day).
e) Gestational: (iron is lost by mother during pregnancy. About 300 mg of iron is transferred to the foetus).
f) Lactational: (0.5 - 0.7 mg, if 400 - 600 ml milk is lactated).

Besides the above, iron loss also occurs through hair clippings, combing and nail clippings which amounts to nearly 1.2 mg per year (1 to 5 µg/day).

Plasma Iron level and its variations

a) Males: 80 to 175 µg per 100 ml
b) Females: 60 to 160 µg per 100 ml

An increase in the concentration is often found in **haemochromatosis,** acute infective hepatitis, etc. whereas its low values are found in iron-deficiency anaemias.

Biological functions:

It plays indispensable role in human body. Its main functions are:

(i) It is involved in the transport of oxygen by haemoglobin and haemoerythrin.
(ii) It is involved in the electron transfer reactions including oxidative phosphorylation.
(iii) It is involved in the synthesis of DNA (as an essential component of ribonucleotide reductase).
(iv) It is involved in the catalysis of oxidation by oxygen and hydrogen peroxide.
(v) It is involved in the decomposition of harmful derivatives of oxygen notably peroxide and superoxide.

(vi) Besides, it also plays a very important role in the fixation of nitrogen and hydrogen.

(vii) It is a component of several proteins such as haemoglobin, myoglobin, peroxidases, catalases, cytochromes and iron requiring enzymes, e.g. xanthine oxidase, acyl CoA **dehydrogenase** and NADH reductase.

(viii) It is also required as a cofactor for various enzymes like aconitase, succinic dehydrogenase, ribonucleotide reductase, etc.

Body Iron: It remains present in the body as a part of several compounds which play role in respiration. Its total amount varies from 2-6 g in healthy adults.

Transport: It is transported in the body by a specific iron binding β_1-globulin called as transferrin (siderophilin). It performs the functions of selective removal of iron from reticuloendothelial cells and intestinal mucosa and selective delivery of iron to the erythron and placenta. It is a glycoprotein having a molecular weight of 80,000 and binds two atoms of ferric iron. The average transferrin content of plasma is about 250-350 mg per 100 ml. Since each gram of transferrin can bind about 1.25 mg of iron, therefore, the total iron binding capacity is approximately 250-450 μg/ 100 ml of plasma.

Storage: It is stored intracellularly as **ferritin** and **haemosiderin,** mainly in the liver, spleen and bone marrow. Approximately 25% of iron (600 to 1500 mg) in the body is in the form which does not participate in active metabolic process but represents a reserve which can be mobilised whenever there is acute need.

Hookworm infestation leading to chromic blood loss is an important cause of iron deficiency especially in the rural population engaged in agricultural work. Each worm causes a loss of nearly **0.3 ml blood per day. This may be one of the important causative factors in the tribal areas of India.**

It is stored in the ferric form but the release of iron appears to be in the ferrous form.

Iron toxicity: The presence of the excess of iron in the body results in its deposition as **ferritin** and **haemosiderin** in various tissues such as liver, spleen, bone marrow, skin etc which is called as **haemosiderosis.**

Deficiency disorders (iron deficiency):

It is the result of an imbalance between iron assimilation and its loss. Deficiency of iron leads to anemia which is a common feature in children, adolescent girls and females of the child bearing age, particularly in the developing countries like India.

Bantu siderosis :

In the African tribe Bantus, iron deficiency anaemia even in women is unknown, absorption of food iron is very high and considerable haemosiderin is present in liver (siderosis). This has been explained on the basis of the facts that their staple diet is corn (high iron, low phosphate) **which is cooked in iron pots (high in iron) and they consume lot of alcohol which enhances iron absorption.**

Following are the signs and symptoms of anaemia:

(a) Dullness

(b) Inactiveness

Haemochromatosis :

It is a genetic disease transmitted by autosomal recessive gene in which the afflicted person has inherited ability to absorb much greater percentage of food iron which is then deposited in the **skin, pancreas,** and **liver,** giving rise to **bronze colouration, diabetes mellitus** and **cirrhosis** respectively.

Although breast milk is a poor source of iron. Prolonged lactation results in a serious drain on the **iron reserves.** The output of the breast milk during the first two years of lactation is nearly 400-600 g per day and average iron content is 0.12 mg/100 g which gives a daily excretion of 0.5 - 0.7 mg iron through the milk for several months. Thus menstrual irregularities, repeated pregnancies and prolonged lactations apart from dietary inadequacy are the chief causes of iron deficiency anaemia in Indian women.

(c) Loss of appetite
(d) Poor growth
(e) Fatigueness
(f) Decreased exercise tolerance
(g) Weakness
(h) Palpitations
(i) Irritability, and
(j) Headache

Children become dull, inactive, lose appetite and exhibit poor growth. Deficiency in females reduces their work capacity and feel fatigueness and breathlessness upon doing work.

Significant anaemia is usually notable **for its pallor pale** face which has long been recognised as a sign of severe iron deficiency anaemia which was initially known as **chlorosis.**

Sources: Meat, fish, chicken, liver, green leafy vegetables, etc, are good sources of iron in which its concentration is from 15-20 mg/100g.

Cereals, legumes, potatoes, carrots are also fair sources in which its concentration ranges from 10-15 mg/100g.

Iron deficiency anaemia is ranked second only to protein calorie malnutrition including Kwashiorkor. There are two main functions of iron in the body because it is the active centre of the haem group. It is required for:

(i) The functions of haemoglobin, and

(ii) The functions of cytochromes

Fruits (guava, banana, papaya, etc) generally are poor sources and so are eggs, rice, milk, etc. in which its concentration ranges <5.0 mg per 100 g.

Requirement:

(a)	Adult males	:	10 mg per day
(b)	Adult females	:	15 mg per day
(c)	Pregnant females	:	20 mg per day
(d)	Children	:	8-15 mg per day depending upon age

Infants are born with additional iron reserves to carry them through the nursing period, for milk contains less than 0.1 mg iron per 100 g. Therefore, iron containing foods are required by the time they are one year old.

COPPER

Copper is essential for both plants and animals. It is widely distributed in all human tissues with highest concentrations in liver, brain, heart and kidney.

It is transported by serum albumin, haemocuprein and ceruloplasmin to various tissue stores; excess is excreted via bile and to a small extent via the intestinal wall. **Copper does not ordinarily accumulate in the human body with age.**

Physiological functions

(i) It is required in small amounts for the synthesis of normal haemoglobin.

(ii) It is required for the synthesis *of;*

(a) Phospholipids,

(b) Melanin, and

(c) Collagen.

(iii) It plays role in the formation of bone.

(iv) It maintains the integrity of myelin sheath in the nerve fibres

(v) It is a cofactor of several oxidative

enzymes:

(a) Tyrosinase,
(b) Cytochrome oxidase,
(c) Ascorbic acid oxidase,
(d) Uricase,
(e) Monoamine Oxidase,
(f) Ceruloplasmin (ferroxidase-I)- a blue copper-protein complex,
(g) Non-ceruloplasmin ferroxidase- a yellow copper-protein complex, etc.

(vi) It is also found in some proteins, namely erythrocuprin, cerebrocuprin; and hepatocuprin, which remain present in red blood cells, brain and liver respectively.

Disorders of copper metabolism

Wilson's disease, (hepato-lenticular degeneration) is a rare hereditary disorder of copper metabolism which is caused due to an autosomal recessive genetic defect. Following disorders are observed in this disease:

(a) Absorption of copper from the intestine gets increased (nearly 50 per cent); whereas 2-5 per cent copper is absorbed in normal ones.
(b) Ceruloplasmin formation is very less.
(c) The disease is characterized by low plasma copper, low biliary copper, poor serum ferroxidase activity, high urinary copper, excessive deposition of copper in liver, pancreas, kidney, cornea and brain, and consequent symptoms like abnormal muscular movements **(like Parkinson's disease)**, diabetes mellitus, renal tubular damage, **a visible brown ring *(Kayser-Fleischer ring)* at the margin of the cornea, hepatic cirrhosis; dementia, jaundice etc. The patient may ultimately die of hepatic failure.**

Menke's disease (Kinky hair syndrome) **is characterized by skeletal malformations, immunological deficiency, mental retardation, and defective thermoregulation.**

Hypochromic microcytic anaemia takes place in milk-fed infants due to the deficiency of copper.

Copper deficiency may cause atrophy of myocardium. The elastic tissue of aorta, coronary and pulmonary artery gets deranged; these vessels may rupture as a result of which end comes into death.

Copper Toxicity: Its excess causes Wilson's disease in which there is a positive copper balance due to the deficient synthesis of ceruloplasmin in liver. There is also a defect in the incorporation of Cu into newly synthesized apoceruloplasmin to form ceruloplasmin. Thus excess of copper gets deposited in tissues mainly in liver and basal nuclei of the brain. Besides, it also causes increased excretion of copper which causes renal tubular damage and generalised aminoaciduria.

Sources

Liver, lentils, nuts, dry legumes, fish, oysters, etc. Milk is a poor source of copper.

Daily Requirement

Adults: 2.5 mg; children: 0.5-2.5 mg.

Normal range

Normal range for plasma/serum copper is within the limits of 75 to 160 μg/100 ml.

Treatment

Treatment consists in the administration of some copper chelating agent such as penicillamine which has got the capability of removing excess copper from the tissues.

CALCIUM AND ITS METABOLISM

This element is the most abundant of all the elements found in the human body. A 70 kg normal man contains nearly 1184 gm of calcium. The skeleton contains at least 99 per cent of the total body calcium. Skeletal calcium is constantly exchanging with the calcium of the extracellular fluid. In an adult in balance, the rate of bone mineral deposition is about 400 mg/ day or 10-15 percent of the total skeletal calcium per annum. The rate of bone resorption is similar. **In older subjects, especially in the women bone resorption exceeds bone loss and there is a progressive loss of calcium from the skeleton which leads to 'osteoporosis' in them.** This phenomenon is universal in **Eastern and as well as Western** communities, the exact cause (biochemistry) of it is not yet well understood.

Dietary Calcium: In advanced countries like U.S.A. and Europe, the average daily calcium intake in adults is nearly 800 to 1000 mg, whereas in developing countries it is often considerably lower i.e., 200- 400 mg/ day. The main sources of calcium include:

(i) Milk,

(ii) Cheese,

(iii) Green vegetables and

(iv) Artificially enriched bread (in Britain and the U.S.A.)

In Eastern countries, good sources of it is through eating of betel leaves in which calcium hydroxide is used invariably along with catechu (kattha). A good satisfactory proportion of the society consumes betel leaves in some of the eastern countries.

Drinking water is not a good source of calcium but very hard water may provide up to 200 mg per day.

At one time it was thought that dietary lack of calcium was a factor contributing to poor development of bone and teeth. This may be true in some very underprivileged communities of the World but the body has a remarkable facility for adapting to a low calcium intake and it is unlikely that calcium intake of as little as 200 mg/day may have any harmful effects in otherwise normal subjects. More calcium than usual is required during period of rapid growth (during adolescence), pregnancy and lactation.

Since calcium, phosphorus and magnesium are very important minerals for the humans, hence it's in the interest of us to be aware of their concentrations in different routine edibles per 100 g (Table 14.2).

Table 14.2 : Approximate concentrations of Ca, P and Mg in various routine edibles (per 100 g)

Edibles	Ca (g)	P (g)	Mg (g)
Almonds	0.239	0.465	0.251
Beef (lean)	0.007	0.218	0.024
Beans(dried)	0.160	0.470	0.156
Cheese	0.931	0.680	0.037
Corn meal	0.018	0.190	0.084
Cottonseed meal	0.265	1.193	0.462
Eggs	0.067	0.180	0.011
Egg yolk	0.137	0.524	0.016
Linseed meal	0.413	0.741	0.432
Milk	0.210	0.093	0.012
Oranges	0.045	0.021	0.012
Potatoes	0.014	0.058	0.028
Spinach	0.067	0.068	0.037
Wheat	0.045	0.423	0.133

From the above Table 14.2, it is evident that amongst the routine edibles which we generally take daily, the best sources of calcium are cheese, milk and egg yolk.

Calcium remains distributed in blood as shown below in Table 14.3.

Table 14.3 : Distribution of calcium in blood of humans in milligrams per 100 ml.

Substance	Normal (Mean value)
Total serum calcium	10.3
Diffusible calcium	5.4
Non-diffusible calcium	4.9

Level of calcium in blood remains as shown below in certain pathological conditions which may be of diagnostic value (Table 14.4).

Table 14.4 : Blood calcium level in certain pathological conditions

Disease	mg per 100 ml.
Rickets	9.0
Parathyroid tetany	7.9
Hyperparathyroidism	15.9

Intestinal Absorption:

In an adult in calcium balance, and on a diet containing nearly 1000 mg per day, the faeces contains about 900 mg per day and the urine nearly 100 mg per day. Therefore, the absorption from the diet appears to be 100 mg/day or one tenth of the dietary calcium. In fact the true intestinal absorption is about 350 mg/day but nearly 250 mg/ day is secreted into the gut with the intestinal secretions.

Calcium can be absorbed from all parts of the small intestine by an active transport mechanism. In normal subjects the proportion of dietary calcium absorbed gets greatly increased after a period on a low calcium diet. This **'adaptation'** which becomes evident within a week of the change in diet is not seen in the absence of vitamin D. **Scientist Nicolaysen in the year 1943 suggested that there was an 'endogenous factor', a hormone, which was responsible for regulating calcium absorption as per its need. This factor is 1,25 dihydroxy- cholecalciferol, a recently discovered metabolite of vitamin D.**

Parathyroid hormone in excess also stimulates the absorption of calcium but not in the absence of vitamin D.

Absorption of calcium is enhanced by the presence of vitamin D and gets inhibited by the presence of phytic acid (inositol hexaphosphate), which is found in abundance in cereal grains and froms insoluble salts with Ca^{++} and Mg^{++}. The exact mechanism of action of vitamin D on calcium absorption is not so far very well understood.

Calcium, as the chief consituent of bone remains present as a salt resembling mineral of the hydroxyapatite group: $3Ca_3(PO_4)_2.Ca(OH)_2$. Around 99 percent of the total calcium of the body is found in the bones. Smaller amounts are found in teeth (dentine and tooth enamel). Bone formation (ossification) involves impregnation with calcium salts of organic material, similar to collagen, and held together by **mucopoly-saccharides and mucoproteins.**

Calcium is found exclusively in the plasma portion of blood, where it occurs to the extent of 9 to 11.5 mg% ; its three forms are found in the plasma, namely;

i) ionized calcium,

ii) diffusible, but not ionic- e.g. as calcium citrate.

iii) nondiffusible, combined mostly with the albumin of serum

THE PLASMA CALCIUM:

The maintenance of a steady level of calcium in the blood is necessary because it influences several important properties of the cell. When there is no intake of calcium from the diet, the element is metabolized from the bone under the influence of parathyroid hormone.

Calcium is found exclusively in the plasma portion of blood, where it occurs to the extent of 9 to 11.5 mg%. Three forms of calcium are recognized in the plasma, viz;

(i) ionized calcium,

(ii) diffusible, but not ionic -e.g, as calcium citrate,

(iii) non-diffusible, combined mostly with serum albumin.

It is the ionizable fraction of the total plasma calcium that is the most important physiologically, and that is in equilibrium with calcium in various tissues. It's this fraction which participates in the following very important activities of human body, namely:

(i) Coagulation of blood,
(ii) Neuromuscular activity,
(iii) Muscle contractility, and
(iv) Myocardial activity.

The non diffusible calcium in plasma remains bound to protein and because of this can exist in a soluble form at levels far above that possible in the absence of proteins, since it would ordinarily precipitate in the form of insoluble calcium salt. A decrease in serum calcium **for example in nephrosis leads also to a decrease in plasma calcium.**

Urinary excretion of Calcium

About 15 g calcium daily passes into the glomerular filtrate from the diffusible fractions of the plasma calcium. 50 to 200 mg is reabsorbed in the tubules but the exact amount is not yet known. Calcium reabsorption gets diminished in the deficiency of vitamin D and in the presence of sodium diuresis.

The calcium lost in the sweat is very variable which ranges from 20-350 mg/day.

Factors affecting the Plasma Calcium

A constant and normal concentration of ionized calcium in the extracellular fluid is of great importance for the following activities/functions, namely;

(i) muscular contractions
(ii) neural transmission
(iii) neuromuscular transmission &
(iv) the activity of several enzymes

Low ionized calcium level may lead to **tetanic spasms** which may be fatal. Side by side, if the plasma calcium level is high, then it disturbs cardiac functions and may be deposited in kidney or other tissues.

Physico-chemical factors: If EDTA (Ethylene diamine tetra acetic acid, a calcium complexing agent) is injected intravenously into

For the proper calcification and eruption of teeth, the diet must contain adequate amount of calcium and phosphorus and certain vitamins.

In the developing tooth, dietary deficiency of vitamin C leads to the impairment of the **odontoblasts** and retarded dentine deposition. The pulp becomes haemorrhagic and is filled with calcified tissue.

Vitamin D regulates absorption of calcium.

Normal dental growth requires an adequate supply of thyroxine. Hypothyroidism in children causes retardation in dental development. In hyperthyroidism, in children which is relatively rare in them, there is early shedding of the deciduous teeth and accelerated dentition.

Deficient parathyroid function may interfere with calcium and phosphorus metabolism to such an extent that growing teeth fail to calcify properly.

The pituitary plays an important role in the eruption of the teeth which gets accelerated in hyperpituitarism, whereas in hypopituitarism, the teeth are normal but eruption gets retarded and the teeth get crowded in the arch due to retardation of bone development.

In hypergonadism, the eruption of the teeth is accelerated. Estrogen in the human has no effect on the teeth; **whereas large doses of adrenal steroids favour osteoporosis.**

man or dog then the plasma calcium falls rapidly but returns to normal level within a few hours. If EDTA is given after removal of the parathyroid glands, the plasma calcium again returns to the preinfusion value (7 to 8 mg%), but not so rapidly. Thus chemical equilibrium between the **labile** part of the bone mineral and the interstitial fluid, quite independent of the parathyroid glands, keeps the plasma calcium upto 7 to 8 mg%. In intact animals, parathyroid hormone is responsible for maintaining the normal serum calcium level around 10 mg%

Parathyroid hormone: The parathyroid glands develop from the third and fourth pharyngeal pouches of the embryo. They lie in the neck immediately adjacent to the posterior surface of the thyroid gland with which, however, they have no physiological relationship. As a rule, they consits of four oval bodies about 6 mm long each weighing 20 to 50 mg, but they are variable in number, size and position. Accessory parathyroid tissue is not uncommon lower in the neck or even in the thorax. The secretory cells are arranged in cords, separated into imperfect lobules by the thin septa of connective tissue. There are two types of **chief cells** with large nuclei nearly filling the cells and **oxyntic cells** with small nuclei and acidophil granules in the cytoplasm.

The vascular supply is rich but the nervous connections are scanty.

PTH is a 84 amino acid single chain peptide (M.W. 9,500) that contains no carbohydrate (Fig 14.1). PTH_{1-34} has full biologic activity. The region 25-34 is primarily responsible for receptor binding.

PTH secretion apparently ceases when the plasma calcium exceeds 12 mg%. Plasma calcium appears to be the sole stimulus of PTH secretion. Since the half- life of the hormone in the blood is about 20 minutes, changes in hormone secretion may play an important role in minute to minute regulation of the plasma calcium.

Quite independent of its action on blood calcium, PTH has effects on bone and kidney, and probably also on the gastrointestinal tract and on the mammary glands during lactation. The effects on the bone and intestine, but not on the kidney, require the presence of vitamin D. PTH exerts its action on bone by stimulating osteoblasts to mobilize bone. PTH decreases the reabsorption of phosphate by the kidney tubules, and therefore increases the excretion of phosphate. It also increases the urinary excretion of sodium, potassium and bicarbonate and decreases the excretion of hydrogen ions. In the

1
H_2N–Ala–Val–Ser–Glu–Ile–Gln–Phe–Met–His–Asn–Leu–Gly–Lys–

15
His–Leu–Ser–Ser–Met–Glu–Arg–Val–Glu–Trp–Arg–Lys–Lys–Leu–

30 34
Gln–Asp–Val–His–Asn–Phe–Val–Ala–Leu–Gly–Ala–Ser–Ile–Ala–

45
Tyr–Arg–Asp–Gly–Ser–Ser–Gln–Arg–Pro–Arg–Lys–Lys–Glu–Asp–Asn–

60
Val–Leu–Val–Glu–Ser–His–Gin–Lys–Ser–Leu–Gly–Glu–Ala–Asp–Lys–

75 84
Ala–Asp–Val–Asp–Val–Leu–Ile–Lys–Ala–Lys–Pro–Gln–COOH

Fig. 14.1: Amino acid sequence of bovine PTH. The fragment 1 to 34 is biologically active, in vivo and in vitro, on both bone and kidney receptors

intestine, PTH enhances calcium absorption. The exact mechanism of action of PTH is not very well understood so far but recent evidences suggest the involvement of 3', 5'- AMP.

Clinical disorders of both excess and deficiency of parathyroid activity are known. Actively secreting tumors of the parathyroid glands produce excessive amount of PTH_1 and the resulting disturbance of phosphorus and calcium metabolism leads to withdrawal of large amount of these elements from the bones which therefore become weak and deformed and liable to be fractured (Fig 14.2).

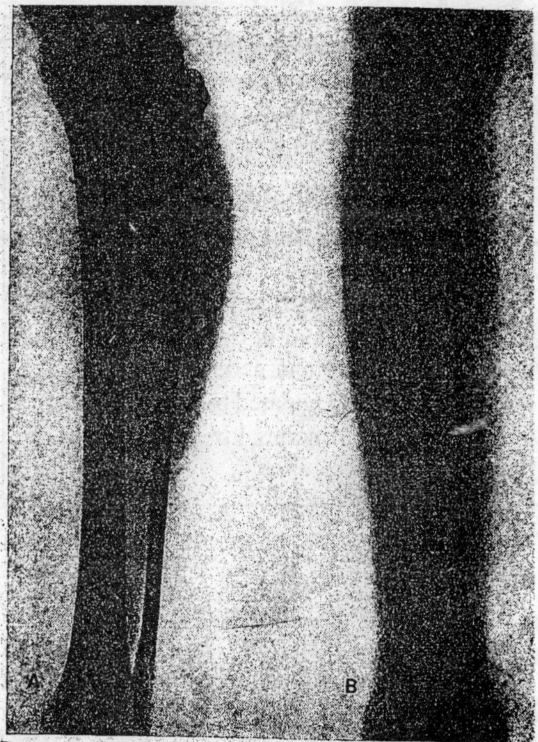

Fig.14.2: X-ray photograph of the right lower legs of the two women, aged 25. A is from a normal subject, B from a patient with a parathyroid tumour. In B the fibula is deformed and both bones cast a poor shadow because of extensive resorption of calcium salts.

The absorption of calcium from the gut is increased. **The serum calcium may reach upto 16 mg% or even more and the urinary excretion may be greatly raised so that stones may form in the kidneys.**

Parathyroid deficiency sometimes occurs after accidental removal of parathyroid glands during thyroidectomy. Neuromuscular excitability and muscular spasm (tetany) are the main symptoms. The condition improves after the administration of PTH but large doses of vitamin D are given for longer period.

Calcitonin: In 1962 Copp and his colleagues produced evidence for the existence of a hormone which lowered the plasma calcium level. He named it as calcitonin. **The hormone is a lipophilic single chain polypeptide of 32 amino acids (Fig 14.3).**

In man calcitonin is secreted by the cells of the thyroid, parathyroids and the thymus. The parafollicular (C cells) of the thyroid have been known since 1932. They contain granules which increase in number during a period of prolonged hypocalcaemia. Calcitonin has been identified within these cells by the immunofluorescent antibody technique.

Calcitonin secretion is stimulated by hypercalcaemia. Calcitonin reduces bone resorption even in the absence of parathormone and promotes phosphate and sodium excretion through the kidneys. Its secretion is also stimulated by gastrin, pancreozymin and glucagon. Therefore, as calcium is absorbed from

```
     S-------------------------------S
     |    2            5             |          10
NH2—Cys—Gly—Asn—leu—Ser—Thr—Cys—Met—Leu—Gly—Thr—Tyr—Thr—

Gln—Asp—Phe—Asn—Lys—Phe—His—Thr—Phe—Pro—Gln—Thr—Ala—Leu—Gly—
     15                  20                      25
Val—Gly—Ala—Pro—CONH2
     30
```

Fig 14.3: Human Calcitonin

Calcium has got very important functions in the body, namely :

(i) It is required for muscle contraction
(ii) It is the major constituent of bone along with the phosphate.
(iii) It is required for blood coagulation.

In high amounts, it is toxic and like K^+ slows down the heart beating. The balance between excess and deficiency of Ca^{2+} in the blood stream is a delicate issue. Its concentration is regulated by the antagonistic action of two hormones, viz; **parathormone** and **calcitonin.**

a meal, thcrc is little or no rise is the level of blood calcium.

As elevation of calcitonin level is found in the patients with medullary- cell carcinomas of the thyroid. So far, no convincing evidence of a syndrome due to calcitonin deficiency is known.

1, 25 - Dihydroxycholecalciferol

This hormone, a metabolite of vitamin D is produced by the kidneys. It promotes the absorption of calcium in the intestine.

Other hormones affecting Calcium Metabolism

An adequate supply of growth hormone from the anterior pituitary is necessary for the proliferation of the cells of the epiphyseal cartilage and therefore, for the growth in length of a long bone. In hypophysectomized animals, epiphyseal activity is much reduced or even absent; which can be restored by the administration of growth hormone (GH)

Increased loss of bone is a feature of Cushing's syndrome due to excessive activity of the adrenal cortex.

The Plasma Calcium in Disease

Hyperparathyroidism causes hypercalcaemia.

Hypercalcaemia may also be caused by:

(i) Tumours which cause rapid bone destruction,
(ii) Tumours secreting a PTH- like substance,
(iii) Vitamin D poisoning
(iv) Excessive ingestion of milk, and
(v) Excessive intake of alkali by patients with peptic ulcer.

Signs of hypercalcaemia include:

(a) thirst
(b) tiredness
(c) weakness
(d) mental disturbances, and if severe, then coma and death

Untreated hypercalcaemia causes renal damage.

Hypocalcaemia is found in:

(a) hypoparathyroidism,
(b) osteomalacia
(c) rickets,
(d) renal failure and
(e) tetany is a prominent feature

The outstanding feature of **tetany** is neuromuscular irritability which manifests itself first as hypertonicity of muscles and then as fibrillary twitchings (tetany) of muscle fasciculi, leading finally to generalized clonic movements especially in children. The muscle hypertonia produces the characteristic attitude of the hand in tetany, the **main d' accoucheur.** Simultaneously the feet are held firmly flexed at the ankles with all the toes planter- flexed. The condition, called carpopedal spasm may be accompanied in infants by spasm of the glottis (**laryngismus stridulus**), which can be severe enough to cause alarming **cyanosis. In the early stages of tetany, sensory phenomena are present, such as widespread tingling feelings and sensations of heat and flushing (paraesthesiae).**

Tapping over the facial nerve in front of the ear produces twitching of the facial muscles **(Chvostek's sign)**, and the motor nerves are unduly excitable to electrical stimulation. Carpal spasm can be induced by inflating a blood pressure cuff round the upper arm to a pressure exceeding the systolic blood pressure and maintaining the occlusion for three minutes **(Trousseau's test).**

The factor most closely related to the onset of tetany is a reduction in the plasma concentration of ionized calcium. This may be caused by a reduced total plasma calcium in the disorders as mentioned above or by a reduced proportion of ionized calcium due to alkalosis caused by vomiting or by over- ventilation. Tetany has very rarely been attributed to a low plasma magnesium, a high plasma potassium or other metabolic changes.

CHLORIDE

It is the main ion of plasma and other extracellular fluids and is responsible for maintaining osmolarity at approximately 0.3 mol/l.

Sources

Sources for chloride include table salt, cheese, butter, pickles, salted fish or meat, salted nuts, etc.

Daily Requirement

Daily requirement of chloride for various categories is as follows:

Adults: 1.5 to 5 g; **infants:** 0.25 to 1 g; **children:** 0.5 to 4 g. **Adult human body contains about 70-80 g chloride** and the excretion of chloride per day is 7-8 g via urine. It is reabsorbed by diffusion from the proximal and distal tubules and the thin segment of the ascending limb along the electrical gradient developed by the reabsorption of Na^+. Apart from this, some Cl^- also gets actively reabsorbed from the thick segment of the ascending limb. Cl^- reabsorption is indirectly helped by aldosterone as Cl^- is always reabsorbed along with Na^+.

Some Cl^- is secreted in saliva, gastric juice, tear, sweat, pancreatic juice, etc. During profuse sweating, Na^+ and Cl^- are lost in greater quantity. Secretion of aldosterone hormone reduces the Na^+ and Cl^- concentrations in sweat.

> **CHLORIDE**
>
> It's the chief anion present in the body, particularly in the extracellular fluid. The excretion in urine is slightly higher than that of Na^+, which would put the average daily intake at about 7g Cl^- (200 meq). However, the kidney is capable of secreting a urine almost free of Na^+ and Cl^-, although this is often an indication of incipient heat exhaustion.

Functions

1. ***Acid-base balance:*** Chloride helps in maintaining acid-base balance. Cl^- has a role in buffering CO_2; some of the HCO_3^- formed from CO_2 in *RBCs* passes out into the plasma in exchange of Cl^- which enters the erythrocytes (chloride-shift phenomenon).
2. **Cl^- in HCl *secretion:*** Plasma Cl^- is the source of Cl^- for the formation of gastric HCl.
3. ***Osmotic-pressure regulation:*** It is also responsible for maintaining osmotic pressure i. e. osmolarity throughout the body which is maintained at about 0.3 mol/l by the joint effect of Na^+, K^+ and Cl^-.

Clinical Condition

Intense vomiting may cause Cl^- depletion due to the loss of Cl^- with the gastric contents as a result of which plasma Cl^- level gets decreased. Some of the lost Cl^- is replaced by HCO_3^- in the ECF

and metabolic alkalosis may result. In several diseases like Addison's disease, primary aldosteronism, Cushing's syndrome, serum Cl^- changes are similar to those of serum Na^+.

PHOSPHORUS

The mean phosphorus content of an adult man is 800 g; four- fifths of this is found in the bones, the remaining being in the cells as phosphates or nucleic acids. The concentration of inorganic phosphorus in the plasma in fasting adults is between 2.5 and 4.5 mg/dl. Higher values are found in infants. Almost all the inorganic phosphate is dialysable, only nearly 12 percent being protein bound. At normal pH i.e., 7.4, 85% of the ionized inorganic phosphate remains present as HPO_4^{--} and 15% as $H_2PO_4^-$. Small amounts of the phosphate may be bound to calcium and magnesium. It has been estimated that the amount of non-ionized phosphate may be 50% of the dialysable phosphate.

Since the greater part of the phosphorus of the body is associated with calcium in bone, the metabolism of these two elements is to a considerable extent parallel to each other.

Phosphorus, however, is abundant also in many of the softer tissues of the body and plays various important roles in life- processes.

Functions:-

It has the following main functions in the human body, namely:

(i) Constituent of bones and teeth: It is a very important mineral for the development of bones and teeth. It is required in greater amount during infancy and childhood when there is growth of every tissue. It is the major constituent of the bone as calcium phosphate or hydroxyapatite.

(ii) Enzyme action: Phosphate remains present in nucleotides, a majority of which functions as coenzymes, for instance pyridoxal phosphate, nicotinamide coenzymes, flavin coenzymes, thiamine pyrophosphate, etc.

(iii) Intermediary metabolism:

(a) Through the intermediary formation of lecithins, it is concerned with fat metabolism

(b) Through the formation of hexosephosphates of adenylic acid, and of creatine phosphate, it plays a primary role in the carbohydrate metabolism of animals as well as in fermentation processes.

(c) It participates in intermediary metabolism in the form of organic phosphates; the most important of these is ATP. Phosphorylation is essential for many reactions like those of glycogenesis, glycolysis, etc.

(iv) Phosphates play a role in the neutrality regulation of the organism.

(v) Phosphates are concerned with the absorption of sugars from the intestine and the reabsorption of glucose in the kidney tubules.

(vi) Phosphorus is a constituent of the phospoholipids present in all tissues. Phospholipids are found in abundance in nervous tissues.

(vii) It remains present in nucleoproteins of the chromatin material of cells and in phosphoproteins such as casein.

(viii) It has been suggested that most of the phosphorus, as well as the fat of milk, arises from the lecithin of the blood of the lactating animal.

(ix) Acid- Base regulation: A very important property. Mixtures of monobasic and disbasic phosphates ($H_2PO^-_4$ and HPO_4^{2-}) constitute the phosphate buffer which plays role in the maintenance of pH of the body fluids.

(x) Energy transfer: Free energy produced by various metabolic reactions is stored as high energy phosphates like adenosine triphosphate and is liberated by their hydrolysis for other energy- requiring pathways/ reactions.

Absorption and Depletion:

Inorganic phosphates are absorbed from the middle third of jejunum. Vitamin D increases the absorption of phosphate. Ninety percent of the phosphorus filtered at the glomerulus is reabsorbed in the tubules.

Depletion of phosphate may occur with tubular defect and a high plasma phosphate may be a consequence of renal i.e., glomerular failure. **Besides, phosphate depletion may also occur in patients who consume excessive amount of aluminium hydroxide (an antacid) which binds phosphorus present in gut.**

Requirement

Indian Council of Medical Research states that the daily allowance of phosphorus should be equal to that of calcium for the children and women during pregnancy and lactation.

Daily requirement of phosphorus for:

(i) adult man/women: 500 mg

(ii) pregnant or lactating women: 1 g

(iii) infants and children : 400- 600 mg

Sources:

(i) Milk is an excellent source of phosphorus, nearly 750 ml of intake a day for children which contains 0.88 g of phosphorus is O.K. in all respects for them. Milk contains 93 mg of phosphorus per 100ml.

(ii) Meat (average 175 mg per 100 g)

(iii) Eggs (200 mg per 100 g)

(iv) Cheese (480 mg per 100 g)

(v) Nuts (400 mg per 100 g)

(vi) Whole cereals (as whole wheat, 375 mg per 100 g)

(vii) Wheat flour (about 90 mg per 100 g)

(viii) Polished rice (about 90 mg per 100 g)

Too high a ratio of calcium to phosphorus in the diet, however, is unfavourable to phosphorus absorption. **Diets high in beryllium or strontium also inhibit the absorption of phosphorus and give rise to rickets.**

Since phosphorus remains present in all animal and vegetable cells, therefore, dietary deficiency of it never occurs in man.

Regulation

Various substances like vitamin D, plasma proteins, hormones like calcitonin and parathormone regulate phosphorus metabolism.

Calcitonin lowers serum calcium and phosphate by reducing their mobilization from bones and thus maintains the bone minerals; whereas parathormone (PTH) has a tendency to increase serum Ca^{2+} and lower serum phosphates.

Clinical Conditions

Phosphate deficiency is not very common as most of the naturally occurring foods contain phosphate in one or the other form. However, **there are some diseases like rickets and osteomalacia which may be caused due to the deficiency of calcium, phosphorus or vitamin D.** These diseases are characterized by reduced calcium and phosphate absorption, low serum Pi, rise in urinary phosphates, demineralization of bones and negative calcium balance.

Serum calcium is, however, almost normal in rickets although it falls sometimes in osteomalacia. Serum calcium level may be elevated by *hypervitaminosis* D; **whereas *hyperparathyroidism* causes demineralization of bones, rise in serum calcium, fall in serum Pi, high urinary calcium and**

phosphate and metastatic calcifications of soft tissues.

***Hypoparathyroidism* is responsible for lowering serum calcium, urinary calcium and urinary Pi; raises serum Pi moderately and produces hypocalcaemic tetany.**

Besides the above, X-linked genetic disorders of phosphate metabolism is responsible for the onset of *vitamin D-resistant rickets* and *idiopathic osteomalacia* which eventually lead to reduced intestinal and renal absorptions of phosphates, low serum phosphate, high serum alkaline phosphatase activity, high urinary Pi and poor mineralization of bones.

IODINE

Introduction

The thyroid gland produces two hormones i.e., 3, 5, 3'- triiodothyronine (T_3) and 3, 5, 3', 5'-tetraiodothyronine (T_4, thyroxine) which have long been recognized for their importance in regulating general metabolism, development and tissue differentiation. These hormones, whose structures are as given below (Fig 14.4) regulate gene expression using mechanisms similar to those employed by steroid hormones.

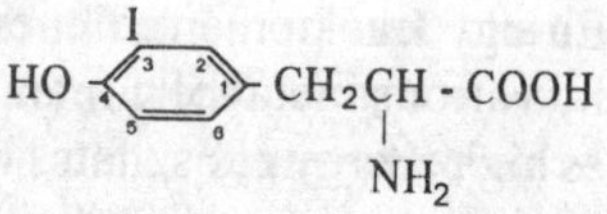

3 - Monoiodotyrosine (MIT)

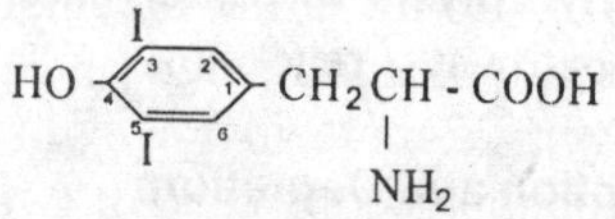

3, 5 - Diiodotyrosine (DIT)

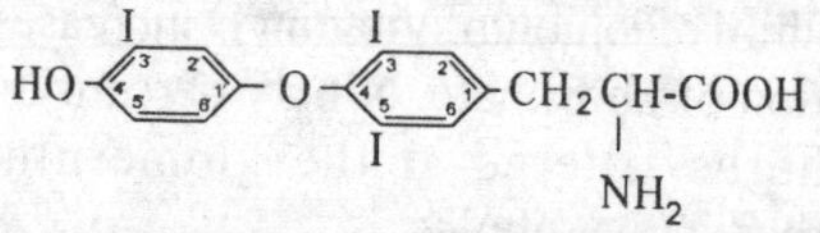

3,5,3' - Triiodotyrosine (T_3)

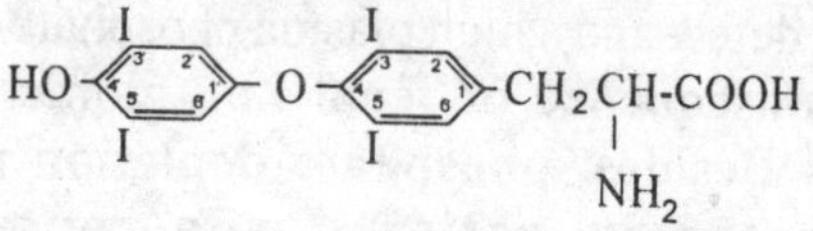

3,5,3',5' - Tetraiiodotyrosine (thyroxine,T_4)

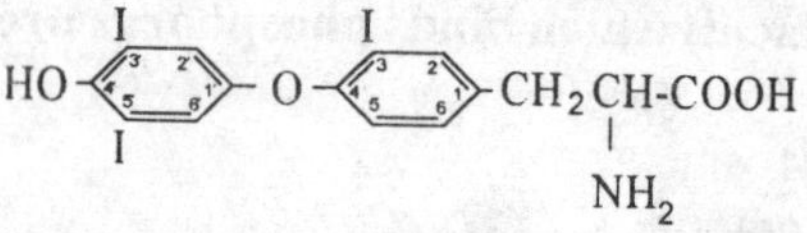

3,3',5' - Triiodothyronine [reverseT_3(rT_3)]

Fig.14.4: Structures of thyroid hormones and related compounds.

About 20 mg of iodine remains present in adult human body and nearly two- third of it remains present in the thyroid gland. Small doses of it are important in the prevention of **'goitre'** in areas where it is endemic.

Iodine remains present in thyroxine. Under normal conditions almost all the blood iodine is in the plasma, less than a third of this remains present as inorganic iodine compounds, the remainder being organic which remains bound to the protein known as protein bound iodine i.e., PBI.

This element for the first time was discovered by **Courtois** in seaweed and as early as in 1820, it was postulated that iodine was a curative factor of **'goitre'.** Since at that time iodine deficiency goitres were common in many parts of the world, the news spread like a wild fire as a result of which the use of iodine and iodine-containing substances like burnt sponge, etc. became very popular for the treatment of goitres. With the time as the knowledge advanced, discrimination in the use of this **'wonder drug'** came forward as a consequence of which, the beneficial effect of salts rich in iodine advanced the prophylactic and therapeutic treatment of goitre.

The thyroid gland in the adults lies at the neck infront of the upper rings of the trachea which sometimes is prolonged into the thorax behind the sternum. Weight of the thyroid gland is nearly 25 g in a healthy adult. This gland is not essential to life but it contributes a lot to physical and mental well- being. In humans, it is necessary for growth and development. The thyroid begins to trap iodine from about the third month of foetal life but the normal synthesis of its hormones does take place only after fourth or fifth month.

Thyroglobulin is the precursor of T_3 and T_4. It is a large, iodinated and glycosylated protein with a molecular weight of 660,000. Thyroglobulin is composed of two subunits. It contains 115 tyrosine residues, each of which is a potential site of of iodination. **About 70% of the iodide in thyroglobulin exists in the form of inactive precursors known as monoiodotyrosine (MIT) and diiodotyrosine (DIT), while 30% is in the iodotyronyl residues i.e., T_3 and T_4.**

The thyroid gland contains a large amount of iodine (0.06 percent), almost all of which remains firmly bound to a protein called as **thyroglobulin.** On hydrolysis thyroglobulin yields:.

(i) Several iodine- containing derivatives of tyrosine
(ii) Monoiodotyrosine
(iii) Diiodotyrosine
(iv) T_3, &
(v) T_4

Biosynthesis

The biosynthesis of thyroid hormones proceeds as shown below in Figure 14.5. The first step in their synthesis is the concentration of inorganic iodide within the thyroid gland (iodide trapping). The next major steps involve **oxidation** and **organic iodination.** The thyroid iodide is oxidized to iodine via a peroxidase enzyme. In the next reaction tyrosine in the presence of iodine (iodination occurs) forms monoiodotyrosine(MIT) and then diiodotyrosine (DIT).

Now, two molecules of diiodotyrosine are coupled to form one molecule of thyroxine (T_4) with the loss of one alanine side chain. Triiodothyronine (T_3) is synthesized either by the

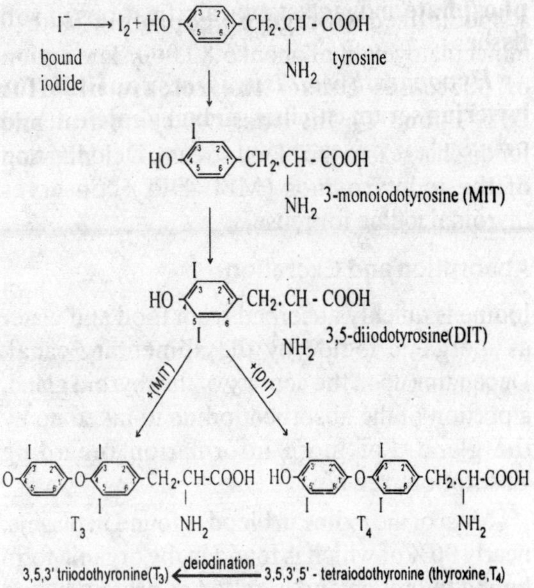

Fig. 14.5 : Biosynthesis of thyroid hormones

coupling of diiodotyrosine with one molecule of monoiodotyrosine (Fig 14.5) or from the deiodination of thyroxine.

All the compounds taking part in the synthesis of thyroid hormones are found in thyroglobulin,

T_3 possesses all the biological properties of T_4 and is 3-5 times more potent than T_4 in raising the oxygen consumption of patients with hypothyroidism and this action occurs within four hours.

As iodide is absorbed by the acinar cells, it is oxidized to iodine ($2\,I^- \rightarrow I_2 + 2e$) by the enzyme peroxidase. The iodine never appears as such in the free state but is immediately taken up by the tyrosine of the glandular protein to form MIT and DIT (Fig 14.5) which upon oxidative coupling remove one side chain so as to form derivatives of thyronine, T_4 being formed from two DIT units and T_4 from one MIT and one DIT unit.

Antithyroid agents include thiouracil, thiourea etc.

a specialized storage glycoprotein with a molecular weight of about 6,80,000. The **action of protcases causes the release of MIT, DIT, T_3 and T_4;** the latter two being available for discharge into the blood stream. Deiodination of the iodotyrosines (MIT, DIT) conserves thyroidal iodine for reuse.

Absorption and Excretion

Iodine is quickly absorbed from food and water as inorganic iodide by the alimentary canal. Depending upon the activity of the thyroid gland, a portion of the absorbed iodide in taken up by the gland. For more information regarding 'absorption', see box.

Most of the iodine in blood is found in plasma, nearly 90% of which is found in the organic form bound to protein and is called as protein bound iodine (PBI).

Inorganic iodine is mostly excreted via urine whereas nearly 10% of the circulating organic iodine is excreted via faeces.

Requirement

100-150 μg/day is sufficient to prevent goitre.

Sources

Its requirement is mostly fullfilled by drinking water and iodized salt. Seafoods generally prevalent in the cities located along sea- shores are very good sources of iodine. Other good sources are fruits, vegetables, cereals, meat, etc.

The iodine content of the food depends upon the iodine content of the soil in which these are grown/ cultivated.

Deficiency disorders :

Its deficiency results in the enlargement of the thyroid gland causing **hypothyroidism, goitre** and **myxedema** (characterized by a low BMR, thickness and puffing of the skin, coarse and brittle hair and fingernails and a general mental and physical lethargy).

In hypothyroidism, the child becomes a **dwarf** or **cretin** who grows slowly (stunted growth) and has a low mental status (low IQ), his/ her hair are scanty and coarse and his skin is thick and dry and low BMR.

Toxicity of iodine may result in **thyrotoxicosis (hyperthyroidism),** one of the most severe condition of which is **Grave's disease (exophthalmic goitre).** It results in weight loss, typical protrusion of the eye-balls and elevated BMR.

> Chemical Name of the goitrogenic substance (goitrin) isolated from rutabagas is 1-5- vinyl - 2 thiooxazolidone.

Goitrogenic foods:

Vegetables / foods which if consumed in abundance may cause **goitre,** these are the following:

(i) Cauliflower,
(ii) Brocooli,
(iii) Cabbage,
(iv) Rutabagas,
(v) Turnip, etc.

FLUORINE (Fluoride)

Traces of fluoride (F) are present in human tissues mainly in bones, teeth, thyroid gland, skin, etc.

Physiological functions

1. This element is essential for the growth of teeth and bones and is required in minute quantities.
2. Fluoroacetate is a powerful inhibitor (it virtually blocks) of TCA cycle.
3. In combination with vitamin D, it is required for the treatment of bone disease i.e. osteoporosis which is characterized by softening of bone as a result of

excessive absorption of bone elements.

4. Sodium fluoride acts as a powerful inhibitor of the glycolytic enzyme enolase, therefore, it's used as a blocker of glycolytic pathway while collecting blood samples for the determination of sugar.
5. It forms a protective layer of acid-resistant fluoroapatite with hydroxyapatite crystals of the enamel.
6. Fluoride ions inhibit the metabolism of oral bacterial enzymes and also restrict the local production of acids which are responsible for dental caries.

Sources

1. Drinking water is the chief source for the human beings.
2. Tea and sea-fishes are the only other significant sources of fluorine in the diet.

Distribution and daily requirement

Fluorine remains present in animal soft tissues in amounts ranging from 0.2 to 1.5 mg per 100 g of the dry material. Bones and teeth contain larger amounts (20 to 30 mg per 100 g ash); whereas dentine may contain more than the enamel of teeth. Drinking water containing 1 to 2 parts per million of fluorine is sufficient to meet all the requirements of the body and thus prevents dental caries without producing any ill effect.

Absorption

Soluble fluorides are rapidly absorbed by the small intestine.

Excretion

It's excreted via: (a) sweat, (b) urine, and (c) intestinal mucosa.

Abnormalities

1. Excessive intake of fluoride (3 to 5 parts per million) in childhood is responsible for "**dental fluorosis** (mottled enamel), in which enamel of the teeth loses its lustre and becomes rough. Chalky white patches with yellow or brown staining do appear over the surface of the teeth which may be easily distinguished by naked eyes. In this disease, enamel becomes weak and in severe cases there is found great loss of enamel with 'pitting' and other depressions **give the surface a corroded appearance.**
2. Highly excessive intake of fluorine (over 10 ppm) may be responsible for increased density and hypercalcification of the bone of spine, pelvis and limbs. The attack most of the times is so serious that even the ligaments of the spine and the collagen in the bone become calcified. Its severity is fatal and may cause neurological disturbances as a result of which such individuals become crippled and can not do normal daily routine work, such as, bending, squatting etc; as the joints become stiff; this is all due to fluoride toxicity which is not very common but its patients may be seen once in a while.
3. Drinking water containing less than 0.5 ppm fluorine causes dental caries amongst children. **Therefore, fluorine is considered to be a caries preventive agent, that is why these days the manufacturers of tooth-paste indiscriminately add it.**

Prevention of fluorosis

It can be prevented by removing excessive fluorides from the water by treating it with activated carbon or by some other appropriate absorbents. Local district water department/ health department may be informed and consulted without any delay in cases of suspicion.

Mechanism

The mechanism by which fluorine inhibits caries

production is not very well understood.

Fluoridation

It is a very important aspect if by chance it comes to knowledge that the drinking water contains less fluorine than the recommended standards; the fact must be brought to the notice of local water/health/competent authorities so that such water gets fluoridated. **Deliberate fluoridation of water supply in such cases is very useful.**

Fluoride Toxicity:

Fluoride toxicity results in **fluorosis** which is common in many parts of the world where its concentration in water is found over 5 PPM. **In India, fluorosis is common in north where water contains over 10 PPM of fluoride.**

In fluorosis, there is mottling of teeth. The dental enamel loses its lustre and becomes rough. Bands of brown pigmentation are seen. Mottling is best seen on the incisors of the upper jaw. There is also loss of appetite and osteoporosis of the bones particularly of the spine, pelvis and limbs. In addition ligaments of the spine become calcified.

SULPHUR

In the diet, greater part of sulphur remains present in proteins in the form of two well known amino acids namely cystine and methionine. Besides, it's also found in some non-protein organic sulphur compounds. It may also be found in inorganic sulphur compounds as sulphates. Most of the sulphur present in proteins is finally converted to **inorganic sulphate;** some of which gets excreted in that form and some as **ethereal sulphates** and the remainder in the *form* of **phenolic compounds such as indoxyl and skatoxyl sulphates** which are formed from indole and skatole produced in the intestine by the action of microorganisms on proteins. Important compounds of the body which contain sulphur are:

(a) Insulin,

(b) Glutathione, and

(c) Thiamine

In blood, sulphur remains distributed in the following forms:

(a) inorganic sulphur: About 1mg per 100ml;

(b) ethereal sulphate sulphur: 0.5mg per 100ml; and

(c) neutral sulphur: 1.9 mg per 100 ml

In this way total sulphur in blood averages nearly 3.4 mg per 100 ml.

Determination of these sulphur compounds in blood has not so far found any diagnostic application in the diseased state. Some types of sulphur compounds are found in urine where also they are not of any diagnostic significance.

ZINC

The importance of zinc as a micronutrient has received increasing attention. Normal animals absorb only 3-10 percent of dietary zinc.

Sources

Liver, legumes, milk, unmilled cereals, maize, meat, spinach, lettuce, yeast, oysters and egg etc.

Daily requirement

(i) Adult men/women: 15 mg;

(ii) Pregnant/lactating women: 20-25 mg; .

(iii) Infants and children; 3-10 mg.

Deficiency

(i) Its deficiency in man causes poor growth and hypogonadism (retarded genital development).

(ii) It is also responsible for low carbonic anhydrase activity in red blood cells.

(iii) It also causes **alopoecia.**

(iv) Its deficiency **lowers spermatogenesis in males and menstrual cycle gets also disturbed in the females.**

(v) Its deficiency is characterized by lesions in the (a) skin (b) mucocutaneous junctions and (c) epithelial structures.

Absorption and Excretion

Nearly 20% of the dietary zinc is absorbed. Its absorption takes place in duodenum and ileum. Phytates and other components of the dietary fibre affect its absorption by increasing the faecal excretion.

Zinc toxicity : When consumed in excess, it causes toxicity which depresses growth and interferes with the utilisation and functions of copper and causes anaemia.

Physiological functions

(i) Role in enzyme action: It is a cofactor for many metalloenzymes like carboxypeptidase A, cytoplasmic superoxide dismutase, carbonic anhydrase, alcohol dehydrogenase phosphatases, etc.

(ii) Role in vitamin A metabolism: Zn^{2+} may stimulate the release of vitamin A from the liver into the blood, thus plays a role in vitamin A metabolism.

(iii) Zinc therapy has been found to be useful in some cases of atherosclerosis.

(iv) It has been found to play a vital role in the healing of wounds.

(v) It is essential for normal growth and reproduction in animals.

(vi) It is required in the commercial preparation of **'insulin'** hormone. It increases the duration of insulin action in diabetics when given to them by injection, that is why, preparations of zinc-insulins (also known as crystalline insulins) or **zinç-protamine insulin is more common and popular.**

(vii) Perhaps, its most vital function may be concerned with the synthesis of **ribonucleic acids.**

(viii) It is also required for the maturation of spermatozoa.

MANGANESE

The kidney and the liver are the chief storage places for manganese in the body. In blood it varies from 0.004 to 0.020 mg per 100 ml. It is largely excreted via faeces.

Sources

It is also an essential element required by the body. Average diet contains nearly 4 mg manganese. Its important sources include cereals, vegetables, nuts, tea, fruits, whole grains, etc.

Daily requirement

Adult men/women: 2.5-5 mg; infants and children: 0.5-3 mg.

Functions

1. **Enzyme action.:** Manganese acts as a cofactor in a number of enzymic reactions. It's also a constituent of number of enzymes, e.g. arginase, isocitrate dehydrogenase, cholinesterase, pyruvate carboxylase, acetyl-CoA carboxylase, glycosyl transferases, etc.
2. **Proteoglycan synthesis:** It plays some role in the synthesis and deposition of proteoglycans in many tissues including bones.
3. **Porphyrin synthesis:** It may help aminolevulinic acid (Am Lev) synthetase **in porphyrin synthesis.**
4. It is also required for the **biosynthesis of long chain fatty acids.**
5. It has been reported to exhibit **lipotropic effect.**

6. It also stimulates the biosynthesis of cholesterol and fatty acids. For example, the biosynthesis of cholesterol from acetate depends upon the presence of a manganese containing enzyme i.e., mevalonic kinase.

Normal Range

4-20 μg per 100 ml blood.

Deficiency symptoms:

Its deficiency leads to bone deformities, poor growth and ataxia in several animal species. Its deficiency has also been shown to affect the synthesis of oligosaccharides, glycoproteins and proteoglycans.

Manganese Toxicity: Manganese toxicity may occur in the mine workers of manganese who then develop **madness with severe psychotic symptoms and parkinsonism.**

COBALT

Not much is known about the metabolism of cobalt. Adult human body contains only about 1-2 mg cobalt.

Functions

1. It may act as a cofactor for several enzymes, e.g. glycylglycine dipeptidase which is found in intestinal juice.
2. It forms a component of vitamin B_{12}.
3. It also occurs in cobamide coenzymes.
4. It helps in erythropoiesis. Cattles grazing in cobalt-deficient fields are found to develop macrocytic anaemia which is easily curable either by vitamin B_{12} or cobalt sulfate administration. It may also increase the production of erythropoietin **and may be a cofactor- for aminolevulinic acid synthetase in the synthesis of heme.**

Cobalt toxicity

Cobalt, if administered to man/animals in large quantity, becomes toxic as a result of which polycythaemia (increased number of red blood cells in blood) takes place.

Sources

It is found in daily edible routine items.

Daily requirement

It is required by the human beings in very less quantity. It is required in the form of vitamin B_{12}. As little as 1-2 μg of B_{12}, containing 0.045-0.09 μg cobalt is sufficient to maintain normal bone marrow functioning in pernicious anaemia.

MOLYBDENUM

The element is readily absorbed as molybdate, excreted mainly in the urine, like other anions, concentrated in liver, kidney and adrenal. Human serum contains about 3 mcg per 100 ml and urine about 56 mcg per day.

Sources

Cereals and dry legumes supply more than 50 μg per day. Liver and kidney are also good sources.

Daily requirement

(i) Adults : Nearly 0.5 mg
(ii) Children: 0.05 - 0.3 mg.

Functions

1. Role in enzyme action: Some of the flavoproteins, such as xanthine oxidase and aldehyde oxidase contain traces of molybdenum in their prosthetic group where it is believed to play an important role in the electron transport.

2. A trace of molybdenum may help in the utilization of copper.

Toxicity

Excess intake of it is responsible for toxicity known as **"molybdinosis"**, in which there occurs anaemia, growth retardation, loss of weight, diarrhoea, skeletal deformities, etc.

SELENIUM

Sources

It is found in different daily edible routine foodstuffs. The variation depends upon the differences of selenium content of the soil of that particular place. Fish, meat and cereals are the rich sources of selenium.

Daily requirement

(i) Adults : 0.2 mg
(ii) Children: 0.02 - 0.1 mg.

Absorption and Excretion

It is mainly absorbed in the duodenum and is taken up by β-lipoproteins, myoglobin, cytochrome C and nucleoproteins. It is excreted mainly in the faeces and expired air.

Functions:

1. It is constituent of **glutathione peroxidase** which catalyzes the breakdown of hydrogen peroxide in RBCs. Deficiency of selenium in human beings is not yet well established.
2. **Tocopherol sparing action**: Se has got close metabolic relationship with vitamin E. It reduces the requirement of vitamin E in more than one way (i) Se-containing glutathione peroxidase destroys acyl hydroperoxides, thus, lowers the need for antioxidant action of vitamin E in preventing peroxidative damages. (ii) Se may probably help in retaining vitamin E in lipoproteins.
3. It is involved in the mitochondrial ATP synthesis, ubiquinone synthesis and immune mechanisms.
4. It has been reported to be a **cancer protecting agent**.

Deficiency symptoms: Selenium deficiency may lead to liver necrosis, muscular atrophy, necrosis of the cardiac muscle and dilatation of the heart.

Toxicity

(i) Its toxicity is fatal which generally occurs in the workers of paint, electronics, ceramic industries and glass factories etc.
(ii) Areas of high selenium have higher prevalence of dental caries.

CHROMIUM

Very small amounts of chromium i.e. 0.01 mcg with insulin promote the conversion of acetate into glucose and fat. It is poorly absorbed from foods. Human serum contains about 6-20 mcg% and daily urinary excretion varies from <0.05 to 1 mcg.

Sources

Cereals, meat, yeast, milk, liver and other dietary foods.

Daily requirement

0.02 - 0.15 mg

Functions:

(i) Chromium plays an important role in carbohydrate, lipid and protein metabolism.
(ii) It is responsible for increasing sugar tolerance, probably by increasing the sensitivity of the peripheral tissues to insulin. **It is known as a *glucose***

tolerance factor.

(iii) It maintains the normal cholesterol level in blood in rats.

(iv) It regulates the incorporation of certain amino acids, mainly α-amino, isobutyric acid, glycine, serine and methionine in heart muscle in rats.

So far, no specific chromium deficiency disease in human beings is known today.

Absorption and Excretion:

Chromium is absorbed in the small intestine and combines with β- globulin in plasma. It's mainly excreted via urine.

Chromium Toxicity: Toxicity of chromium may be observed in occupational exposure to chromium dust **which is responsible for the cancer of lungs.**

WATER AND MINERALS

Everybody, whether plants or animals or human beings, is very familiar with the water from the day life starts in them. **Human body contains about 60- 70% water and nearly 8.5% minerals.** Minerals required relatively in larger quantities are sodium, potassium, calcium, magnesium, phosphorus, chlorine and sulphur; whereas those required comparatively in small amounts are iron, copper, cobalt, manganese, zinc, selenium, iodine, fluorine, chromium, cadmium, molybdenum etc.

Water Metabolism

Importance of water than the food is evident from the fact that the deprivation of water brings about death much more rapidly than the deprivation of food. When water is completely withheld, death takes place in a few days after the body has lost only 10 to 20 per cent of its water content. If, however, water is given but no food, life may continue for several weeks inspite of the loss of most of the body fat and about 50 per cent of the tissue proteins.

Water is so important that its importance can not be ignored as most tissues contain more than 70 per cent water; even bone possesses nearly one third water and adipose tissue (fat) contains large quantity of water in the connective tissue and in the spaces between the fat cells. About half of the body water is to be found in muscle which accounts for about one-third of the body mass.

Sources

Body water comes through main three channels:

1. *Food water:* Nearly 700 - 1000 ml of water comes from food daily.
2. *Water in drinks:* Human beings receive at least 600 ml of water daily through various kinds of drinks like water itself, tea, coffee, milk, beverages etc. On an average, the amount comes around 1200 ml per day.
3. *Metabolic water:* Nearly 300-400 ml of water is formed daily within the body itself by way of oxidation. Each gram of carbohydrate, lipid and protein yields 0.55, 1.06, and 0.45 g of water respectively on complete oxidation.

Losses

Water is lost daily by several ways:

1. **Insensible losses;** About 1000-1200 ml of water may be unconsciously lost daily from the human body. These *obligatory losses* occur irrespective of the availability of water.

(a) **Insensible cutaneous evaporation:** Man loses nearly 600 ml of water daily by way of cutaneous diffusion and evaporation, excluding that by sweating.

(b) **Pulmonary evaporation:** Normally about 400 ml of water gets evaporated from pulmonary alveoli and respiratory passages and eliminated with expired air every day.

2. ***Loss via sweat:*** In extreme hot circumstances, a man may lose upto 10 litres per day of sweat containing as much as 30 g of salt. If water and salt are not taken at frequent intervals under such hot circumstances, then the blood becomes concentrated which eventually affects the circulation, which may even fail. On an average, the loss is nearly 700 ml per day.

   Sweat is a slightly acidic, watery fluid of variable composition but always hypotonic with respect to blood plasma. It contains 0.5 per cent solids only, mainly sodium chloride. The sodium content of sweat is also affected by aldosterone.

3. ***Faecal loss:*** Normally, about 100-200 ml may be *obligatorily* lost via faeces due to osmotic effects of faecal constituents. Diarrhoea increases the faecal loss.

4. ***Renal loss;*** About 14 litres of fluid is filtered by the renal tubules in 24- hours, but nearly 99% of the water is reabsorbed leaving behind 1000-1500 ml of urine only.

Water balance

An equilibrium is maintained by different factors between the intake and output of water in the body (Table 14.5). In addition to other factors, certain hormones like anti-diuretic hormone (ADH), vasopressin, oxytocin and aldosterone also influence the regulatory mechanism of the body water.

An animal is said to be in *water equilibrium* when the total loss of water is in toto replaced by the amount obtained from various sources. When more water is eliminated from the body than what is taken in, the body is said to be in negative water balance, e.g., in less consumption of water, diarrhoea, excessive and frequent vomiting and excessive sweating. If the loss of water is less than the amount received from various sources, the body is said to be in ***positive water balance,* e.g., during growth and pregnancy.** The balance sheet of water is as given in Table 14.5.

Physiological functions of water

1. ***Solvent action:*** The most important role of water is that it acts as a solvent both around and inside the cells. That is why, both, the extracellular and intracellular fluids are aqueous solutions. Water acts as a solvent for many biomolecules and also forms the medium where they may intermix and interact easily. Water donates H^+ and OH^- for many biochemical reactions, a beautiful property of water. It is also a reactant in hydrolysis and hydration.

2. ***Ionization:*** This property is very important from the point of view that water itself ionizes into H^+ and OH^- to provide a specific H^+ concentration in the biological fluids: Besides this, ionization of mineral salts in aqueous body fluids provides mineral ions like Na^+, K^+ and Cl^-, which are required for electrical

Table 14.5 : Balance sheet of water (per day)

Water intake			Water loss		
(a)	By food water	850 ml	(a)	By lungs	400 ml
(b)	By drinks	1,200 ml	(b)	By skin	700 ml
(c)	By oxidation of foods	400 ml	(c)	By urine	1,250 ml
			(d)	By faeces	100 ml
Total		**2,450 ml**	**Total**		**2,450 ml**

conductivity of body fluids and membrane polarization and depolarization.

3. ***Homeostasis:*** Homeostasis or constancy of internal environment is largely maintained with the help of body water.
4. ***Fluid exchange:*** Small molecules and polar nature of water enable its molecules to pass through the hydrophilic pores of membranes.
5. ***Lubricating action:*** Water also acts as a lubricant in the body so as to prevent friction in joints, pleura, peritoneum and conjunctiva.
6. ***Latent heat of evaporation:*** Water has the highest latent heat of evaporation than any other liquid. A certain amount of water can, therefore, cause maximum cooling by evaporation; so that the temperature of body does not rise so easily.

Regulation of Water Metabolism

There are several factors which regulate the water metabolism in the body; they are as follows:

1. *Antidiuretic hormone or Vasopressin:* Posterior pituitary releases ADH which has got the property to enhance water reabsorption in the distal tubules and collecting ducts. Water permeability gets increased.
2. *Hypothalamus:* There is a centre in hypothalamus known as a *thirst centre;* whenever there is dehydration in the body, osmoconcentration of plasma takes place which eventually stimulates the thirst centre producing thirst as a result of which animal gets provoked to drink the required amount of water. Besides this, osmoconcentration of plasma also stimulates supraoptic and paraventricular nuclei of hypothalamus; nerve impulses from them are responsible to increase the release of vasopressin from neurohypophysis into the blood. Lesions in the supraopticoparaventricular region or in the neurohypophysis produce ***diabetes insipidus*** in which large volume of dilute (hypotonic) urine is passed, may be 10 litres or so a day. ***Diabetes insipidus* is due to the abnormalities in the ADH secretion. In primary diabetes insipidus, there is less secretion of the ADH hormone** which is usually due to the destruction of the hypothalamic-hypophyseal tract either from a basal skull fracture, or tumor, or infection. **Besides, diabetes insipidus may be hereditary also.**
3. *Adrenal Cortex and Water loss:* Loss of electrolytes and the loss of water from the body are closely interlinked. Adrenal cortex plays a very important role in governing the reabsorption of water by the renal tubules. **The excretion of sodium and potassium by the kidneys is controlled by a steroid hormone called *aldosterone* which is secreted by the zona glomerulosa of the adrenal cortex.** In man, aldosterone first increases the elimination of potassium and hydrogen ions and then decreases the excretion of sodium without any change in GFR. Aldosterone acts mainly at the distal tubule but its effect on sodium reabsorption may be partly at the proximal tubule. Apart from its action on the renal tubule, aldosterone increases the reabsorption of sodium from the secretions of the intestinal mucosa and of the salivary and sweat glands. Thus, the body content of Na^+ rises and that of K^+ decreases.

   Aldosterone is not the only cortical hormone affecting water balance. The diuretic response to a water load gets impaired in patients whose adrenal glands are destroyed by diseases like Addison's disease or are removed after operation. The ability to deal normally with water is, however, restored by the administration of cortisone or hydrocortisone.

4. *Renin-Angiotensin system:* **This system is also involved in the regulation of blood pressure and electrolyte metabolism. The primary hormone involved - is *angiotensin II,* an octapeptide formed from angiotensiongen.** A decrease in circulating blood volume stimulates renin secretion from kidneys which in turn promotes angiotensin formation in plasma. Angiotensin II stimulates the synthesis and secretion of aldosterone and the release of vasopressin, and thereby increases renal absorption of Na^+ and H_2O.
5. *Prostaglandins:* They are also believed to help maintain glomerular filtration inspite of hypotension, by causing renal vasodilation. They may also increase urinary loss of water by inhibiting the antidiuretic effect of vasopressin and by increasing the urinary sodium.
6. *Solutes:* Osmotic effect of Na^+ helps to retain water in extracellular fluids. Elevation in plasma Na^+ raises the ECF volume in primary aldosteronism while an increase in urinary Na^+ raises the urinary water output in Addison's disease. K^+ helps to retain water in the cells, whereas, plasma proteins do help to retain water in the body by their osmotic effects. Increase in urinary urea or excretion of glucose in urine increases osmotically the urinary loss of water **(osmotic diuresis).**

Dehydration

Dehydration may be defined as a state in which loss of water exceeds that of intake, as a result of which body's water content gets reduced. In this state, the body is in negative water balance.

Causes

1. *Primary- dehydration:* There is purely water depletion and no salt depletion. It occurs in following states:
   (a) Due to deprivation of water as generally happens during desert travelling.
   (b) In mental patients who refuse to drink water/fluids.
   (c) In those who keep such a 'fast' in which water/fluid is completely restricted.
   (d) It occurs more quickly during fever or in the high temperature of the environment.
   (e) Excessive water loss due to vomiting, prolonged diarrhoea, gastroenteritis.
   (f) Due to excretion of large quantities of urine or sweat.

   This type of dehydration raises the concentration and osmotic pressure of extracellular fluid as a result of which there is consequent outflow of the intracellular water to the ECF; thus, ECF volume gets largely restored but there becomes deficiency of water inside the cells as a result of which they suffer from osmoconcentration; symptoms of which include dry tongue, poor salivation, dry shrunken skin, nausea, reduced sweating and intense thirst.

   When the blood becomes hypertonic, it lowers the urinary output and also makes the urine concentrated as a result of which there is less elimination of NPN and other acids which leads to acidosis and eventually coma. Death occurs in man due to renal failure, acidosis, intracellular hyperosmolarity, circulatory collapse or neural depression, when body water falls by 20%.

Drinking of concentrated saline like sea-water or failure of Na^+ excretion (e.g., in Cushing's syndrome and Primary aldosteronism) may cause hypertonicity of ECF which in turn is responsible for withdrawal of water from tissue cells, dehydration of tissues, but a rise in ECF volume. Mg^{2+} of sea-water may be responsible for an increased intestinal loss of water due to its osmotic effect in the intestinal lumen.

2. *Secondary dehydration:* The concentration of the electrolytes of the body fluids is maintained constant either through the elimination or retention of water. The reduction or elevation in the total electrolytes, which affects the basic radicals chiefly i.e. Na (extracellular) and K (intracellular) and the acid radicals HCO_3 and Cl are accompanied by a corresponding increase or decrease in the volume of body water which is eventually the cause of intracellular edema; as a result of which there is slowing of circulation and impairment of urinary functions. All this causes an individual to become weak bodily.
3. *Dehydration due to injection of hypertonic solution:* When a highly concentrated solution of sugar or salt is injected into the body of an individual, the osmotic pressure of blood will increase which results in the flow of fluid from the tissues into the blood unless an equilibrium is reached. Consequently, the blood volume increases. This increased blood volume soon returns to normal by the loss of excess material through excretion which finally causes a net loss of body water producing dehydration.

Effects of dehydration

There are various side effects of dehydration as follows, which may be overcome as soon as the body gets hydrated; otherwise the consequences are serious and may even lead to death.

1. Disturbance in acid-base balance.
2. Loss of body weight due to the reduction in tissue water.
3. Rise in nonprotein nitrogen (NPN) of blood.
4. Dryness, wrinkling and looseness of the skin.
5. Elevation in the plasma protein concentration and chloride.
6. Rise in the temperature of body due to reduction of circulating fluid.
7. Increased pulse rate and reduced cardiac output.
8. Exhaustion and collapse i.e. death.

Correction of dehydration

1. Ordinarily, sodium chloride solution may be given parenterally to compensate the loss.
2. In several disorders like diarrhoea, gastroenteritis, pancreatic or biliary fistulas, etc., a mixture of two-thirds isotonic saline solution and one-third sodium lactate solution (M/6) should be administered intravenously.
3. **Dehydration is a burning problem in several disorders like diabetes mellitus, Addison's disease, uremia, shock and extensive burns** which is difficult to correct by the above two ways.

Water Intoxication

This condition is generally caused due to the retention of excess water in the body and can occur due to renal failure, excessive administration of fluids parenterally and hypersecretion of ADH. Symptoms of water intoxication include nausea, headache, muscular weakness, etc.

CHAPTER 15

BIOENERGETICS/BIOLOGICAL OXIDATIONS

THE OXIDOREDUCTASE

Living organisms require continuous nonstop supply of energy to carry out different types of functions of living matter (Fig. 15.1). In most of the cases, the energy is obtained by the oxidation of metabolites which are formed from the digestion of food. There are three ways by which such oxidations can take place. All the ways are basically the same and involve the loss of electrons from the compound being oxidized (Fig. 15.2).

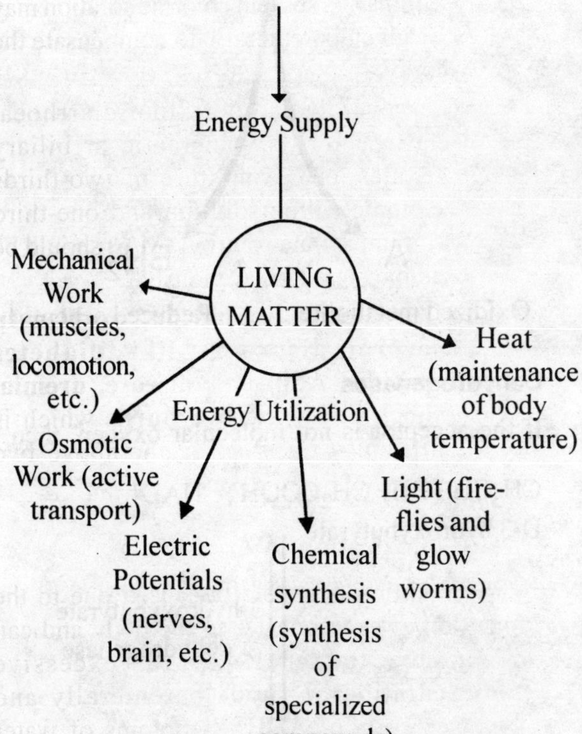

Fig. 15.1: Energy turnover in living organisms

Addition of Oxygen

$$CH_3CHO + ½O_2 \longrightarrow CH_3COOH$$

acetaldehyde → acetic acid

Removal of Hydrogen

$$\begin{array}{l} CH(OH).COOH \\ | \\ CH_2COOH \end{array} \longrightarrow \begin{array}{l} CO.COOH \\ | \\ CH_2COOH \end{array} + 2H$$

malic acid → oxaloacetic acid (H to acceptor)

Removal of Electrons

Cytochrome (Fe^{++})

↓

Cytochrome (Fe^{+++}) + Electron (to acceptor)

Fig. 15.2 : Methods of Biological Oxidation

The enzymes responsible for biological oxidation are classified in group 1, the oxidoreductases. Trivial names are still used for enzymes in this group which are as considered below in brief:

Oxygenases and Hydroxylases

A few metabolites are oxidized by the direct addition of molecular oxygen, but this is the exception rather than the rule for biological oxidations.

Oxygenases

These enzymes catalyse the incorporation of both atoms of molecular oxygen directly into the substrate.

catechol + O_2 —(catecho-1,2-oxygenase)→ cis-cis-muconate

Hydroxylases

These are similar to the oxygenases except that only the atom of molecular oxygen is introduced into the substrate instead of two. The other oxygen atom is incorporated into water by reaction with a reduced acceptor which therefore acts as a co-substrate. The overall reaction is as given above:

aniline (NH_2) + NADPH + H^+ + O_2 —(aryl-4-hydroxylase)→ p- hydroxyaniline (NH_2, OH) + $NADP^+$ + H_2O

Dehydrogenases and Oxidases

Nearly all biological oxidations take place by the removal of hydrogen from the substrate. Hydrogen atoms are removed from a metabolite (AH_2) and passed on to an acceptor (B).

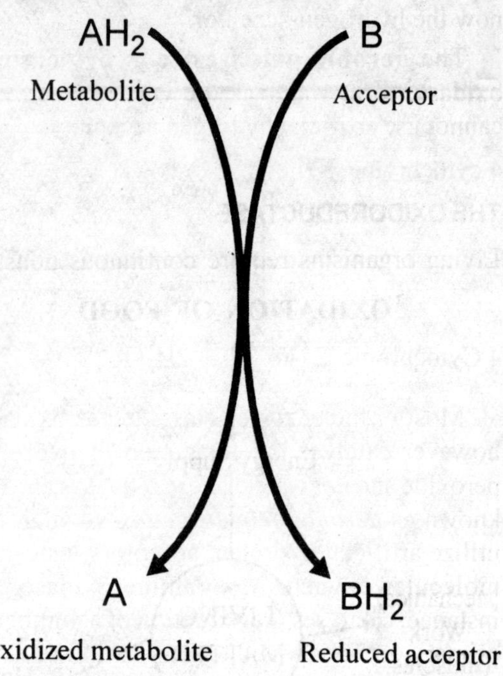

Dehydrogenases

If the acceptor is not molecular oxygen, then

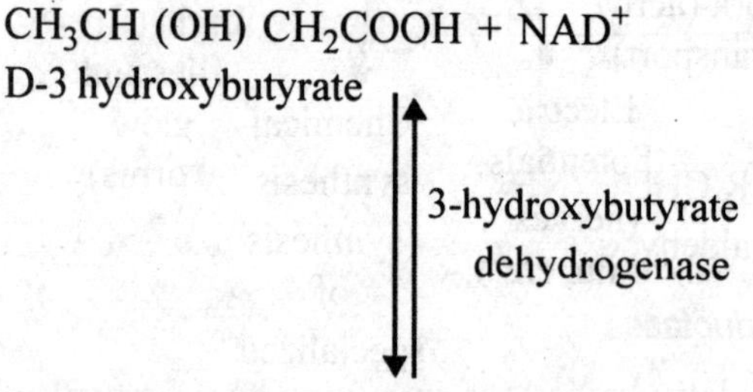

the enzymes are known as **dehydrogenases.** For the purpose of studying a dehydrogenase catalysed reaction in the laboratory, artificial hydrogen acceptors can be used instead of the 'natural' coenzymes of the cell.

Oxidases

These are conjugated proteins and usually contain a metal; they catalyse the same type of reaction as the dehydrogenases, but molecular oxygen is now the hydrogen acceptor.

The **aerobic oxidases:** e.g. cytochrome oxidase, form water as the end product. and cannot use artificial hydrogen acceptors.

$$4 \text{ cytochrome C } (Fe^{++}) + O_2 + 4H^+ \xrightarrow{\text{cytochrome oxidase}} 4 \text{ Cytochrome C } (Fe^{+++}) + 2H_2O$$

Most of the enzymes classified as oxidases however catalyse the formation of hydrogen peroxide and *not* water. These oxidases are also known as ***aerobic dehydrogenases*** which can utilize artificial hydrogen acceptors instead of molecular oxygen. Monoamine oxidase, for instance, catalyses the oxidation of a number of primary, secondary and tertiary amines.

$$\underset{\text{primary amine}}{RCH_2NH_2} + H_2O + O_2 \xrightarrow{\text{monoamine oxidase}} \underset{\text{aldehyde}}{R.CHO} + NH_3 + H_2O_2$$

Reductases

Oxidative reactions involving the removal of electrons but not hydrogen ions from the substrate are catalysed by enzymes which are known as **reductases.** Some plants and micro-organisms are known to contain an enzyme which catalyses the reduction of nitrate.

$$-NO_3^- + NADH + H^+ \underset{\text{Nitrate reductase}}{\rightleftharpoons} -NO_2^- + NAD^+ + H_2O$$

Catalase and peroxidase

Hydrogen peroxide formed by the catalytic action of the **aerobic dehydrogenases** is highly toxic to living cells but does not accumulate due to the rapid action of catalase or a peroxidase. Catalase is found in both the animals and the plants, whereas peroxidases are found in plants only.

$$2H_2O_2 \xrightarrow{\text{catalase}} 2H_2O + O_2$$

$$\underset{\text{donor}}{AH_2} + \underset{\text{peroxide}}{H_2O_2} \xrightarrow{\text{peroxidase}} 2H_2O + \underset{\text{oxidized donor}}{A}$$

ELECTRON TRANSPORT CHAIN (RESPIRATORY CHAIN)

Components of the Chain

Pyridine nucleotides

Dehydrogenase enzymes cannot catalyse the removal of hydrogen from a substrate unless low molecular weight cofactors are also present to act as hydrogen acceptors. The compounds that are most frequently found as coenzymes for dehydrogenases are the two pyridine nucleotides, nicotinamide adenine dinucleotide (NAD) and nicotinamide adenine dinucleotide phosphate (NADP); both are freely soluble. These have a typical nucleotide type of structure, as given below:

Nicotinamide — D — ribofuranose-phosphale
|
Adenine — D — ribofuranose-phosphate

Nicotinamide adenine dinucleotide (NAD)

The nicotinamide part of the molecule is only involved in the reaction, therefore, the structure can be simplified to ;

NAD$^+$ or NADP$^+$ [pyridinium ring with $CONH_2$ at position 3, N^+–R]

Nicotinamide

where R represents the rest of the molecule. Work with isotopes has revealed that the hydrogen atoms from the substrate add on the 1 and 4 positions of the nicotinamide ring but, at neutral pH, the hydrogen at position 1 dissociates as an hydrogen ion.

NAD$^+$ (oxidized form) + 2H ⇌ NADH (reduced form) + H^+

This reaction is usually abbreviated as :

$$NAD + 2H \rightleftharpoons NADH_2$$

or

$$NAD^+ + 2H \rightleftharpoons NADH + H^+$$

Flavoproteins

Another major group of reversible hydrogen acceptors are the flavoproteins, which consist of a protein moiety and a prosthetic group containing riboflavin. These compounds are often called nucleotides although the sugar component linked to the isoalloxazine ring is present as the alcohol ribitol and not the sugar ribose, and the link between base and 'sugar' is not glycosidic. The two flavin prosthetic groups are flavin mononucleotide (FMN) and flavin adenine dinucleotide (FAD).

6,7 - Dimethyl isoalloxazine-D-ribitol-phosphate

riboflavin

Flavin mononucleotide (FMN)

6,7 - Dimethyl-isoalloxazine- D-ribitol-phosphate

Adenine-D-ribose-phosphate

Flavin adenine dinucleotide (FAD)

The hydrogen atoms react with the isoalloxazine part of the molecule so that the prosthetic groups, can be conveniently represented as shown below where R is the rest of the molecule.

FP [yellow oxidised form of flavoprotein]

+2H ⇌

FPH_2 [colourless reduced form of flavoprotein]

Coenzyme Q

An important part of the chain of compounds involved in cellular respiration is coenzyme Q, which is associated with the lipoprotein part of the mitochondria. Coenzyme Q is found widely in living materials and has therefore been given the name of **ubiquinone** ***(Latin ubique, everywhere).***

CH_3O, CH_3, CH_3, CH_3O, $(CH_2-CH=C-CH_2)_n-H$ + 2H

oxidized or quinone form of ubiquinone

In animals and higher plants, n = 10

CH_3O, OH, CH_3, CH_3, CH_3O, OH, $(CH_2-CH=C-CH_2)_n-H$

reduced or quinol form of ubiquinone

Cytochromes

The word cytochrome means cellular pigment, and the name is derived from the fact that all living cells exhibit characteristic absorption bands in the visible region of the spectrum due to these iron porphyrin compounds. The cytochromes are redox catalysts of major importance in cellular respiration. Unlike the compounds previously considered, they act by reversibly donating and accepting electrons, not hydrogen atoms. Electrons are transported by the haem iron which undergoes a change of valency in the process.

$$\text{Cytochrome } (Fe^{+++}) + e \rightleftharpoons \text{Cytochrome } (Fe^{++})$$

Oxidized form Electron Reduced form

Cytochromes were first discovered by McMunn in 1886, then rediscovered by Keilin in 1925. On the basis of spectroscopic data, Keilin demonstrated the existence of three cytochromes designated a, b and c and later cytochrome d was also discovered. Classification of a cytochrome into one of these 4 groups is on the basis of the absorption spectra of the haem prosthetic group and certain chemical properties.

In the mitochondria, cytochromes act together as a coordinated system for electron transfer. Most cytochromes are intimately associated with membranes and are extremely difficult to isolate. Cytochrome c, a low molecular weight protein (12,000) with one atom of iron per molecule, is the only cytochrome which is readily soluble.

The Function of the Chain

Formation of water

In the mitochondria, above compounds, i.e, pyridine nucleotides, flavoproteins, coenzyme Q (ubiquinone) and cytochromes act together as an integrated chain during biological oxidations. This sequence of redox compounds is known as the electron transport chain or respiratory chain. Reducing equivalents from most metabolites are transferred to NAD, pass down the chain and finally react with molecular oxygen to form water (Fig. 15.3). The first part of the chain involves the transfer of a pair of hydrogen atoms, while the cytochromes transfer only a single electron.

Water is probably formed from H^+ discharged at the CoQ-Cyt b step and OH^- arising from the reaction of molecular oxygen with cytochrome a_3.

$$CoQ.2H + 2Cyt.b^{+++} \rightarrow 2\,Cyt.b^{++} + 2H^+ + CoQ$$

$$\downarrow$$

$$2H_2O$$

$$\uparrow$$

$$2Cyt.a_3^{++} + \tfrac{1}{2}O_2 + HOH \rightarrow 2Cyt.a_3^{+++} + 2OH^-$$

Arrangement of components of the chain

The major components of the respiratory chain are arranged sequentially in order of increasing redox potentials (Table 15.1).

Table 15.1: Some redox potentials in oxidation systems

System	Eo' volts
H^+/N_2	-0.42
$NAD^+/NADH$	-0.32
Flavoprotein-old yellow enzyme, ox/red	-0.12
Cytochrome b; Fe^{+++}/Fe^{++}	+0.08
Ubiquinone; ox/red	+0.10
Cytochrome c; Fe^{+++}/Fe^{++}	+0.22
Cytochrome a; Fe^{+++}/Fe^{++}	+0.29
Oxygen/Water	+0.82

Hydrogen **or electron flows** through the chain in a step-wise **manner from** the more electro-negative components to the more electro-positive oxygen through a redox span of 1.1 volts from NAD/NADH to $O_2/2H_2O$.

Role of Respiratory Chain Enzymes

All of useful energy, which is released during oxidation of amino acids and fatty acids and nearly all of that liberated from oxidation of carbohydrates is made available as reducing equivalents (-H^+ or electrons) within the mitochondria. **Mitochondria are well known to contain various key enzymes which are important for the energy production (as shown ahead in 1st Box). These enzymes perform various important functions such as :**

(i) **collection and transport of reducing equivalents,**

(ii) **trapping the liberated free energy as high energy phosphates, and**

(iii) **production of most of reducing equivalents in earlier stages i.e. β-oxidation and tricarboxylic acid cycle.**

OXIDATIVE PHOSPHORYLATION

Introduction

At first sight, the chain appears to be a rather complicated way of producing water, but this sequence of carriers has a more important function than that.

The transfer of hydrogen from a substrate (AH_2) to NAD generally involves a relatively small change in free energy:

$$AH_2 + NAD^+ \rightleftharpoons A + NADH + H^+ \qquad \Delta G \text{ small}$$

The oxidation of reduced coenzyme by molecular oxygen however releases a large amount of energy:

$$NADH + H^+ + \tfrac{1}{2}O_2 \rightleftharpoons NAD^+ + H_2O \qquad \Delta G = -52 \text{ kcal}$$

The release of this energy does not take place in one step, as suggested by the overall equation, but in a series of different stages. This is the difference between stepping out of a first floor window to reach the ground and going down the stairs; the overall energy change is the same in both cases, but using the stairs is less traumatic and also more reversible. In the electron transport chain, the energy is not only released in different steps but at certain points is converted into a form which can be used by cell. **Adenosine triphosphate (ATP) is the *'energy currency'* of the cell** and the formation of 1 mol from ADP and inorganic phosphate (P_i) requires 7.5 kcal.

$$ADP + Pi \rightarrow ATP + H_2O \qquad \Delta G = +7.5 \text{ kcal}$$

At certain points in the chain, enough energy is available to form ATP and 3 molecules of this compound are believed to be formed for each pair of hydrogen atoms oxidized. The means whereby this is accomplished are, to say the least, obscure but some form of **'coupling'** exists between oxidation and the phosphorylation of ADP. In the case of dehydrogenases with NAD as coenzyme, 3 molecules of phosphate (P) are incorporated into ATP for each atom of oxygen (O) utilized, so that a P/O ratio of 3 is obtained. Some substrates such as succinate and fatty acyl CoA react directly with flavoproteins and therefore bypass the step involving NAD; in these cases, a P/O ratio of 2 is found (Fig. 15.3).

Definition

The oxidation of a substrate with accompanying phosphorylation of ADP to ATP is known as oxidative *phosphorylation.* This process takes place in mitochondria as the enzymes concerned with **"Citric acid cycle"** are located in the space between the cristae and the enzymes concerned with **"electron transport"** (Fig 15.3) are arranged in an appropriate pattern in cristae themselves.

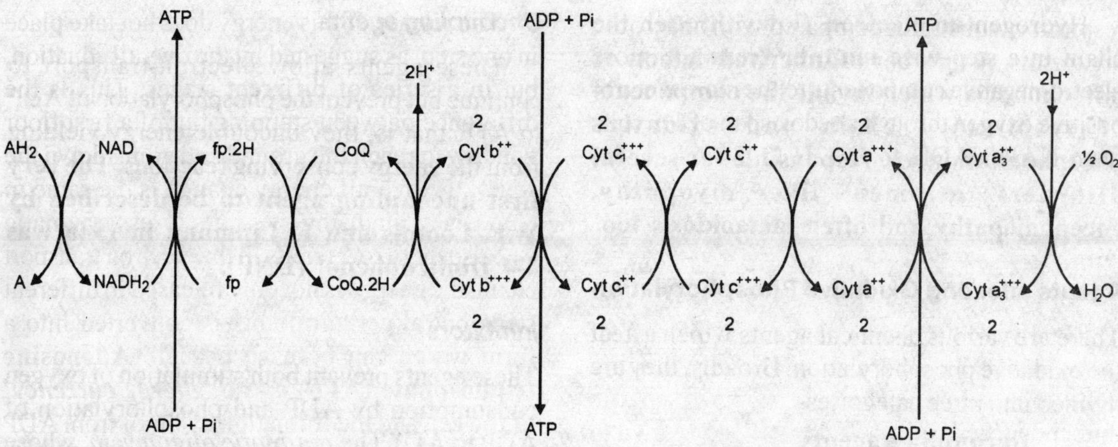

AH_2 = most substrates

ATP = adenosine triphosphate

NAD = nicotinamide adenine dinucleotide

ADP = adenosine diphosphate

fp = flavoproteins

Pi = inorganic phosphate

Cyt = cytochromes

Fig. 15.3 : The electron transport chain

Biomedical Importance

Oxidative phosphorylation is fundamental to all *aspects of cellular life* in *aerobic organisms since it is their main source of useful energy.* It enables aerobic organisms to capture a far greater proportion of available free energy of

LOCATION OF SOME ENZYMES IN RAT LIVER MITOCHONDRIA

Outer membrane

- MAO (mono amine oxidase)
- Kynurenine-3-monooxygenase
- NADH dehydrogenase (Antimycin insensitive)
- Acyl CoA synthetases
- Phospholipase A_2
- Nucleoside diphosphate kinase

Space between the membranes

- Adenylate kinase

Inner membrane

- NADH dehydrogenase (Antimycin sensitive)
- Iron-sulphur proteins
- Cytochrome b, c, c_1 and a a_3
- F_1 ATPase
- Succinate dehydrogenase
- D-β Hydroxybutyrate dehydrogenase
- Carnitine acyl transferase

Matrix

- Citrate synthetase
- Isocitrate dehydrogenase
- Fumarase
- Malate dehydrogemse
- Glutamate dehydrogenase
- Asparate transaminase
- Fatty acyl-CoA oxidation enzyme

respiratory substrates compared with anaerobic organisms. **A number of inherited defects of mitochondria which invade the components of respiratory chain and oxidative phosphorylation are responsible for several disorders in men like myopathy, encephalopathy and often lactacidosis too.**

Agents affecting Oxidative Phosphorylation

There are various chemical agents which affect the oxidative phosphorylation. Broadly, they are divided into three categories-

1. **Uncoupling agents**
2. **Inhibitors**
3. **Ionophores**

TYPES OF AGENTS AFFECTING OXIDATIVE PHOSPHORYLATION

Uncoupling agents

2, 4-Dinitrophenol

Dicumarol

Carbonylcyanide phenylhydrazone

Salicylanilides

Arsenate

Inhibitors of ATP formation

Oligomycin

Rutamycin

Aurovertin

Triethyltin

Ionophores (Carriers of cations)

Valinomycin

Gramicidin

Nonactin

Nigericin

Uncoupling agents

These agents allow electron-transport to continue but prevent the phosphorylation of ADP to ATP, that is, they uncouple energy yielding from the energy conserving reactions. **The very first uncoupling agent to be described by W.F. Loomis and F. Lipmann in 1948 was 2-4 Dinitrophenol (DNP).**

Inhibitors

These agents prevent both stimulation of oxygen consumption by ADP and phosphorylation of ADP to ATP. The *antibiotic oligomycin,* whose action for the first time was described by H.A. Lardy and his colleagues, *is the prototype of this class.*

Ionophores

These agents cause breakdown of high energy intermediate state only if certain monovalent cations are present. The *prototype of this group is the antibiotic Valinomycin* which requires K^+ for its inhibitory effect, other agents include ***Nigericin*** and ***Nonactin.***

Mechanism of Oxidative Phosphorylation

(Formation of ATP by Oxidative Phosphorylation)

Despite all the complexities of (a) glycolysis, (b) citric acid cycle, (c) dehydrogenation and (d) decarboxylation, only small amounts of ATP (two ATP molecules in glycolysis and another two ATP molecules in the citric acid cycle) are formed during all these processes. Instead 90 per cent of the total ATP formed by glucose metabolism is formed during subsequent oxidation of the hydrogen atoms that are released during these earlier stages of glucose degradation. Truly speaking, the main function of all these earlier stages is to make the hydrogen of the glucose molecule in forms that can be utilized for oxidation.

Oxidation of hydrogen is completed by a series of enzymatically catalyzed reactions in the mitochondria which (a) split each hydrogen atom into a hydrogen ion and an electron i.e., $H \rightarrow H^+ + e^-$, and (b) use the electrons finally to change the dissolved oxygen of the fluids into hydroxyl ions, i.e. $O_2 \xrightarrow{e} OH^-$. Then the hydrogen and hydroxyl ions combine with each other to form water i.e., $H^+ + OH^- \longrightarrow H_2O$. During the sequence of oxidative reactions, large amount of energy is released to form ATP. Formation of ATP in this way is called ***'oxidative phosphorylation'***. This occurs exclusively in the mitochondria by a highly specialized process called the ***'chemiosmotic mechanism'***.

In all there are three hypotheses regarding the mechanism of oxidative phosphorylation:

(i) **Chemical coupling hypothesis**

(ii) **Conformational coupling hypothesis**

(iii) **Chemiosmotic hypothesis**

Chemical Coupling Hypothesis

It proposes that electron transport is coupled to ATP synthesis by a sequence of consecutive reactions in which a high energy covalent intermediate is formed by electron transport and subsequently is cleaved and donates its energy to generate ATP.

Conformational Coupling Hypothesis

It postulates that the transfer of electrons along the respiratory chain causes a conformational change in protein components of inner membrane to yield a high-energy form. The conformational change so produced is transmitted to the F_0F_1 ATPase molecule, causing it to become energized. Relaxation of the energized F_0F_1 ATPase to its normal conformation has proposed to provide energy for the synthesis of ATP and its release from the enzyme.

Chemiosmotic Hypothesis

It was for the first time proposed by the *British Biochemist* named *Peter Mitchell,* which postulates that **'electron transport'** pumps H^+ form the matrix across the inner mitochondrial membrane to the outer aqueous phase, thus generating a H^+ gradient across the inner membrance. The osmotic energy inherent in its gradient was postulated to drive the energy requiring synthesis of ATP.

This mechanism mainly involves the following three important stages:

(i) **Ionization of Hydrogen,**

(ii) **Electron Transport Chain, and**

(iii) **Formation of Water.**

The first step in the oxidative phosphorylation in the mitochondria is to ionize the hydrogen atoms that are removed from the food substrates. These hydrogen atoms are removed in pairs; one immediately becomes a hydrogen ion, H^+, and the other combines with NAD^+ to produce NADH. The upper portion of Figure 8.4 reveals the subsequent fate of the NADH and H^+. The initial effect is to release the other hydrogen atom bound with NAD to form another hydrogen ion, H^+; this process also re-forms NAD^+ that will be reused again and again.

Now, the electrons that are removed from the hydrogen atoms to cause the ionization immediately enter an *electron transport chain* (ETC) which is an integral part of the inner membrane of the mitochondria. This transport chain (Fig. 15.4) consists of a series of electron acceptors which can be reversibly reduced or oxidized by accepting or giving up electrons. The important members of this ETC include flavoprotein, several iron sulfide proteins, ubiquinone and the cytochromes B, C_1, C, A and A_3. Each electron gets shuttled from one of these acceptors to the next until it finally reaches cytochrome A_3, **which is called *cytochrome oxidase*** because it is capable, by giving up two electrons, of causing elemental oxygen to combine with hydrogen ions to form water.

Figures 15.3 and 15.4 illustrate transport of electrons through the electron chain and then

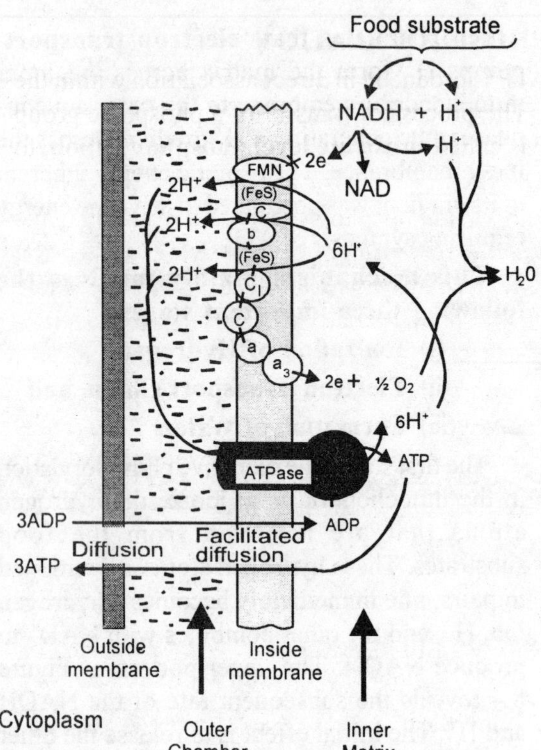

Fig. 15.4: The chemiosmotic theory of oxidative phosphorylation for the generation of large amount of ATP

ultimate use of these electrons by *cytochrome oxidase* to cause the formation of water molecules. During the transport of these electrons through the electron transport chain, energy is released which is later on used for the generation of ATP.

Pumping of hydrogen ions into the outer chamber of the mitochondrion is caused by the electron transport chain. **As the electrons pass through the ETC,** large amount of energy is released which is eventually used to pump hydrogen ions from the inner matrix of the mitochondrion into the outer chamber between the inner and outer mitochondrial membranes. This creates a high concentration of hydrogen ions in this chamber; besides, it also creates a strong negative electrical potential in the inner matrix.

Generation of ATP

The next step in the oxidative phosphorylation is to convert ADP into ATP, which occurs in the large protein molecule that protrudes all the way through the inner mitochondrial membrane and projects with a knob like head into the inner matrix. This protein molecule is known as ATPase (Fig 15.4), which is also called as ATP synthetase. It is believed that the high concentration of hydrogen ions in the outer chamber and the large electrical potential difference across the inner membrane are responsible for the flow of hydrogen ions into the mitrochondrial matrix through the substance of the ATPase molecule. In doing so, energy derived from the hydrogen ion flow is utilized by the ATPase to convert ADP into ATP in the presence of inorganic phosphate (Pi), thus forming an additional high energy phosphate bond.

The last step in this process is the transfer of the ATP from the inside of the mitochondrion back to the cytoplasm which is accomplished by facilitated diffusion outward through the inner membrane and then by simple diffusion through the very permeable outer mitochondrial membrane. In turn, ADP gets continuously transferred in a like manner back into the mitochondrial matrix for continuous conversion into ATP.

For each two electrons which pass through the entire ETC (representing the ionization of two hydrogen atoms), upto three ATP molecules get synthesized.

> Central role of transmembrane gradient of H^+ in providing energy for different cell activities
>
> ΔH^+ membrane gradient →
> - **ATP synthesis**
> - **Transport of Ca^{++}**
> - **Transport of PO_4**
> - **Transport of ADP and ATP**
> - **Heat**
> - **Rotation of bacteria flagella**

SUBSTRATE LEVEL PHOSPHORYLATION

In addition to oxidative phosphorylation, some ATP is produced in direct association within the individual steps of certain metabolic pathways. The process of transfer of a phosphate group from a very high energy phophate donor to ADP is called **substrate level phosphorylation,** to cite few examples:

(i) The enzyme phosphoglycerate kinase acts on 1, 3-diphosphoglyceric acid resulting in the synthesis of ATP and formation of 3-phosphoglyceric acid **(step of glycolysis).** This step is a good example of **substrate level phosphorylation;** since ATP is synthesized from the substrate without the involvement of electron transport chain. Phosphoglycerate kinase reaction is reversible, a rare example among the kinase reactions.

(ii) The enzyme pyruvate kinase catalyses the transfer of high energy phosphate from phosphoenolpyruvate to ADP, leading to the formation of ATP **(step of glycolysis).** This step is another example of **substrate level phosphorylation. This reaction is irreversible.**

Unsaturated fatty acid residues of membrane lipids form a-hydroperoxyalkenes by reacting with oxygen:

$$>C=C-\overset{|}{\underset{|}{C}}- + O_2 \longrightarrow >C=C-\overset{OOH}{\underset{|}{\overset{|}{C}}}-$$

These hydroperoxides undergo cleavage to give rise to short-chain aldehydes. **Peroxidation can also cause damage to DNA and proteins.**

$$2\,GSH + \begin{matrix} | \\ HC-O \\ | \quad | \\ HC-O \\ | \end{matrix} \longrightarrow GSSG + \begin{matrix} | \\ HC \\ \| \\ HC \\ | \end{matrix} + H_2O_2$$

glutathione — oxidized glutathione

In the latter, sulfhydryl groups give rise to disulfide linkages. **Vitamin E** functions as an **antioxidant** and can prevent **oxygen toxicity. Glutathione peroxidase,** a selenium containing enzyme, inactivates peroxides:

Glutathione, which protects sulfhydryl groups of proteins, is regenerated by glutathione reductase, which uses reducing equivalents from NADPH.

$$GSSG + NADPH + H^+ \longrightarrow 2GSH + NADP^+$$

The hydrogen peroxide formed above is decomposed by catalase:

$$2H_2O_2 \longrightarrow 2H_2O + O_2$$

Aerobic organisms are protected from oxygen toxicity by three enzymes namely: glutathione peroxidase, catalase and superoxide dismutase.

CHAPTER 16

HORMONES

By S.P. Singh* and Anshuman Singh**

The term *'hormone'* for the first time was given by Bayliss and Starling in 1902. It was derived from the Greek word "Hormaein" which means to excite or to arouse. Hormone is a chemical substance which is produced in one part of the body, enters the circulation and is carried to distant organs and tissues to modify their structures and functions.

Hormones have three major functions in the body, namely:

1. **Integrative,**
2. **Regulative and**
3. **Morphological**

A particular hormone is involved in only one function. The integrative action is possible because hormones travel through blood from the source to the site of their action and enable the body to function accordingly in response to stimuli.

Regulatory actions of hormones are related to all or almost all the *homeokinetic reactions of metabolism.* Homeokinetic refers to the dynamic maintenance of the **constant** body environment.

Chemical nature

Hormones are grouped according to their chemical similarities, such as :

A. *Phenol derivatives*
- — Adrenaline
- — Nor-adrenaline
- — Thyroxine

B. *Proteins*
- — Anterior pituitary hormones
- — Insulin
- — Human chorionic gonadotropin
- — Gonadotropin, thyroglobulin and secretin

C. *Peptides*
- — ACTH
- — Vasopressin (ADH or Pitressin)
- — Oxytocin (Pitocin)

D. *Steroids*
- — Estrogens
- — Androgens
- — Progesterone
- — Adrenal corticoides

* *The Author;*

** *Senior Medical Officer; Primary Health Centre, Phursatganj, Raibareli, U.P.*

Hypothalamic releasing hormones

Hormones from the anterior pituitary is under the control of *hypothalamus* which lies in brain and forms its integral part. The stimuli are received by neuro-receptors present in hypothalamus which in turn secretes humoral substances into the *hypothalamic-hypophyseal portal circulation.* The humoral substances on reaching the adenohypophysis cause release of specific trophic hormones from the anterior pituitary gland (described under anterior pituitary gland).

ENDOCRINE ORGANS

1. Pituitary gland (or hypophysis)

It is the most important endocrine organ. This is also called as a ***master gland.*** This gland is divided into three functionally distinct parts as mentioned below:

(i) Anterior lobe,
(ii) Posterior lobe, and
(iii) Intermediate part

Anterior lobe

It secretes

1. Growth hormone (GH, or somatotrophin),
2. Thyroid stimulating hormone (TSH),
3. Adrenocorticotrophic hormone (ACTH),
4. Luteinizing hormone (LH),
5. Follicle stimulating hormone (FSH) and
6. Prolactin

Functions

Functions of the above mentioned hormones (known as *trophic* hormones, i.e., **nourishing hormones)** are to stimulate the growth and the functions of other endocrine organs, such as:

(i) Thyroid gland by TSH
(ii) Adrenal gland by ACTH
(iii) Gonands by LH and FSH

GH stimulates the growth of cells in general, especially those of bone and other types of connective tissue. Secretion of trophic hormones is controlled by **'releasing hormones'** (and by *'release-inhibiting* hormones), secreted by *hypothalamus.*

Posterior lobe

It secretes

1. Antidiuretic hormone (ADH or vasopressin), and
2. Oxytocin

These hormones are synthesized in the hypothalamus, and pass directly to the posterior lobe of the pituitary gland by *axonal* transport.

Functions

ADH stimulates the reabsorption of water in the kidney. Oxytocin stimulates the contraction of certain smooth muscles.

Intermediate part

It secretes melanophore stimulating hormone (MSH) only.

Functions

Its only function is in the darkening of the skin.

2. Adrenal glands

Each adrenal gland is divided into two parts as:

(i) Cortex
(ii) Medulla

Cortex

It secretes

1. Glucocorticoids and
2. Mineralocorticoids

Functions

Glucocorticoids,such as *cortisol* stimulate

the breakdown of protein into carbohydrate and have an anti-inflammatory action.

Mineralocorticoids such as *aldosterone* stimulate the reabsorption of Na^+ in the kidney, and thus control the ionic composition of plasma.

Medulla

It secretes catecholamines.

Functions

Catecholamines, such as, adrenaline (also called epinephrine) stimulate the breakdown of glycogen and triglycerides in their respective stores, and increase the blood flow. Thus, by such means, extra glucose and fatty acids are made available to the muscles and other cells for the production of ATP.

3. The Male and Female Gonads

They secrete sex hormones, **which are responsible to stimulate primary and sexual characteristics.**

Testes secrete androgens (such as testosterone). Ovaries secrete oestrogens (such as oestradiol and oestrone).

4. Thyroid gland

It secretes thyroid hormones as mentioned below:

(i) Thyroxine (T_4) and triiodothyronine (T_3). **They stimulate the overall metabolic rate,** i.e., the oxidation of foodstuffs throughout the body.

(ii) Caicitonin. **It has a tendency to lower plasma concentration of Ca^{2+}** by inhibiting Ca^{2+} release from the bone.

5. Parathyroid gland

It is the neighbouring gland of the thyroid gland and secretes a hormone known as parathormone which has the capability to raise Ca^{2+} levels in blood by stimulating Ca^{2+} release from bone.

6. Secretion by cells

Besides glands, hormones are also secreted by specific cells present in certain organs that have a predominantly non-endocrine function, for instance, **pancreas secretes insulin and glucagon.** Insulin has a tendency to stimulate an uptake of glucose from the plasma into the muscle and other cells, as a result of which blood sugar level gets reduced, whereas the role of *glucagon* is just opposite to insulin which means that glucagon has a tendency to stimulate release of glucose from liver glycogen into the blood-stream.

Kidney secretes ***renin,*** which through another hormone stimulates the secretion of aldosterone from the adrenal cortex. Likewise, *gastrointestinal tract* also secretes a number of hormones which have a tendency to stimulate the secretion of ***hydrochloric acid*** **and digestive enzymes.**

Types of hormones

1. GH, TSH, LH, FSH, ACTH, prolactin, insulin, glucagon, calcitonin, parathormone, renin, MSH, ADH, and oxytocin are **polypeptides.**

Catecholamines and thyroid hormones are amino acid derivatives. All these hormones are stored in the cells in which they are synthesized in the form of small vesicles. Release of hormones, by stimulation of the cells in which they are stored, is by **'exocytosis'** of the vesicular contents.

2. *Prostaglandins,* a class of **'local hormones'** not produced by specific cells, are in fact *derivatives of polyunsaturated fatty acids* which control smooth muscle contraction.
3. Glucocorticoids, mineralocorticoids, androgens and oestrogens are steroids in nature and are derived from cholesterol.

Mechanism of Action

Hormones act in two ways, either

(i) at the cell surface, e.g., most polypeptide hormones and catecholamines. Action at the cell surface is through an activation of enzyme **adenyl cyclase** which leads to an increase in the concentration of intracellular cyclic AMP, either through increased Ca^{2+} concentration, or through increased nutrient (glucose and amino acids) entrance.

(ii) in the interior of cells, e.g., most steroidal hormones act in this fashion. Action within the cells is on *transcription* of specific genes (within the nucleus) or on *translation* of mRNA in the cytoplasm.

Disease

A decrease or increase in the synthesis of a particular hormone leads to an imbalance of metabolism for instance **diabetes mellitus, Cushing's syndrome, thyrotoxicosis, Addison's disease etc.** An increase is often due to an endocrine tumor.

Mechanism of hormone action (in detail)

The exact mechanism of a number of hormones is not yet very well understood, though, the net result is known, for instance, testosterone and oestrogens stimulate protein synthesis in target organs, but how does it happen? Thirdly, more than one biochemical action has been attributed to several hormones, for instance, insulin stimulates glucose uptake and glycolysis by muscles, glycogenesis and protein synthesis in liver, and lipogenesis in fat cells, whereas it inhibits gluconeogenesis in liver and glycolysis in fat cells. Now, the question arises, which is the action primarily concerned to its hypoglycaemic (reduction in blood glucose)function?

It has been observed that all hormones have one property in common. They interact with a specific receptor at the target cell, and as a result of that interaction, the cell responds in one or more ways. For convenience, the interactions may be easily divided into two types:

(i) interaction with a receptor at the cell surface and

(ii) interaction with a receptor inside the cells.

Interaction at the cell surface

A majority of the hormones is polypeptide in nature, such hormones are incapable of crossing the plasma membrane. This suggests that they interact with a receptor at the cell surface. It has been confirmed by several ways, that proteins, and even bigger molecules, are taken up by cells either by :

(a) Pinocytosis or

(b) Phagocytosis

But the entry of a substance by pinocytosis or phagocytosis is not the same as entry across the plasma membrane. Actually, what happens, the contents of a pinocytotic or phagocytotic vesicle become hydrolysed by lysosomal action as soon as they enter a cell, meaning to say; the molecules ingested in this manner cannot exert any specific action within the cell (viruses are an exception; their nucleocapsids (protein-RNA or protein-DNA complexes), which become exposed once they are inside a cell, are so arranged as to make them relatively resistant to the lysosomal hydrolysis).

It has been studied that not only polypeptides, but also **amino acid derived hormones such as the catecholamines and also fatty acid-derived hormones such as the prostaglandins,** act at the cell surface. In general, non-steroid hormones act at the cell surface, while the steroid hormones (and possibly thyroid hormones too) act intracellularly. Following three types of surface responses are known:

(i) Adenyl cyclase,

(ii) Calcium entry,
(iii) Other mechanisms

Role of Adenyl Cyclase

The enzyme adenyl cyclase catalyses the conversion of ATP to cyclic AMP (c-AMP). This enzyme, remains situated on the plasma membrane, 'facing inwards': in other words, reactant and product remain in the cytoplasm. Many hormones like adrenaline, glucagon, ACTH, FSH, LH, ADH,catecholamines etc., have a tendency to stimulate the enzyme, **as a result of which c-AMP has been termed as a *"second messenger"*, the first messenger being the hormone itself (cyclic GMP, which tends to be increased in situations that depress cyclic AMP, and vice versa, may be another type of second messenger).** Binding of hormone is not directly to the enzyme, but rather to a protein receptor on the plasma membrane that 'faces outwards'. Receptor and enzyme then interact, as a result of which enzyme activity is increased.

The c-AMP that is formed has several important actions, out of which the main one is to stimulate the phosphorylation of proteins. Structural proteins such as histones, and enzymes like glycogen phosphorylase, triglyceride lipase, and glycogen synthetase, exist in two forms i.e. phosphorylated and unphosphorylated. It has been studied that the phosphorylation, which is catalysed by a specific ***protein kinase,*** generally takes place on the hydroxyl group of a serine residue. The two forms have different activities. Histones, for instance, bind DNA less effectively in the phosphorylated form, and thus in some way 'free' DNA to enable replication and transcription to take place. Glycogen phosphorylase and triglyceride lipase are more active in the phosphorylated form, whereas glycogen synthetase is less active.

Thus, **activation of enzyme adenyl cyclase can lead to DNA replication and transcription,** to glycogen and triglycerides breakdown, and to inhibition of glycogen synthesis as well. Exactly how c-AMP that is produced near the plasma membrane reaches the nucleus to affect histone phosphorylation is not clear. There is possibility of a second type of adenyl cyclase situated at the nuclear membrane, which actually controls nuclear events. How protein hormones that do not enter cells stimulate DNA replication and transcription is also not well understood.

It has further been studied that cells possess other c-AMP-sensitive proteins, but then the cells respond to hormones in more than one way. ACTH, for example, stimulates gene activity and protein synthesis in adrenal cortex cells as well as steroidogenesis (it's a trophic hormone), and glucagon stimulates gluconeogenesis as well as glycogen breakdown in liver. In short, hormones do not stimulate one or the other metabolic event inside a cell. *Hormones* stimulate cells, the response depends upon the cell type. An endocrine cell, such as an adrenal cortex, thyroid, or gonad cell, which is programmed to grow and divide as well as to synthesize specific hormones, will respond by increasing all these activities. Side by side, a non - endocrine cell, such as a liver cell, will respond by mobilizing the pathways leading to increased glucose output namely glycogen degradation, gluconeogenesis, conversion of glucose-6-phosphate to glucose, inhibition of glycogen synthesis, and so forth.

Insulin is the main hormone responsible for a decrease of c-AMP, but how does it happen, is not yet clear; it is not by the inhibition of adenyl cyclase, as the insulin receptor does not interact with adenyl cyclase.

The effect of hormones such as adrenaline in causing an increase in intracellular c-AMP may not be as direct as one hopes. The increase may be caused by factors other than the activity of adenyl cyclase e.g., Ca^{2+}. There is ample evidence that adrenaline and other hormones stimulate cells through an increased uptake of Ca^{2+}.

Calcium Entry

The mechanism by which Ca^{2+} enters cells is not clear as yet. As the cytoplasmic concentration of Ca^{2+} is several times lower than the plasma concentration of Ca^{2+}, it is likely that the entry is positive but whether this entry is caused by opening of a Ca^{2+} 'channel', or by inhibition of the normal Ca^{2+}- exit mechanism, is not clear.

Many metabolic processes are modulated by Ca^{2+} ions e.g., degradation of glycogen. Other enzymes, such as the phosphodiesterase that degrades c-AMP to AMP, are inhibited by Ca^{2+}. Several hormones that were originally thought to act entirely by stimulating adenyl cyclase have now been shown to stimulate the *entry* of Ca^{2+} into cells. Exactly, how much of the hormonal effect is due to Ca^{2+} entry and how much due to the activation of adenyl cyclase is not clear at present.

Other mechanisms

There is a third type of mechanism, which is not yet very clear, by which interaction between hormone and the receptor at the cell surface leads to an intracellular change. This change is brought about by a stimulation of **nutrient uptake**. One hormone that acts in this manner is insulin. Muscle and fat cells are relatively impermeable to glucose and amino acids, entry of which is facilitated by diffusion, that is to say, that the specific transport proteins catalyze the entry process. The activity of the proteins is stimulated by the binding of insulin to a cell surface receptor.

Interaction with a receptor inside the cells i.e. Intracellular receptor

The theory of hormonal action at the cell surface proves to be quite satisfactory for the mechanism of action of most of the polypeptide, amino acid-derived and fatty acid-derived hormones. On the other hand steroid hormones, which readily cross the plasma membrane, act within the cells, the mechanism of entry is as follows:

The specificity of steroid hormone action is achieved through the presence of specific receptor proteins in the cytoplasm of target cells. Because there is little barrier to their permeability, steroid hormones enter all cells. In the absence of an intracellular receptor, however, the equilibrium between intracellular and extracellular hormone lies in favour of extracellular hormone (where it is bound by plasma globulins). In target cells, on the other hand, the equilibrium lies in favour of intracellular binding to the receptor proteins. These receptors readily pass into the nucleus. During passage, the size of the receptor gets altered which is evident from the fact that initially its sedimentation coefficient is approximately 9 S whereas in the nucleus it is approximately 4 S. When *steroid hormones* enter the nucleus, they become rather tightly bound to the chromatin; binding is most likely to the acidic proteins of chromatin. The receptor protein returns to the cytoplasm. Therefore, if a radioactive steroid hormone, such as oestradiol, is injected into the blood stream, the net result is that the radioactivity becomes concentrated in the nucleus of target cells.

Hormones of the anterior pituitary gland

Anterior lobe of pituitary gland is also known as adenohypophysis which secretes a number of hormones for vital importance and all are low molecular weight proteins. Secretion of most of the hormones of the anterior pituitary is under the control of the hypothalamus. Adenohypophyseal secretion is also controlled by the rate of secretion of endocrine gland through negative feed back mechanism (Fig. 16.1).

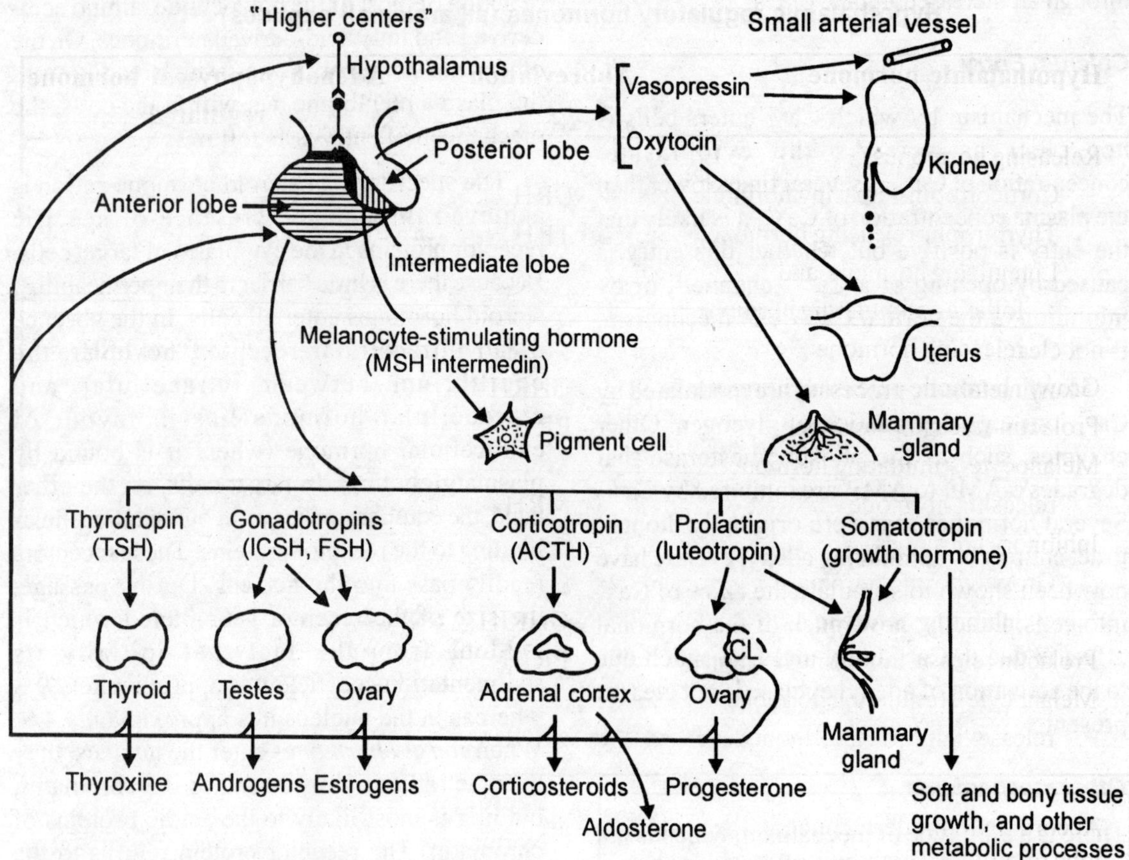

Fig. 16.1 : Scheme illustrating the relationships among the anterior and posterior pituitary glands and their target structures.

Anterior pituitary hormones

Hormones	Structure	Approx. M. Wt.	No. of Amino Acids
1. GH	Single chain polypeptide	21,500	191
2. Prolactin	Single chain polypeptide		
3. TSH (Thyroid stimulating hormone)	Double chain glycoprotein	28,000	209
4. FSH (follicle stimulating hormone)	Double chain glycoprotein	28,000	-
5. ACTH	Single chain polypeptide	4,500	39
6. LH	Double chain glycoprotein	28,000	-
7. MSH	α-Single chain	1,820	13
	β-(Polypeptide)	2,730	22

Hypothalamic regulatory hormones (all are small peptides)

Hypothalamic hormone	Abbreviation	Adenohypophyseal hormone regulated
Releasing hormones		
Corticotropin-releasing hormone	CRH	ACTH
Thyrotropin-releasing hormone	TRH	TSH
Luteinizing hormone-and follicle - stimulating hormone-releasing hormone	LHRH/FSHRH	LH and FSH
Growth hormone-releasing hormone	GHRH	GH
Prolactin-releasing hormone	PRH	PRL
Melanocyte-stimulating hormone releasing hormone	MRH	β - MSH
Inhibitory hormones		
Growth hormone release inhibiting hormone	GHRIH	GH
Prolactin release-inhibiting hormone	PRIH	PRL
Melanocyte-stimulating hormone release- inhibiting hormone	MRIH	β - MSH

According to modern concept, the middle lobe of pituitary gland is nothing but it is a part of anterior lobe.

Growth hormones

This hormone affects the growth. The hyposecretion of this hormone causes the *dwarfism* and the hypersecretion causes the *gigantism.* Growth hormone is also known as *somatotrophic hormone* or *somatotrophin hormone.* It causes the growth of all tissues of the body that are capable of growing. It promotes both, i.e., the size of the cells and increased mitosis with the development of increased number of cells.

Chemical nature

Growth hormone is a protein-molecule containing 191 amino acids in a single chain and possesses a molecular weight of about 22,005.

Secretion

Normal concentration of growth hormone in plasma of an adult is about 3 mμg/ml and in children about 5 mμg/ml. However, these values may often increase to as high as 50 mμg/ml after depletion of the body stores of proteins or carbohydrates.

Biochemical functions of growth hormone

1. Growth hormone does not affect directly the cartilages and the bones. However, growth hormone indirectly stimulates their growth with the help of several small proteins, collectively known as ***somatomedin*** which is mainly synthesized in liver and perhaps in the muscles, kidneys and placenta as well.

Somatomedin acts directly on cartilages and bones to promote their growth.

Somatomedin is required for the deposition of chondroitin sulphates and collagen, both of which are necessary for the growth of cartilages and bones.

2. GH increases protein synthesis of all cells of the body by increasing the amino acids transport through the cell membrane. This increases the concentration of amino acids in the cells (this control of amino acids transport is similar to the effect of insulin in controlling glucose transport through the membrane) .
3. GH increases the formation of RNA. GH also stimulates the transcription process in the nucleus for a longer time, causing the formation of increased quantity of RNA. This in turn promotes the protein synthesis and thus, promotes the growth. Sufficient amino acids, energy, vitamins and other necessary factors for growth are, thus, available.
4. GH is also responsible to increase fat utilization for energy purposes. It increases the fatty acids concentration in body fluids by releasing them from adipose tissue. In addition, in tissues it enhances the conversion of fatty acids to acetyl CoA with subsequent utilization. Thus, under the influence of GH, fat is utilized for energy in preference to both the carbohydrates and the proteins.
5. GH has got a tendency to convert more glucose into glycogen which is stored in the tissues for emergency period.
6. GH reduces the uptake of glucose by the cells and thus increases blood glucose concentration.
7. GH fails to cause growth in an animal lacking pancreas and it also fails to cause growth if the carbohydrates are excluded from the diet.

Factors affecting GH secretion

Stimulants

1. Exercise
2. Onset of deep sleep
3. Hypoglycaemia
4. Protein meal
5. I.V. infusion of amino acids
6. Stress induced by :
   (a) arterial puncture
   (b) surgery
   (c) endotoxins
   (d) vasopressin
7. Glucagon
8. Laevo (-) dopa
9. Malnutrition
10. Chronic hepatic and renal diseases
11. β-Adrenergic blockade

Inhibitants

1. Hyperglycaemia
2. Obesity
3. Hypothyroidism
4. Third trimester of pregnancy
5. High dose of glucocorticoids
6. Chlorpromazine
7. Medroxy progesterone
8. α-Adrenergic blockade

HYPO AND HYPER SECRETION OF GROWTH HORMONE:

Deficiency of growth hormone developing during the growth phase produces ***pituitary dwarfism.*** On the other hand, excessive growth hormone secretion produces ***pituitary gigantism,*** if hypersecretion occurs before the epiphyses have united and ***acromegaly*** when hypersecretion occurs after the epiphyses have united.

Thyroid stimulating hormone : TSH

Chemical nature

TSH is a glycoprotein secreted by basophilic

staining cells of the anterior-pituitary (Fig. 16.2). It has a molecular weight of about 30,000.

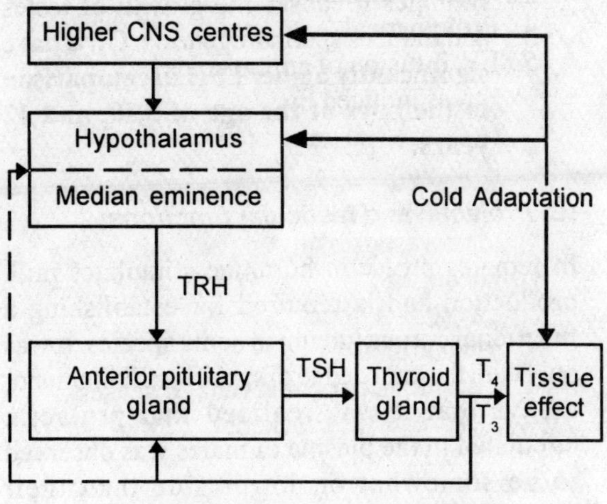

Fig. 16.2 : Scheme showing major regulatory influences on thyroid glands i.e., CNS, TRH & TSH

Actions.

(i) TSH stimulates the secretion of thyroxine and other iodothyronines.

(ii) TSH increases oxygen utilization, glucose uptake and oxidation processes. Nicotinamide adenine dinucleotide phosphate levels also rise in association with stimulus to glucose oxidation.

(iii) TSH stimulates adenyl cyclase activity in isolated thyroid cell membrane and also increases the tissue levels of c-AMP.

ADRENOCORTICOTROPIC HORMONE (ACTH)

Chemical nature

This hormone is also known as Corneotropin. The hormone ACTH is a polypeptide consisting of 39 amino acids. It is secreted from the anterior pituitary gland under the control of the corticotrophin releasing hormone of the hypothalamus (Fig 16.3).

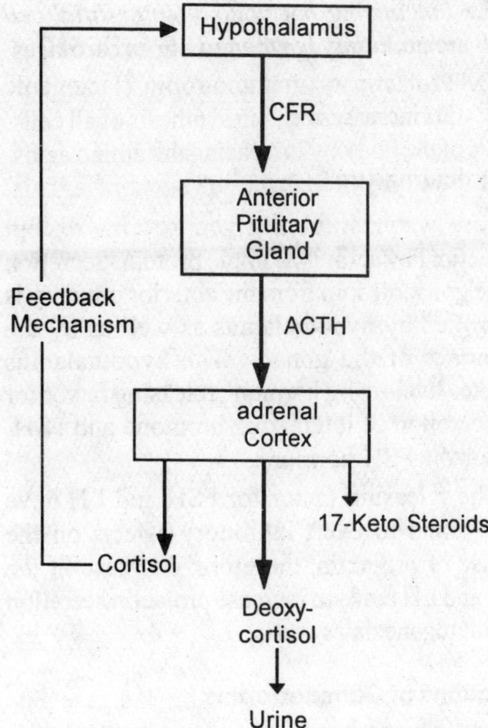

Fig 16.3 : A diagram of the normal hypothalamic pituitary adrenal axis showing regulation of adrenal cortex.

Actions

(i) It stimulates the synthesis of cortisol and 17-ketosteroids by the adrenal cortex. It has little or no effect on aldosterone secretion.

(ii) ACTH is also necessary to maintain adrenocortical size, structure, and vascularity.

(iii) The action of ACTH is mediated by c-AMP.

(iv) ACTH promotes insulin secretion from β– cells of pancreas.

Gonadotrophic hormones

Anterior pituitary secretes three gonadotrophic hormones.

1. Follicle stimulating hormone, i.e. FSH - (follicle stimulator thylokentin)

2. *Luteinizing hormone or interstitial cell stimulating hormone* (LH or ICSH).
3. Prolactin or mammotropin (lactogenic hormone).

Chemical nature

All are water soluble glycoproteins except prolactin. Prolactin is a simple protein. Secretion of the gonadotropin from the anterior pituitary is controlled by hypothalamus as well as by the hormones of the gonads. The hypothalamus secretes luteinizing hormone releasing factor for the secretion of luteinizing hormone and FSH-RF for the FSH hormone.

The releasing factor for FSH and LH have been found to exert inhibitory effects on the release of prolactin, therefore, decrease in the FSH and LH tends to increase prolactin secretion and lactogenesis as well.

Functions of Gonadotropins

(A) Luteinizing hormone

Both LH and FSH are required for the spermatogenesis. It is currently held that all the effects of LH are mediated by way of testosterone. Testosterone and FSH are hormones which act directly on the seminiferous tubular epithilium. In the immature animal, initiation of spermatogenesis requires both testosterone (or LH) and FSH.

(B) Follicle stimulating hormone : FSH

The early work of Smithzohndek and Aschhiem indicated that the sex functions are controlled by the secretion of pituitary gland. **FSH was shown to cause spermatogenic activity in testes.**

Purified preparations of FSH have been made but the actual structure of this hormone is still not known.

— In mammals FSH stimulates the maturation and growth of ovarian follicles. Cyclic AMP formation in target tissues is also found to be increased.

— In males it causes the growth of testes and induces spermatogenesis. **Girls have significantly higher FSH in comparison to the boys at the age of 5,10, and 12 years.**

(C) Prolactin and testicular functions

In females prolactin hormone stimulates milk production and is required for establishing a functional corpus luteum in some species. It was only with the knowledge of specific radioimmuno-assays that it was realized that prolactin circulated in the plasma of males was observed to be somewhat on lower side than their counterparts, i.e., females. *Plasma level of prolactin in males increases with puberty and decreases following castration and can be restored by treatment with gonadal steroids.*

Hyperprolactinemia : Considerable number of studies suggest that prolactin synergizes with LH and testosterone to increase the reproductive functions in males. The prolactin producing tumors result in testicular involution and decreased testosterone levels. All men with small prolactin producing pituitary tumors are impotent regardless of their plasma testosterone levels.

In addition, sexual function is restored by lowering prolactin level with ***Bromergocryptine*** or by surgical removal of the pituitary tumor. The later observation suggests that prolactin can produce impotence independent of its action on testosterone secretion. **Although the mechanism by which prolactin influences sexual desire is not known.**

Hormones of the middle lobe of the pituitary gland

Middle lobe of pituitary secretes MSH (melanocyte stimulating hormone). This is also known as *intermedin.*

Chemical nature

Two forms of MSH have been reported, i.e. α-MSH and β -MSH (Fig 16.4):

α- MSH is a single chain having a molecular weight of about 1,820 and contains 13 amino acids.

β-MSH is a polypeptide having 22 amino acids and a molecular weight of about 2,730. Its structure is as shown below. MSH secretion is inhibited by corticosteroids and its activity is inhibited by catecholamines.

Actions

1. Both α - and β - MSH increase melanin biosynthesis by stimulating melanocytes present in dermis and epidermis of the skin.
2. MSH promotes the dispersion of the melanin pigment in entire cells making them dark in appearance.
3. 30-60 mg cortisone is given orally to prevent excess deposition of melanin in the skin.
4. Importance of MSH in man has not been fully evaluated but increase in its production accounts for the increase in pigmentation as seen in Addison's disease, some cases of thyrotoxicosis and pregnancy as well.

1. α-MSH **(pig, beef, horse)**

CH_3CO - Ser - Tyr - Ser - Met - Glu - His - Phe - Arg - Trp - Gly - Lys - Pro - Val - NH_2
1 2 3 4 5 6 7 8 9 10 11 12 13

2. β-MSH

Ala - Glu - Lys - Lys - Asp - Glu - Gly - Pro - Tyr - Arg - Met - Glu - His - Phe -
1 2 3 4 5 6 7 8 9 10 11 12 13 14

Arg - Trp - Gly - Ser - Pro - Pro - Lys - Asp.
15 16 17 18 19 20 21 22

Fig. 16.4: Structures of α - MSH and β - MSH

NEUROHYPOPHYSIS (HORMONES OF THE POSTERIOR LOBE OF PITUITARY)

(Please refer to Figure 16.1)

Posterior lobe of pituitary gland secretes following two important hormones:

(a) Vasopressin (Pitressin, Antidiuretic hormone i.e., ADH) and

(b) Oxytocin (Pitocin)

Vasopressin (Antidiuretic hormone i.e. ADH)

Chemical nature

This hormone is a cyclic octapeptide (nonapeptide if cystine is considered as *two* cysteines). The sequence of amino acids in different preparations of vasopressin has been found to be the same except one amino acid. Vasopressin isolated from most of the mammals, i.e. human, beef, sheep etc., possesses arginine amino acid (hence, called arginine vasopressin) whereas vasopressin isolated from pigs contains amino acid lysine in place of arginine, hence, called as lysine vasopressin. Chemical structures are as shown on the next page.

Factors that stimulate its secretion

(i) Pain,

(ii) Emotional state,

(iii) Haemorrhage,

(iv) Dehydration,

(v) Salt intake,

(vi) Acetylcholine,
(vii) Anaesthetic drugs,
(ix) Morphine, nicotine and barbiturates.

Factors that inhibit its secretion

(i) Epinephrine and
(ii) Caffeine

Regulation

Volume receptors (**"stretch receptors"**) are believed to be involved in the regulation of its secretion.

Physiological and biochemical functions

(i) Principal physiological action of ADH is the regulation of water balance by promoting reabsorption of water in the cells of the distal tubules. **Failure of hypothalamus to produce enough ADH or prevention of release by damage of the nerve tracts causes an important disorder known as *'diabetes insipidus'*, in which volume of urine increases to as much as 20 litres per day. Therefore, in this disorder, the specific gravity of urine, decreases to very low (1.001). Normal secretion and the release of ADH are regulated by the osmoreceptors in the diencephalon of the brain.**

(ii) The specific biochemical action of ADH is probably by the stimulation of the synthesis of cyclic 3', 5'- AMP, which promotes reabsorption of water through the membranes of epithelial cells constituting the distal tubules.

(iii) Its powerful action is in raising blood pressure.

Oxytocin (pitocin)

Chemical nature

Oxytocin is also a octapeptide - (nonapeptide if cystine is considered as two cysteines). Its secretion from the posterior hypophysis is under the control of hypothalamus. The structure of oxytocin is as shown on the next page.

Oxytocin differs from vasopressin (ADH) in the content of two amino acids, whereas the rest six amino acids are the same. Oxytocin contains isoleucine and leucine in place of phenylalanine and arginine present in ADH, therefore, functions of the two hormones are somewhat different and not the same. Close similarity of the structures of the two is reflected in some overlapping of action: vasopressin has 6% of the oxytocin and 20% of the milk-ejecting power of oxytocin; in contrast, oxytocin has only 1 % and 0.5%, respectively, of the pressor and antidiuretic activity of vasopressin.

Factors that stimulate its secretion

(i) **Release of oxytocin from the neuro-hypophysis is stimulated by efferent impulses from the nipple induced by suckling (tactile stimulation).**

(ii) **In most species, tactile stimulation of female genitalia during coitus stimulates release of oxytocin, thereby, inducing uterine contractions which promote ascent of sperm in the fallopian tubes.**

Physiological and biochemical functions

(i) **This hormone is a powerful stimulant of uterine contraction. The pregnant uterus is more susceptible to it than the virgin uterus; this effect is utilized in obstetrics to stimulate inert uterus, and to provoke quick delivery as well as to stop *uterine bleeding*. Due to this very property, its name has been derived (Greek word, *oxytocin = rapid birth*).**

(ii) **Oxytocin appears to be the natural (physiological) initiator of *labour*.** It

$$\begin{array}{l} S\text{—————————————}S \\ H-Cys-Tyr-Phe-Glu\,(NH_2)-Asp-(NH_2)-Cys-Pro-Arg-Gly-NH_2 \\ \quad 1 \quad\; 2 \quad\; 3 \quad\; 4 \qquad\qquad 5 \qquad\qquad\quad 6 \quad\; 7 \quad\; 8 \quad\; 9 \end{array}$$

Arginine Vasopressin (most mammals)

$$\begin{array}{l} S\text{—————————————}S \\ H-Cys-Tyr-Phe-Glu\,(NH_2)-Asp\,(NH_2)-Cys-Pro-Lys-Gly-NH_2 \\ \quad 1 \quad\; 2 \quad\; 3 \quad\; 4 \qquad\qquad 5 \qquad\qquad 6 \quad\; 7 \quad\; 8 \quad\; 9 \end{array}$$

Lysine Vasopressin (pigs)

has been observed that even the minute dose of it induces the *labour.*

(iii) **It also facilitates upward movement of spermatozoa in the vagina and the fallopian tubes, even non-motile sperms ascend the female genital tract.**

(iv) It also stimulates the contraction of the myoepithelial tissue around the ducts of the lactating mammary gland, thereby, stimulates the ejection of milk **(milk "let-down" action).**

Hormones of the pineal body

Pineal body is a small protuberance, shaped like a pine cone, from the base of the third ventricle of the brain. In human beings, its weight ranges from 50 to 400 mg; average being 170 mg.

Physiological and biochemical functions

(i) Since secretion of melatonin follows a circadian rhythm, the pineal may function as a neuroendocrine transducer (device for changing the variations of quantity), mediating the effects of light on gonads.

(ii) Pineal contains high concentration of serotonin (5-hydroxytryptamine) and an enzyme called as hydroxyindole-o-methyl transferase **(HIOMT)** which converts it (serotonin) to melatonin and methoxy-tryptophol.

(iii) Pineal probably secretes adrenoglomerulotropin, which stimulates the secretion of aldosterone by the adrenal cortex.

(iv) The function of pineal in adult humans is yet unknown, since it usually undergoes involution (curling inwards) in children who are older than seven years.

(v) Tumors of the pineal sometimes cause early sexual characteristics, usually in males, as well as increased intracranial pressure.

(vi) In mammals it inhibits vaginal estrus and

$$\begin{array}{l} S\text{—————————————}S \\ H-Cys-Tyr-Phe-Glu\,(NH_2)-Asp-(NH_2)-Cys-Pro-Leu-Gly-NH_2 \\ \quad 1 \quad\; 2 \quad\; 3 \quad\; 4 \qquad\qquad 5 \qquad\qquad\quad 6 \quad\; 7 \quad\; 8 \quad\; 9 \end{array}$$

Oxytocin (mammals, birds)

is also responsible to reduce testicular or ovarian weight.

(vii) It also inhibits thyroid and adrenal cortical hormone secretions.

The only known hormone released from the pineal is **melatonin** (N-acetyl-5 methoxytryptamine). This compound blocks the action of MSH, causing aggregation of melanin granules (dark pigments of skin and hair) in the skin and hair.

MSH concentrates melanin pigments in the melanophore cells and is known as ***darkening hormone.*** On the other hand, melatonin helps in the disposal of the pigment from such cells and is therefore known as ***lightening hormone.***

Biosynthesis

It takes place from tryptophan as shown in schematic diagram (Fig. 16.5).

THYROID HORMONES

Iodine has long been known to be associated with thyroid gland. Bauman in 1895 observed that iodine was 10 times more abundant in thyroid gland than any other tissue and that it was in organic combinations.

Kendall succeeded in isolating the substance in a state of purity. The constitution of the hormone was established by Harington in 1926 and confirmed by synthesis in 1927 by Harington and Berger. Principal hormones of the thyroid gland are thyroxine and triiodothyronine.

Chemistry

Natural form is L-thyroxine which is twice as active as D-thyroxine. Thyroxine is an iodo-derivative of hydroxyphenyl tyrosine. A part of iodine present in thyroid gland remains present as diiodotyrosine.

If a solution of di-iodotyrosine is kept at pH 8.8 at 70°C for several days, thyroxine is formed. **Human thyroid gland weighs about 20-25 g**

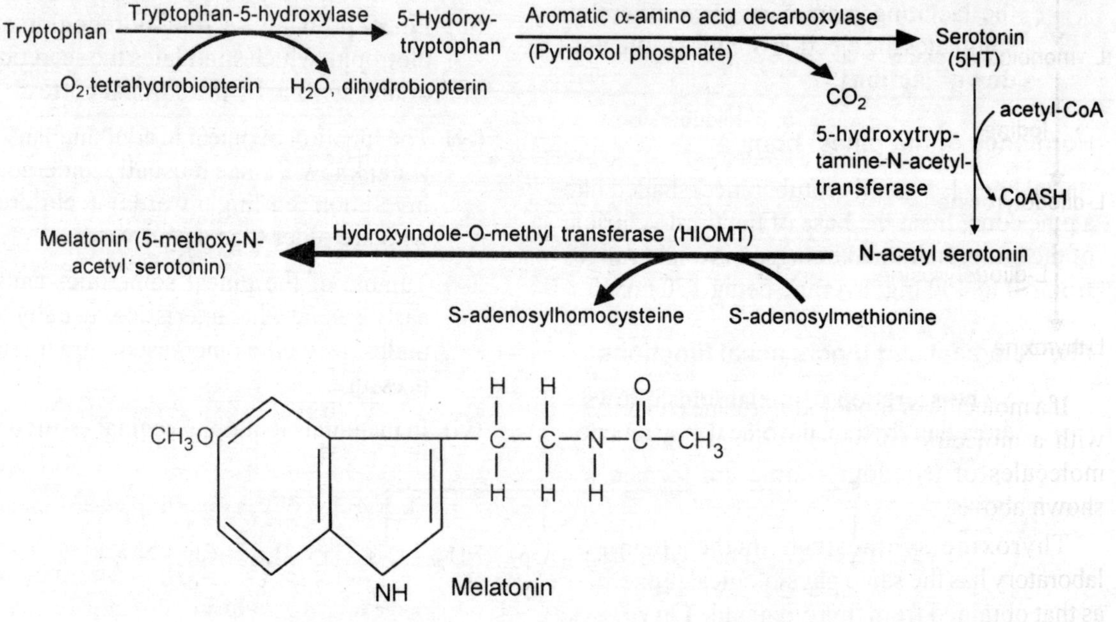

Fig. 16.5 : Biosynthesis of melatonin in Pineal gland

and contains about 25mg thyroxine and 40mg diiodothyronine. The triiodothyronine is also formed in the peripheral tissues by the deiodination of thyroxine. Structures of thyroxine and triiodothyronine are as given below:

HO–(ring with I, I)–O–(ring with I, I)–CH_2-$CH(NH_2)$-COOH

Thyroxine (T_4)

HO–(ring with I, I)–O–(ring with I)–CH_2-$CH(NH_2)$-COOH

3, 5, 3′-Triiodothyronine (T_3)

Biosynthesis of Hormones

Biosynthesis of thyroid hormones involves several fairly well defined steps, the first of which is the "trapping" of iodide in the thyroid gland. Now, synthesis of L-thyroxine (3, 5, 3', 5' i.e. tetraiodothyronine) begins with the iodination of tyrosine as shown below in the schematic diagram resulting in the formation of L-monoiodotyrosine. Now, further iodination of L-monoiodotyrosine takes place forming L-diiodotyrosine, which in the presence of one molecule of L-diiodotyrosine gives rise to L-thyroxine.

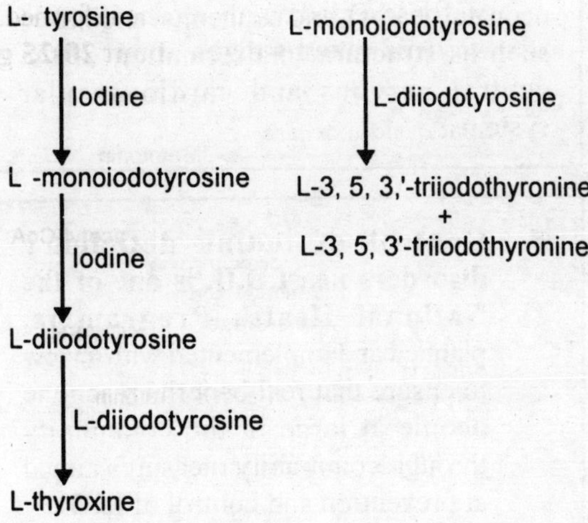

If a molecule of monoiodotyrosine condenses with a molecule of diiodotyrosine, then, two molecules of triiodothyronine are formed as shown above.

Thyroxine synthesized in the chemical laboratory has the same physiological properties as that obtained from thyroid gland. **Thyroxine remains present in the thyroid glund in a protein called thyroglobulin, which is the principal "colloid" of the gland.**

> Thyroglobulin is the storage form in the follicles and the principal form in the circulating blood is thyroxine or a derivative bound to an *alpha-globulin* known as thyroxine-binding protein (TBP). Small amounts are also bound to albumin. As the demand for the hormone arises, it is freed from the protein carriers.
>
> In addition to thyroxine, the blood and tissues also contain T_3, which is 4 to 10 times as potent as T_4.

Iodine metabolism

Iodine is a raw material essential for the synthesis of thyroid hormones. Ingested iodine is converted into iodide and is absorbed.

Simple goiter (goitre)

The most common type of goiter is known as simple or endemic goiter. In this condition there is an enlargement of the thyroid gland, which is very clęar by a swelling in the neck (Fig. 16.11 to 16.17 & 16.21). In simple goiter, the basal metabolic rate (BMR) is normal or below normal. **Simple goiter is a condition of hypofunction rather than hyperfunction of**

the thyroid gland. In fact, the enlargement of the thyroid may be looked upon as a compensatory attempt to produce the required amount of thyroid hormones. The increase in the size of the gland results from an increase in the amount of colloid present; therefore, this type of goiter is sometimes called as **"colloid goiter".** The administration of iodine in the form of iodides is beneficial and the right choice of treatment but it should be carried out in consultation with some physician. **Simple goiter may be treated as the first stage of exophthalmic goiter.**

Iodine and its relation to goiter

Since the active principle of the thyroid gland is rich in iodine, it appears that an adequate supply of this element via food is essential for the proper functioning of the gland. Iodine is often widely distributed in a variety of edible items, may be in smaller or larger amount. It also remains present in water but it has been observed that in many regions, the amount present in edibles (vegetables, fruits, corns, etc) and as well as water is extremely low. Therefore, in such regions, one is unable to get adequate supply of iodine through edibles and water in order to meet out the requirement of the body. It becomes essential to take it through other means such as iodized salt etc. **Sea water is comparatively rich in iodine and therefore, the land along the sea-coast is also rich in iodine content than the interior land. Usage of sea water for irrigation purposes brings about sufficient quantity of iodine in that very particular land/ area and therefore, anything grown in that area contains sufficient iodine. Water and crops from such regions are richer in iodine than those from interior regions. Simple goiter is usually much less common in regions nearer to the sea than the interior regions.**

Scientist **McClendon** has shown that the incidence of goiter is closely associated with the amount of iodine in the drinking water and in the crops grown in that particular locality. **Plants of the cabbage family, such as cauliflower,**

Deficiencies of certain trace elements during pregnancy have been shown to impair the growth and development of the foetus in experimental animals. In both, genetically hypothyroid and thyroidectomized guinea pigs, animals deprived of the trace iodine - containing thyroid hormones, there is noticed a three to four fold increase in **still births.** In the former group, thyroxine supplementation during pregnancy almost eliminated the excess of still births and of foetal resorptions and abortions.

Iodine deficiency in man, therefore, might well be expected to increase the incidence of spontaneous abortions, perinatal deaths (comprising still births and neonatal deaths), and congenital anomalies such as structural malformation of the central nervous and cardiovascular systems.

- **Control of iodine deficiency disorders i.e., I.D.D. is one of the National Health Programme,** planned and implemented with a view to ensure that real benefits reach the people at large in the community through community measures aimed at prevention and control of IDD.
- In India IDD is responsible for many physical and mental abnormalities with various motor disfunction problems.
- In India, it is estimated that nearly 167 million persons are prone to the risk of IDD.
- Out of the persons at the risk of IDD, 54 millions are having *Goitre,* 2.2

millions are ***cretins,*** and 6.6 millions have mild ***neurological disorders.***

- It is estimated that every passing hour, 10 children are being born in this country who will not attain their optimum mental and physical potential due to neonatal hypothyroidism caused by iodine deficiency.
- With continuous depletion of ***Iodine*** from natural resources, the situation is expected to worsen in the coming years unless measures are taken to control the situation.
- IDD are highly prevalent in the sub-himalayan belt as well as in the plains of **Uttar Pradesh.** The deficiency presents wide spectrum of disabilities which includes ***Goitre, deaf-mutism, mental retardation, retardation of physical growth*** and various degrees of impairment of intellectual and motor functions. Because of the magnitude of the problem, IDD **control programme** has been given ***National Priority*** and has been included in the ***Prime Minister's* 20 Point Programme** in our country.

Iodine is a natural element which has been graded as very important for human life. Iodine is very important for the proper development and functioning of body and brain. Its deficiency causes goitre (enlargement of thyroid gland) which results in the loss of smartness; one feels dullness, laziness and tiredness. Such people feel tired after doing work in comparison to a normal person.

Moreover, its deficiency may be responsible for permanent interruption in the development of body and brain of nascent children, therefore, it's very important for the children, adults and pregnant women. If a pregnant woman has got low iodine, then her child may be abnormal one. If such children are not treated immediately after birth, then as the age advances, their physical and mental condition shall be highly affected.

On an average, the daily requirement of iodine is very less which is equivalent to the head of a needle i.e. nearly 150 μg. It means that an individual requires even less than a teaspoonful of iodine throughout his/her life. Its daily intake is very essential which one can do by using iodized salt in the diet.

"Iodine deficiency is so easy to prevent that it is a crime to let a single child be born mentally handicapped for that reason."

- Lack of iodine in the environment has serious consequences for both human and animals.

  The wide spectrum of disorders by inadequate iodine consumption are known collectively as iodine deficiency disorders (IDD), which include:

  (i) Lowering of IQ and impaired learning.

  (ii) Energy loss.

  (iii) Reproductive losses e.g. increased miscarriages, increased still births.

  (iv) Cretinism

  - Mental retardation,
  - Deaf-mutism, squint,
  - Dysplegia (spastic paralysis of the lower limbs),
  - Dwarfism, coordination abnormalities.

  (v) Goitre - the most visible manifestation but it is less dangerous than the above mentioned losses.

(vi) Reduced milk, egg, meat and wool *yields* in animals.

(vii) Reproduction failure in animals.

- Deficiency of iodine in pregnant women can cause irreversible brain damage in the unborn baby (Fig 16.10).
- The world's single most significant cause of preventable brain damage and mental retardation is deficiency of iodine.
- Current research indicates that iodine deficiency results in lowering the average intelligence of entire school age population by as much as 10 to 15 I.Q. points.
- The number of primary school age children in endemic areas is estimated to be 40 millions. The total I.Q. points lost in these children amount to be 400 millions.
- No state in India is free trom IDD. In India, out of the 216 districts surveyed (in 29 states and union territories), 186 districts have goitre prevalence rate ranging trom 10% to over 65%.
- With every passing hour, 10 children are being born in India who will not attain their optimum physical and mental potential due to iodine deficiency.

broccoli (a variety of cauliflower with greenish flower-head), **cabbage, may be goitrogenic when eaten raw, as they contain antithyroid compounds which are destroyed by cooking.**

Iodized salt should never be left open in air as it causes loss of iodine (Fig 16.24). Iodine evaporates when it comes in contact with air.

Prevention

- Preventing iodine deficiency raises the learning capacity of school children and improves school performance.
- IDD is preventable.
- Daily consumption of iodlised salt prevents the spectrum of disorders caused due to the deficiency of iodine.
- Consumption of iodised salt is safe.
- Iodisation of salt is a low cost, highly effective mean of preventing iodine deficiency.
- The cost of iodising salt is only about 30 paise per person per year.
- Within just 12 months of iodised salt becoming available and used in a community, no more ***cretins*** will be born, **no more babies will suffer from retarded mental and physical development** attributed to iodine deficiency.

Regions Affected from the Deficiency of Iodine in India (Fig. 16.23).

Maximum deficiency of iodine is found in the water/ soil of the cities and villages located in the foot of Himalaya mountain. Regions affected from it include from Jammu-Kashmir in North to 2,500 sq. km. area in North-East but the incidence is found to be

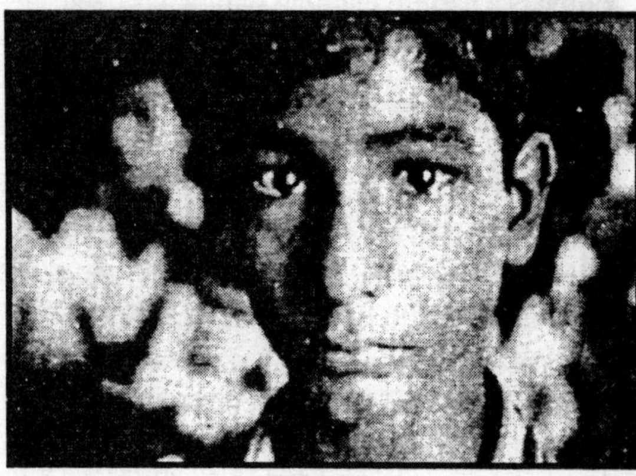

Fig. 16.6: A child having low I.Q. and impaired learning

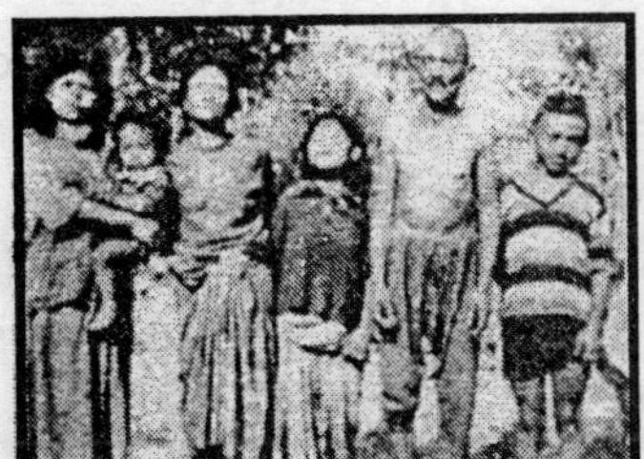

Fig. 16.7 : Sufferers of goitre, dwarfism and mental retardation.

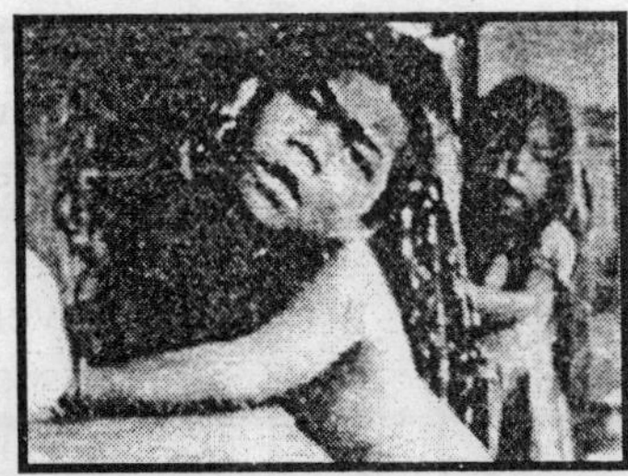

Fig. 16.8 : A cretin child.

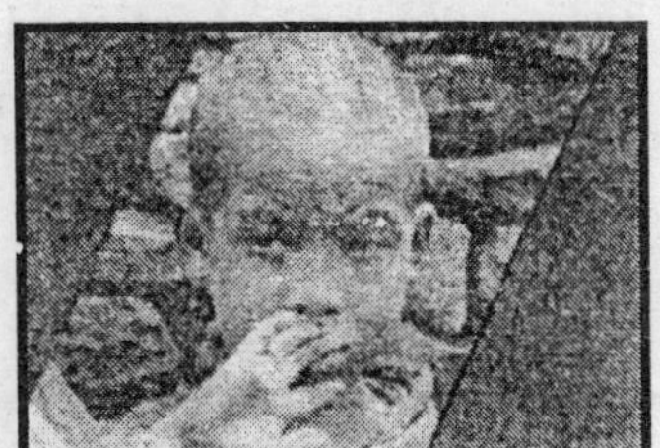

Fig. 16.9 : A cretin child.

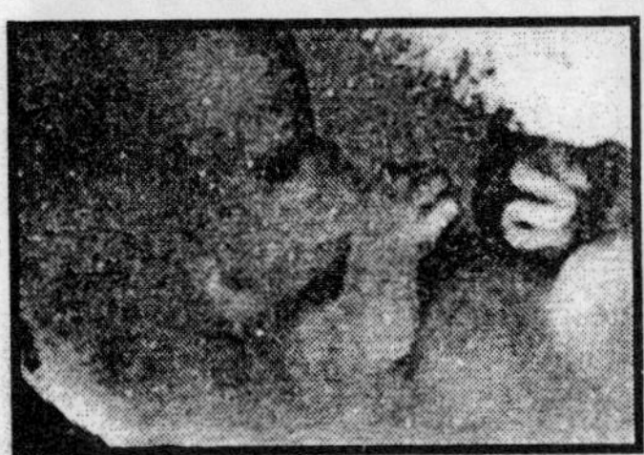

Fig. 16.10 : Deficiency of iodine in pregnant women can cause irreversible brain damage in the unborn baby.

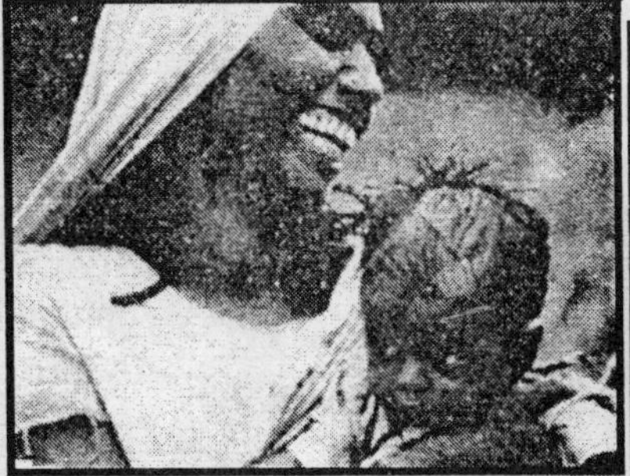

Fig. 16.11 : A 'goitre' lady with her child.

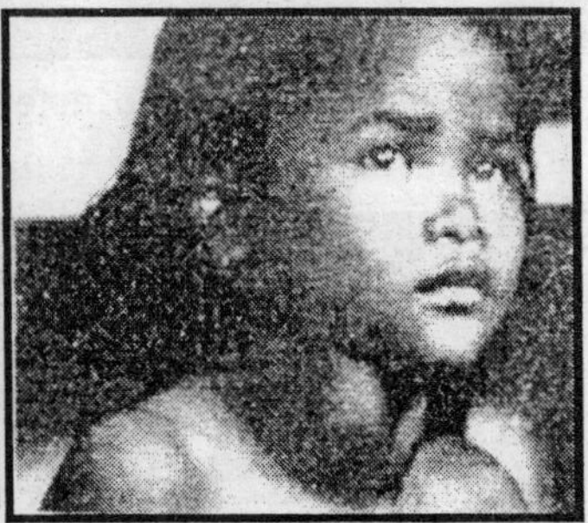

Fig. 16.12 : A child having 'goitre'

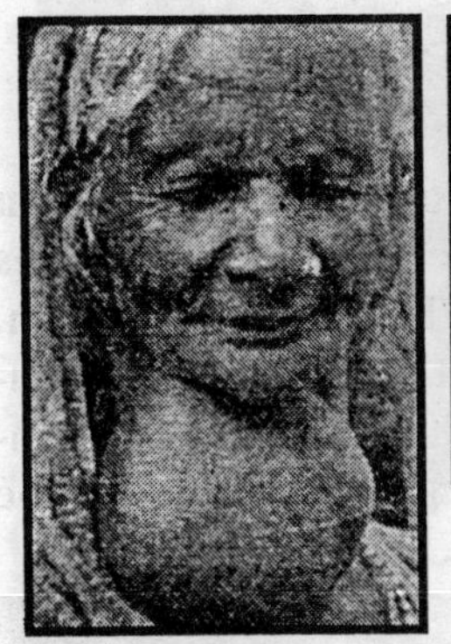

Fig. 16.13

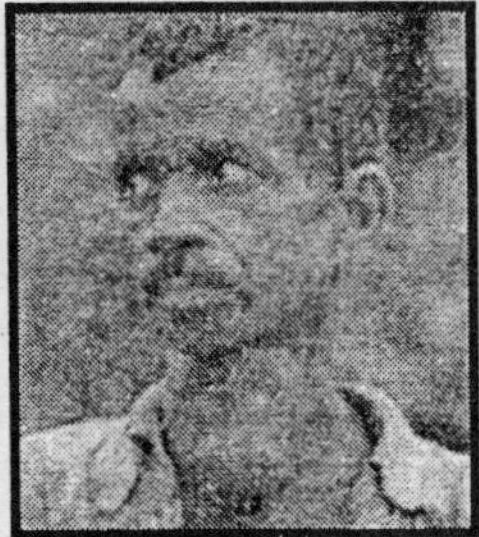

Fig. 16.14

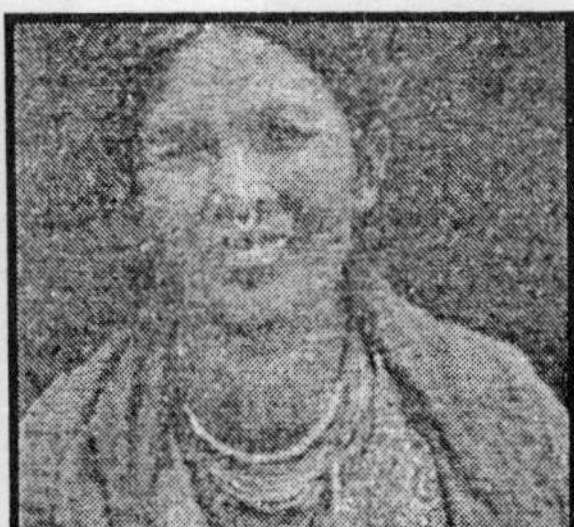

Fig. 16.15

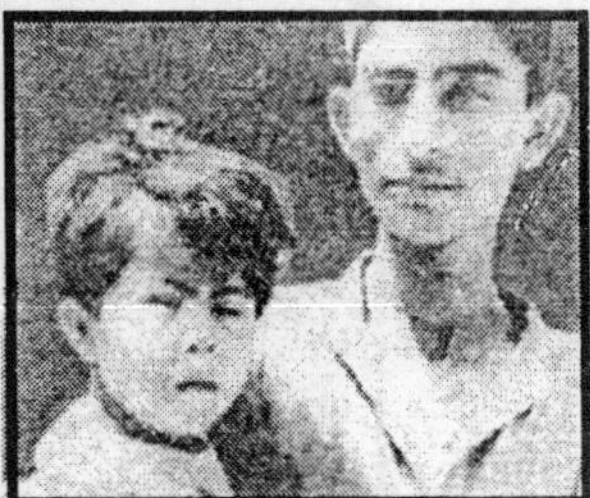

Fig. 16.18 : Children having low I.Q. and mental retardation

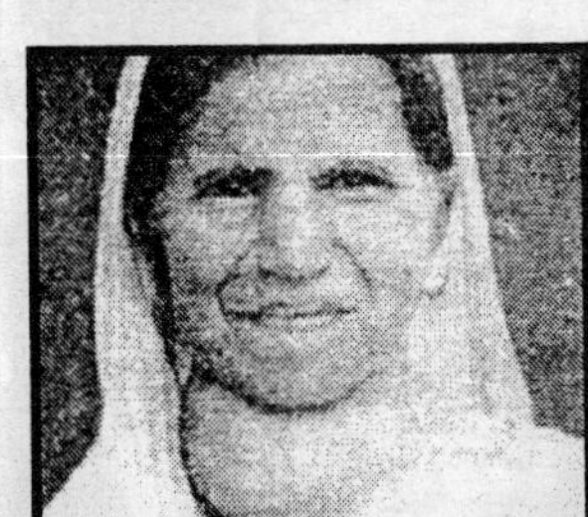

Fig. 16.16

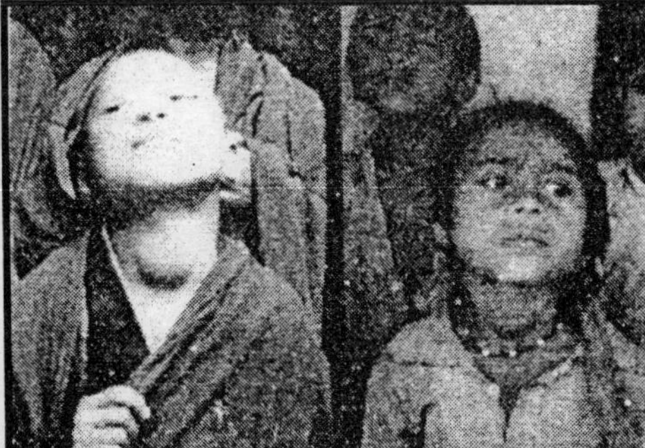

Fig. 16.17

Figures 16.13, 16.14, 16.15, 16.16 & 16.17 : Sufferers of 'goitre'

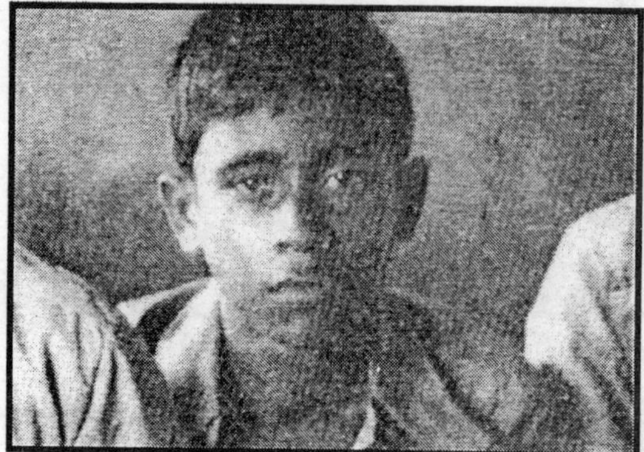

Fig. 16.19 : A hypothyroid child; note the vacant look

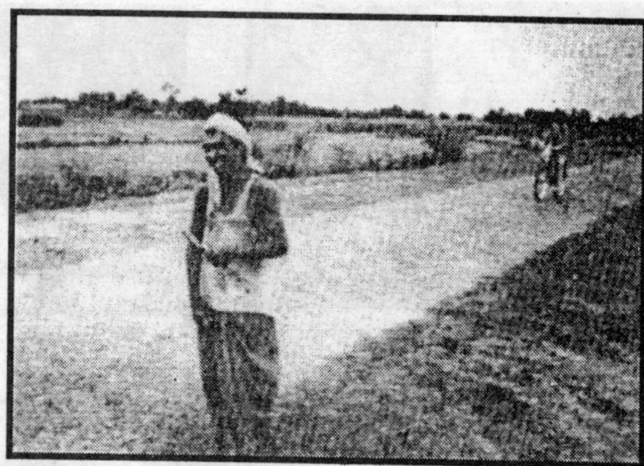

Fig. 16.20 : Stunted growth; note the unnaturally short legs.

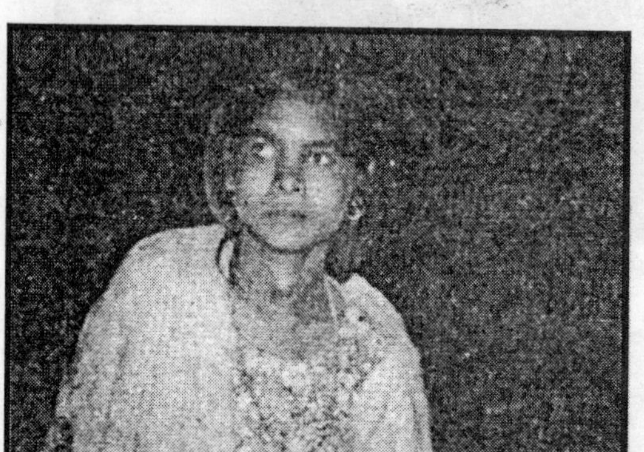

Fig. 16.21 : A deaf-mute with squint and goitre

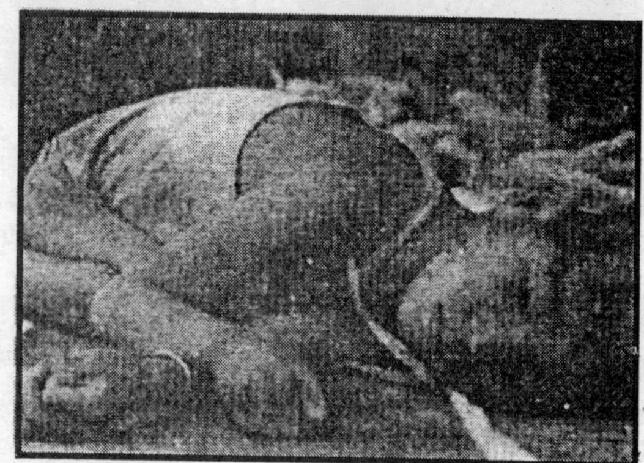

Fig. 16.22 : A 12 year old cretin

Where goitre has been recorded ●

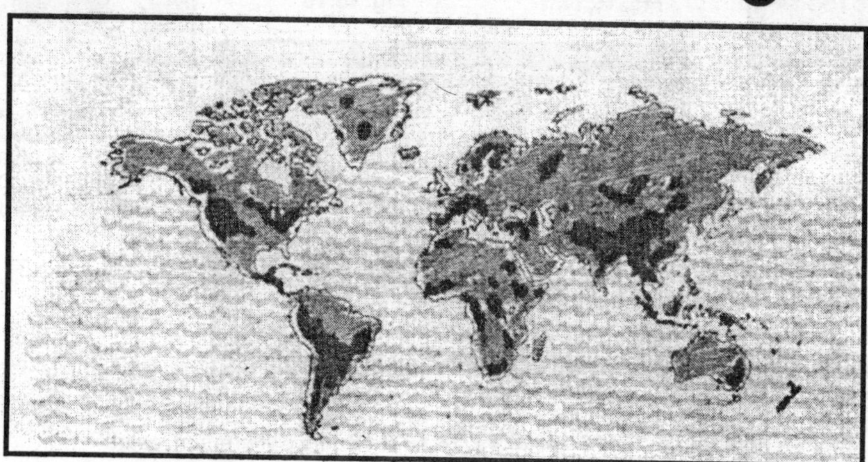

Fig. 16.23 : Regions where goitre has been recorded.

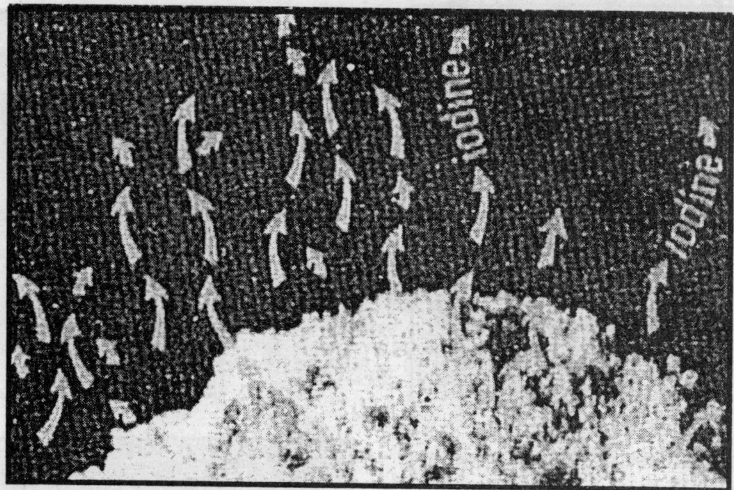

Fig. 16.24 : Loss of iodine from iodised- salt if left open in the air

Deficiency of iodine in diet sometimes occurs in the areas where the water supply and the soil are poor in iodine and produces a condition known as ***simple* or *endemic goiter* or *colloid goiter.*** In this type of goiter, there is enlargement of thyroid gland, the obvious sign of which is swelling in neck. This condition is relieved by ensuring adequate supply of *inorganic iodides* in the diet.

Goitrogenic foods (in raw state harmful otherwise not)

1. **Cauliflower,**
2. **Broccoli (a variety of cauliflower with greenish flower head)** and
3. **Cabbage, etc.**

Iodine is essential not only for the human beings but also for the animals.

comparatively very less in Maharashtra, Gujarat, Madhya Pradesh, Andhra Pradesh, Orissa, Karnataka, Kerala, Tamil Nadu, Goa, Rajasthan, West Bengal and Delhi. In India, there is no state/union territory where there is not found any deficiency of iodine in the soil/water. Every day we are being informed about new pockets of IDD.

Hypothyroidism (Fig. 16.19)

It is a state in which there is not sufficient development of thyroid gland, in the embryonic life, the child becomes a *dwarf* or *cretin* (Fig. 16.7, 16.8, 16.9 and 16.22). **A *cretin* grows slowly (stunted growth) and has a low mentality and low I.Q. (figures 16.6, 16.7 and 16.18); his hair is scanty and coarse, and his skin is thick and dry. His BMR is also low. If such a child is given thyroid extract or thyroxine, he or she does not remain a *cretin* but develops normally. This treatment, however, must be continued indefinitely in consultation with a physician in order to prevent the child from developing into a *cretin*** (Fig. 16.20).

If the gland is removed or if it becomes subnormal in activity in an adult, myxoedema develops (Fig. 16.25) in which the skin becomes thick and dry, the hair coarsen and fall out, and there is a disinclination towards work, either physically or mentally. There

IODINE-CONTENT OF COMMONLY CONSUMED FOODS

Iodine is an important trace element, the deficiency of which in food and water leads to iodine deficiency disorders including goiter.

Green leafy vegetables have relatively higher concentration of iodine if compared to fruits, spices and beverages. Fruits like apple and sweet lime have almost negligible amount of iodine.

Among pulses like lentil, bengal gram, green gram (Moong), red gram (Arhar), black gram (Urad) and horse gram (Chana), **the iodine content in horse gram is the highest** (58 μg/kg) and that of red gram is the lowest (30 μg/kg).

becomes a tendency to *put on weight.* The metabolic rate is reduced, nitrogen metabolism gets lowered, and the body's temperature is subnormal. Further, ossification of the bones is delayed; density of the carpals in the wrist is often used as a criterion of thyroid activity or physiological age in a prepubertal child. Stimulation of ossification by T_4 and T_3 may be offset by thyrocalcitonin, which has a tendency to decrease blood Ca^{++} level.

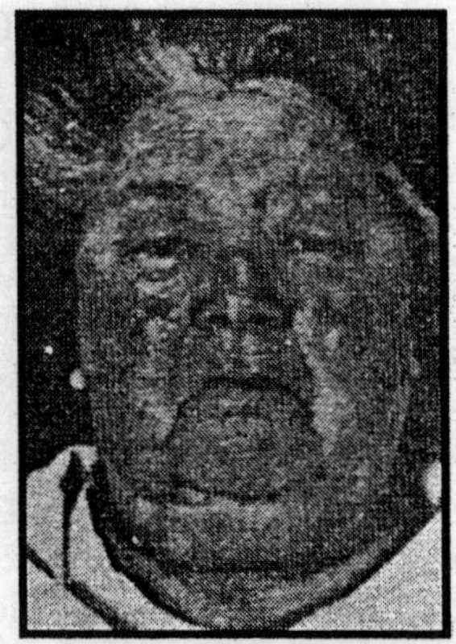

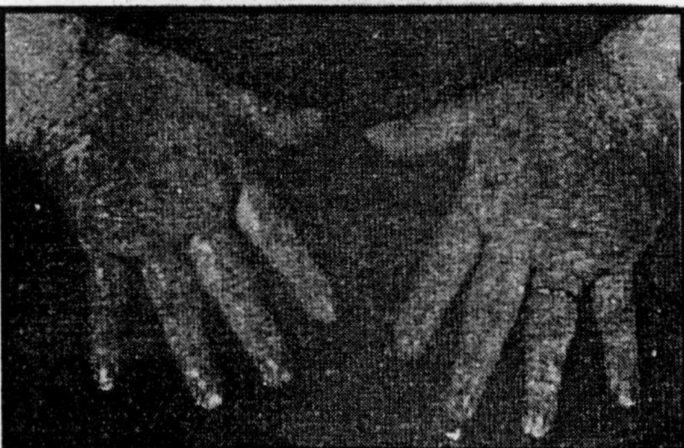

Fig. 16.25 : Photographs of the face and hands of a woman, aged 70, suffering from myxoedema. Note the dull expression, scanty eyebrows and dilated vessels on the cheeks. The face and hands are puffy and the skin of the hands is dry and wrinkled.

Hyperthyroidism

It is a state in which thyroid gland is too active, as a result of which a condition known as **exophthalmic goiter occurs.** A common symptom of this disease is the bulging of the eyes; hence the name. The disease is also known as **'Graves'** or **'Basedow's disease.** The symptoms of exophthalmic goiter are just the opposite of myxoedema which mean that the basal metabolic rate (BMR) is high instead of low, nitrogen metabolism is increased instead of low, the hair is fine instead of coarse, the body temperature is above instead of below normal. The patient is nervous and irritable instead of sluggish; his mentality is above rather than below normal and he or she is underweight. His/her heart beat is generally fast and irregular.

Usually, but not always, the thyroid gland is enlarged in exophthalmic goiter. **Such a condition**

Normally, **PBI content** is found to be in the range of 4 to 8 μg/100ml of blood; however, **in myxoedema** it is found to be in the range of 0.2 to 2.5 μg/100ml of blood.

In **'Graves' disease,** there is hyperfunction of the gland and increased BMR is seen. In this disease; PBI content is found in the range of 8-18 μg/100ml of blood which is a good index of hyperthyroidism.

```
NH2                NH — C = O
|                  |     |
C = S          S = C     CH
|                  |     |||
NH2               HN  —  CH

Thiourea          Thiouracil
```

can be easily treated by removing part of the thyroid gland; the improvement produced in the patient by this method is wonderful. Radioactive I^{131} sometimes is efficacious in decreasing the secretion of the thyroid gland.

Hyperparathyroidism may also be treated by the use of drugs such as thiourea, thiouracil, propylthiouracil, and the sulfa drugs. These are thought to act by inhibiting either the uptake of iodine by the thyroid gland or the formation of thyroxine from diiodotyrosine.

PARATHYROID GLANDS

Parathyroid glands were discovered by **Sandstrom** in 1880. They are minute glands, weighing about 0.1 g each and remain closely associated with the thyroid gland. In man they are four in number: two of them are embedded in the posterior surface of the thyroid gland; whereas the remaining two lie close to and behind the thyroid. They are yellowish-brown, egg shaped bodies.

Since, these remain so closely attached with the thyroid gland, it becomes very difficult to remove the thyroid without also removing them (parathyroids).

Two hormones namely ***parathormone*** and ***calcitonin*** are known to be secreted by these glands and **both are responsible for controlling calcium and phosphate metabolism in the human beings in a balancing manner.**

PARATHYROID HORMONE

Parathormone (PTH) is a protein having a molecular weight of approximately 9,500. It consists of a straight chain of 83 amino acid residues composed of 17 different amino acids.

Secretion of **parathormone (PTH)** is believed to be regulated by the level of circulating ionic calcium. Low ionic calcium level stimulates whereas high ionic calcium level inhibits PTH secretion. However, more recent studies have shown that the secretion of PTH is regulated by both, i.e. calcium and magnesium. PTH secretion is impaired when the concentration of magnesium is very low. Since, PTH is a proteolytic hormone, therefore, it can be digested by the proteolytic enzymes.

Physiological and Biochemical Functions and Mode of Action

PTH plays various important roles in the body:

1. **It is perhaps the single very important factor in the fine regulation of blood calcium level.**
2. **It has a tendency to raise plasma calcium level.**
3. It has a tendency to increase proximal tubular reabsorption of calcium by the kidneys, thus decreases Ca^{2+} excretion via urine.
4. **It decreases reabsorption of phosphate by the kidneys.**
5. It promotes the intestinal absorption of calcium.
6. It increases Ca^{2+} reabsorption from bone.
7. It increases the production of 1, 25-dihydroxy- cholecalciferol (an active metabolite of vitamin D) by the kidneys. This active metabolite, in turn, is a very good substance as it (a) increases Ca^{2+} absorption from gut (b) increases Ca^{2+} reabsorption from bone.

HYPERPARATHYROIDISM

Hyperparathyroidism causes a syndrome known as ***osteitis fibrosa cystica*** **or** ***von Reckling-***

***hausen's disease* which is characterized by hypercalcemia, hypophosphatemia, and raised serum activity of alkaline phosphatase. Excessive demineralization of the**

> After complete removal of parathyroids, blood shows a decided ***decrease in its calcium*** and an ***increase in its phosphorus content.*** Whereas normal serum contains about 10 mg of Ca^{2+} per 100 ml; after removal of the parathyroids, the amount may be reduced to as little as 5 mg. This lowering of the blood Ca^{2+} is undoubtedly the cause of ***tetany.***
>
> Parathormone influences excretion of phosphate by the kidneys and as well as mobilization of calcium from bones. Specific effects are inhibition of phosphate reabsorption by the kidney tubules and inhibition of osteoblasts as well as stimulation of osteoclasts, thereby, releasing calcium from bone cells. The hormone also facilitates intestinal absorption and renal tubular reabsorption of Ca^{2+}. **Muscle spasm develops only when the blood Ca^{2+} level falls below 7 mg%.**
>
> Renal threshold for Ca^{2+} ranges from 7.5 to 9.0 mg per 100 ml serum.

bones causes pain in them, deformities, and spontaneous fractures too. Because of the high levels of calcium in the serum, deposition of calcium salts takes place in soft tissues and **calculi may also be formed in the kidneys.** The main cause of hyperparathyroidism is the development of a tumor in the parathyroid glands. Other symptoms of this disorder (hyperparathyroidism) also include muscular asthenia, peptic ulcers, and constipation. Depression of the central nervous system may sometimes be encountered.

HYPOPARATHYROIDISM

Injury to the parathyroids may lead to hypoparathyroidism, other major possibility is the destruction or removal of the parathyroids during surgical operation of the thyroid. Hypoparathyroidism is more common than the excessive secretion.

Less secretion of PTH causes hypocalcemia leading to muscle spasms, lenticular cataracts and calcification of the basal ganglia in the brain. There may also be hypocalciuria, since the blood concentration is usually below the renal threshold for Ca^{++} (renal threshold for Ca^{2+} is between 7.5 and 9 mg per 100 ml). Therapeutic measures are usually taken to maintain serum Ca^{2+} level at or somewhat above renal threshold values. **Be it known that excessive concentration of blood Ca^{++} is as dangerous as low.** A simple criterion and control in Ca^{++} therapy, therefore, is the urinary excretion of minimal amount of Ca^{++} just enough to indicate a blood level of Ca^{++} slightly above 7.5 mg per 100 ml. A simple test for urinary Ca^{2+} is the ***Sulkowitch reaction,*** which depends upon the degree of turbidity developing in urine two or three minutes after a mixture of oxalic acid, ammonium oxalate and acetic acid is added to the sample. The painful muscle spasms symptomatic of hypoparathyroidism can be eliminated immediately by the administration of simple, water-soluble calcium salts; but for more lasting effects a ***'vitamin D' preparation* and *dihydrotachysterol (AT-10)* are also given.**

CALCITONIN, CT, (THYROCALCITONIN)

Although, parathyroid hormone is the single most important factor in the fine regulation of blood calcium level (extracellularly and intracellularly); **yet there is a *calcium lowering hormone known as calcitonin* (CT), *which is secreted* by the parafollicular or "C" cells of the thyroid gland (hence the name *thyrocalcitonin,* once used by several).** These cells are found in the basement membrane of the thyroid follicle and are partly of neural crest origin.

Chemistry

The structure of human calcitonin has been determined which consists of 32 amino-acid residues, having a molecular weight of nearly 3,000. Human calcitonin has also been synthesized in the laboratory and found to be biologically as active as the natural one.

Factors affecting secretion of Calcitonin

The only known physiological stimulus of CT secretion is a rise in plasma Ca^{2+} level. Secretion of calcitonin is also stimulated by glucagon and cyclic-AMP. Its release is directly proportional to the plasma Ca^{2+} concentration.

> Calcitonin in serum is estimated by radio-immunoassay technique. The normal serum concentration in man is less than 100pg/ml (< 29.2 pmol/L). An infusion of calcium raises plasma calcitonin level by 1.5-3 folds, In patients with medullary carcinoma of the thyroid, plasma calcitonin level gets elevated. The half-life of human CT in circulating blood is less than 15 minutes.
>
> Raised serum CT level is found in medullary thyroid carcinoma (MTC). **CT level in MTC is often thousands times greater than the normal.**
>
> CT may be administered in the treatment of **Paget's disease.**
>
> There is no clinical syndrome of the deficiency of calcitonin.
>
> CT in the treatment of osteoporosis is not at all of any value.
>
> Recent studies have shown that two gastrointestinal hormones namely, cholecystokinin-pancreozymin and gastrin are potent stimulators of CT secretion.

Actions of Calcitonin

It has the following actions:

1. Calcitonin has significant effects on phosphate metabolism. It facilitates the entry of phosphate into bone cells and periosteal fluid, thereby decreasing plasma phosphorus level and on the other hand it reduces the movement of calcium from bone to blood plasma, hence, is responsible for lowering blood calcium level.
2. The entry of phosphate into bone cells may be accompanied by calcium, thus, blood calcium level gets lowered.
3. Calcitonin may also exert a small phosphaturic effect.
4. In the human beings, however, the role of calcitonin in calcium homeostasis is obscure.

THE THYMUS

Thymus at birth weighs 10-12 g. It increases in weight during childhood. In adolescence, its weight ranges from 20 to 30 grams. Thereafter it atrophies remarkably until in old age its weight is reduced to 3-6 g.

The mammalian thymus is endodermal in origin, arising from the third branchial pouch. It is composed of a medulla and a cortex. The medulla develops first and consists of reticular-epithelial cells, a few lymphocytes and the concentric corpuscles of Hassall; whereas the cortex is made up of actively multiplying, closely packed lymphocytes and does not contain **Hassall's corpuscles.** The lymphocytes are arranged in packets surrounded by epithelial cells which form a barrier between the capillaries and the lymphocytes. The thymus is therefore, essentially a lymphoid organ and like other lymphoid tissue, it undergoes atrophy in response to adrenal glucocorticoids.

Thymus gland secretes following two types of hormones which are known as thymic hormones, namely:

1. Thymosin

This hormone is secreted by the reticular-epithelial cells of the thymus gland.

Chemistry

It is a peptide with a molecular weight of nearly 1,000.

Actions

(i) It promotes the immunocompetence in young T -lymphocytes.
(ii) It also produces lymphocytosis.
(iii) Maturation of T - lymphocytes

2. Thymopoietin (Thymin)

Action

It has got the capability to inhibit the release of acetylcholine at the endings of motor nerve in the disease called as ***Myasthenia gravis.***

In nutshell, the thymus, **thus promotes the development of immunologically competent T - lymphocytes,** meaning to say, it eventually gives rise to resistance against infection (foreign body) and **thus helps in preparing a strong defence mechanism in the body.** It is also responsible for the maturation of T - lymphocytes.

HORMONES OF THE ADRENAL CORTEX

In the human the *adrenal,* or *suprarenal* glands are a pair of flattened, triangular bodies located adjacent to the superior pole of each kidney. They measure approximately 5 x 3 x 1 cm and have a combined weight of about 10 to 15 g. Each gland is enclosed in a thick, connective tissue capsule.

The glands are composed of two distinct parts, a central one which is known as *medulla* and an outer *cortex.* In the adult, medulla represents about 10 percent of the total weight of the adrenal gland.

Most of the parenchymal cells of the adrenal cortex are under partial control of the adenohypophysis and function in regulating metabolism and maintaining normal electrolyte balance.

Adrenal cortex, in fact, **synthesizes dozens of different types of steroid molecules,** but only a few of them have got biological activity. For convenience, they have been classified into three categories. viz:

(i) Glucocorticoids,
(ii) Mineralocorticoids and
(iii) Androgens (sex hormones)

These hormones initiate their actions by combining with specific intracellular receptors, and this complex binds to specific regions of DNA to regulate gene expression.

Biomedical Importance

1. The hormones of the adrenal cortex, particularly the glucocorticoids, give the body capacity to adjust to stress, such as prolonged exposure to cold or shock.
2. **Mineralocorticoids are required for normal Na^+ and K^+ balance.**
3. Synthetic analogs of both classes i.e., glucocorticoids and mineralocorticoids are used therapeutically. Many glucocorticoid analogs are potent anti-inflammatory agents.
4. Excessive or deficient plasma levels of any of the above mentioned three classes of the hormones, whether due to disease or therapeutic use, result in severe complications leading even to death.
5. Increase blood glucose level and liver glycogen content as well, chiefly by

In young animals, deprivation of cortical hormones delays growth and maturation.

The most potent and physiologically important glucocorticoid is hydrocortisone, 17- hydroxycorticosterone or cortisol (also known as compound 'F' because, it was the sixth compound to be isolated by Kendall as pure crystals from cortical extracts).

Glucocorticoids such as cortisone and cortisol have an anti-inflammatory action, possibly by inhibiting proliferation of fibrous, connective tissue by fibroblasts.

Cortisone has proved of value in many diseases other than rheumatoid arthritis and rheumatic fever. Among these may be mentioned as asthma, hay fever, inflammatory eye diseases and Addison's disease, etc.

stimulating gluconeogenesis but also by decreasing sensitivity to insulin. Synthesis of necessary enzymes gets induced.

6. Decrease synthesis of acid-sulfated mucopolysaccharides in bone and connective tissues.
7. Increase release of fatty acids from adipose tissue, and side by side, decrease synthesis of fat from glucose.
8. They accelerate the rate of catabolism, in general.
9. They inhibit the anabolism of proteins.

Zones of the Adrenal Cortex:

The adult cortex has 3 distinct zones/layers as mentioned (Fig 16.26):

(i) Zona glomerulosa (responsible for the production of mineralocorticoids).

(ii) Zona fasciculata
(iii) Zona reticularis
] responsible for the production of glucocorticoids and androgens

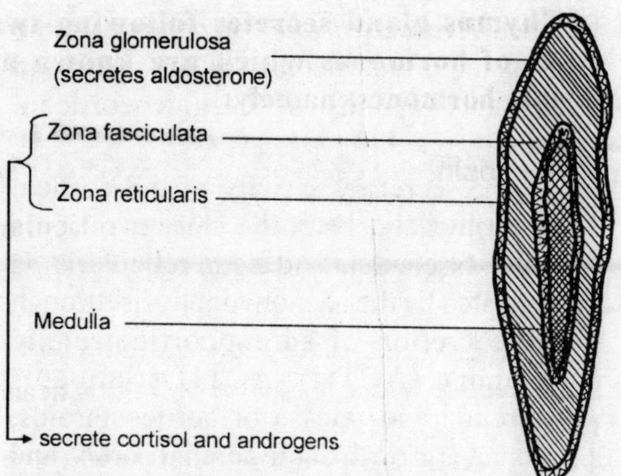

Fig 16.26 : Secretion of adrenocortical hormones by different zones of the adrenal cortex.

Biosynthesis of Adrenal Corticosteroids

The adrenal cortex synthesizes three classes of hormones as described above i.e., **glucocorticoid, mineralocorticoid and sex hormones.** Although, **nearly 50 hormones are**

Parenchymal cells of the adrenal cortex secrete a variety of hormones collectively referred to as *corticosteroids.* Functions of the adrenal cortex are essential for life in contrast to the adrenal medulla which are not so essential. Although, numerous steroids have been extracted from the adrenal, only a few are normally secreted, by the gland. The parenchymal cells of the **zona *glomerulosa*** secrete a class of steroid hormones known as ***mineralocorticoids,*** the function of which is in the maintenance of normal electrolyte balance. *Aldosterone* is the most potent mineralocorticoid and accounts for approximately 95% of the activity of this class.

The parenchymal cells of ***zona fasciculata,*** and to a lesser extent those of *zona* reticularis, secrete a class of steroid hormones known as *glucocorticoids,* which influence carbohydrate metabolism the most. *Hydrocortisone,* or *cortisol* is the most important member of this class and accounts for most of the glucocorticoid activity.

The secretory activity of the cortical parenchymal cells of the inner two layers (Zona fasciculata and Zona reticularis) is regulated by the adenohypophysis through the secretion of adrenocorticotrophic hormone (ACTH). ACTH stimulates secretion and release of corticosteroids, promotes growth of the adrenal cortex, and also increases blood flow through the adrenal gland. The release of ACTH is regulated by a feedback system which involves the adenohypophysis, the hypothalamus, and higher brain centres. The hypothalamus produces corticotropin-releasing factor (CRF) which stimulates cells in the adenohypophysis to release ACTH. The circulating levels of corticosteroids influence the release of both CRF and ACTH. High plasma levels of corticosteroids inhibit CRF and ACTH release; whereas *low levels* of *it trigger the* hypothalamus to release CRF which causes the adenohypophysis to release ACTH. Target cells within the adrenal cortex respond to ACTH and release additional corticosteroids.

synthesized from the adrenal cortex, out of which only a small number are secreted in significant amounts and out of these secreted, only few possess significant hormonal activity. The most important steroids secreted by the normal adult human adrenal cortex are: (Fig. 16.27).

(a) the glucocorticoid, named as cortisol, and

(b) the mineralocorticoid, named as aldosterone.In addition, small quantities of estrogens and steroid precursors, including progesterone are released into the circulation. Adrenal androgens, although secreted in large amount, are of less physiological significance.

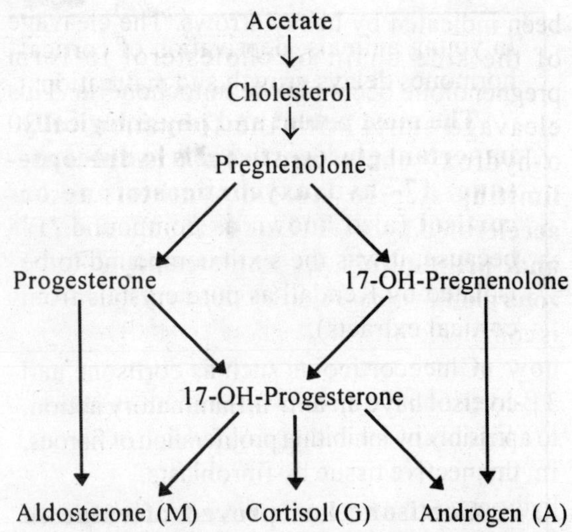

Fig. 16.27: Major steps in the synthesis of the three principal steroids where M denotes mineralocorticoid effect; G for glucocorticoid effect, and A for androgenic effect.

Glucocorticoid (Cortisol)

All hormonal steroids are synthesized from acetyl coenzyme A with cholesterol as their common intermediate. Only a small fraction of the intracellular cholesterol pool is immediately available for steroid synthesis. This small pool appears to be in rapid equilibrium with plasma cholesterol. The uptake of cholesterol from plasma appears to be stimulated by ACTH.

The major reactions in the biosynthesis of adrenal steroids have been given in Fig. 16.28. The exact sequence in which the reactions occur is not known and may depend upon the relative concentrations of substrates, enzymes and cofactors. End products are known and the enzymes catalyzing such reactions are also known. The starting material is cholesterol (Fig. 16.11) which gives rise to a battery of steroidal hormones. The probable major pathways have been indicated by heavy arrows. The cleavage of the side chain of cholesterol to form pregnenolone occurs in the mitochondria. This cleavage starts with the formation of 20 α-hydroxy cholesterol. **This is the rate-limiting step in steroid synthesis and is accelerated by ACTH in the zona fasciculata and, presumably, by angiotensin II in the zona glomerulosa.** Conversion to pregnenolone is completed in the mitochondria. Pregnenolone now moves out of the mitochondria. The 3 β-hydroxyl group of pregnenolone is oxidized to a ketone by the enzyme 3 β-ol dehydrogenase in the presence of NAD which acts as a hydrogen acceptor. The shift of the double bond is catalyzed by Δ^5-3-ketosteroid isomerase as a result of which progesterone is formed.

The remaining reactions in the synthesis of cortisol are all hydroxylations which require various cofactors like molecular oxygen, reduced nicotinamide adenine dinucleotide phosphate (NADPH), flavoproteins, the cytochrome system, a nonhème iron protein, and a special cytochrome known as **cytochrome P-450 because of its sharp absorption peak at 450 nm after exposure to CO.** Since the zona glomerulosa lacks 17α-hydroxylase, progesterone is converted to 17-hydroxy-progesterone only in the zona fasciculata and zona reticularis, where it is then converted to 11-deoxycortisol (Reichstein's "Substance S"), the final relatively inactive precursor of cortisol. Deoxy-cortisol then returns from the smooth endoplasmic reticulum to the mitochondrion for the final 11 β -hydroxylation to cortisol (substance 'F'). **The normal rate of the synthesis of cortisol is 15-30 mg per day.**

> Aldosterone secretion by the cells of the *zona glomerulosa* is regulated by the renin-angiotensin system and the plasma levels of sodium and the potassium. ACTH has little or no direct effect on the secretion of aldosterone. The renin-angiotensin system is believed to be the major controlling system involved in the release of aldosterone.

Mineralocorticoid (Aldosterone)

Since 17 α-hydroxylase remains absent in the zona glomerulosa, progesterone is converted on the smooth endoplasmic reticulum of the glomerulosa first to 11-deoxycorticosterone (DOC) by 21-hydroxylation (Fig. 16.28) and then by 11 β-hydroxylation, within the mitochondrion, to corticosterone, "substance B". Then the mitochondrial enzyme, 18-hydroxylase, catalyzes its conversion to 18-hydroxycorticosterone, which in turn, is later on dehydrogenated to form aldosterone in the presence of an enzyme which is found only in the mitochondria of the zona glomerulosa. It is secreted at a rate of 50 to 200μg per day.

Androgens and Estrogens

The side chain of 17 α-hydroxypregnenolone gets cleaved at the 17-20 carbon bond (Fig. 16.28) to form dehydroisoandrosterone (D) which, with its sulfate, is the major precursor of urinary 17-ketosteroids. Minor quantities of 17-hydroxyprogesterone are converted by a similar reaction to another 17-ketosteroid, Δ^4-androstenedione, which can be further converted to *testosterone* by the reduction of the 17-ketone. Estrogens apparently can be synthesized by adrenal tissue, as evidenced by estradiol and estrone production *in vitro* by feminizing adrenal tumor tissue. The amounts normally produced, if any, are very small, however, and the biosynthetic pathways are not very clear. It is likelihood, they may involve 19-oxidation of testosterone, followed by 19-demethylation and aromatization of the A ring to yield estradiol-17 β. A similar series of reactions might produce ***estrone*** from Δ^4-androstenedione.

The role of the foetal adrenal cortex in the

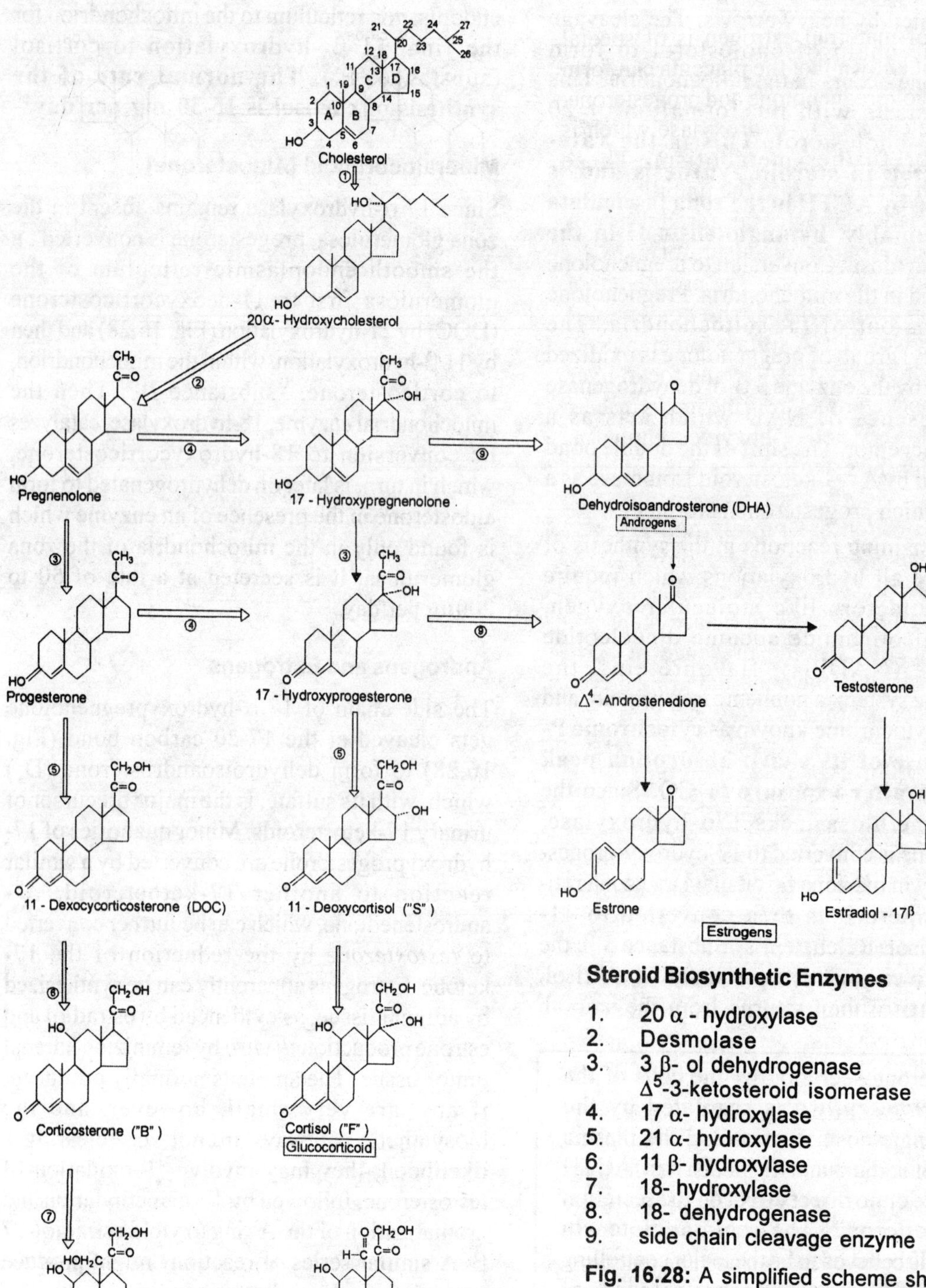

Cholesterol

20α - Hydroxycholesterol

Pregnenolone

17 - Hydroxypregnenolone

Dehydroisoandrosterone (DHA)

Androgens

Progesterone

17 - Hydroxyprogesterone

Δ^4 - Androstenedione

Testosterone

11 - Dexocycorticosterone (DOC)

11 - Deoxycortisol ("S")

Estrone

Estradiol - 17β

Estrogens

Corticosterone ("B")

Cortisol ("F")

Glucocorticoid

18 - Hydroxycorticosterone

Aldosterone

Mineralocorticoid

Steroid Biosynthetic Enzymes

1. 20 α - hydroxylase
2. Desmolase
3. 3 β- ol dehydrogenase
   Δ^5-3-ketosteroid isomerase
4. 17 α- hydroxylase
5. 21 α- hydroxylase
6. 11 β- hydroxylase
7. 18- hydroxylase
8. 18- dehydrogenase
9. side chain cleavage enzyme

Fig. 16.28: A simplified scheme showing the pathways in adrenocortical steroid biosynthesis after formation of cholesterol. The probable major reactions are indicated by heavy arrows.

production of maternal estrogen is of special interest. Be it known that the placenta can form large amount of pregnenolone and progesterone, but lacks the enzyme 17-hydroxylase which is required for further metabolism. These substances are released into the umbilical vein and are carried to the foetal adrenal cortex where progesterone is used to form DOC, corticosterone, and cortisol. The pregnenolone is sulfated, 17-hydroxylated, and converted to DHA sulfate. Now, DHA sulfate is metabolized to form 16 α-hydroxy-DHA by the foetal liver. When the blood returning from the foetus reaches the placenta, very active enzymes known as sulfatases split the ester linkages. Oxidation of DHA gives rise to androstenedione and testosterone, which are rapidly converted to *estrone* and *estradiol.* The 16 α-hydroxy-DHA, which remains present in higher concentration, is also converted to *estriol.* These steps are solely responsible for the presence of large amounts of estriol in the maternal urine during the third trimester of pregnancy.

Metabolism of Adrenal Corticosteroids

Glucocorticoid (Cortisol)

Cortisol is reversibly oxidized to cortisone (substance 'E') in the tissues, predominantly the liver. In plasma, the normal level of cortisol is nearly 2% which circulates in the free state, a small fraction of which remains nonspecifically bound to serum albumin, whereas, greater than 90% fraction remains specifically bound to corticosteroid-binding α_2 - globulin (CBG).

The major pathway of cortisol degradation involves two types of reactions i.e., reduction and conjugation. Reductases present in the liver perform the major, irreversible step in the metabolism of cortisol and cortisone, reducing the 4-5 double bond of the A ring. The reactions require NADPH as cofactor; the predominant products are the 5 β-rather than the 5 α-metabolites as is clear from the figure 16.29.

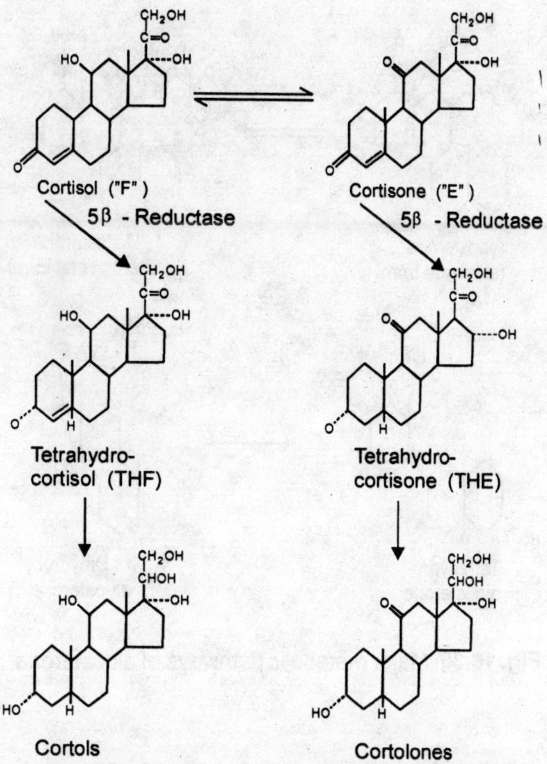

Fig. 16.29 : Major metabolites of cortisol and cortisone

Further reduction of tetrahydrocortisol and tetrahydrocortisone at the C_{20} carbonyl gives rise to the cortols and cortolones. By far, the major portion of the metabolite of cortisol and cortisone are excreted in the urine as the conjugates of glucuronic acid.

Metabolism of Mineralocorticoid (Aldosterone):

Aldosterone is believed to be weakly bound to plasma proteins, perhaps to CBG. Under normal conditions, aldosterone circulates in the hemiacetal form, which is more stable than the aldehyde configuration (Fig. 16.30). The major metabolic pathway for the degradation of aldosterone has been shown below. It has been

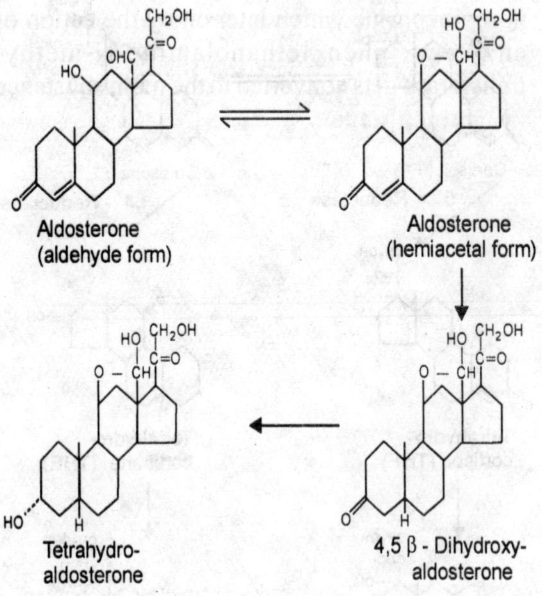

Aldosterone (aldehyde form) ⇌ Aldosterone (hemiacetal form) → 4,5 β - Dihydroxy-aldosterone → Tetrahydro-aldosterone

Fig. 16.30: Major metabolic pathways of aldosterone.

studied that less than 1 % of aldosterone is excreted in the urine unaltered; however, the major portion of it is excreted as tetrahydroaldosterone glucuronide.

Physiological effects of adrenal corticosteroids:

The term, *glucocorticoid,* refers to the sum of a wide range of influences on organic metabolism i.e., the metabolisms of carbohydrate, fat, and protein and includes, among others, effects on the immune and inflammatory responses, vascular permeability, wound healing and muscle integrity.

On the other hand, mineralocorticoid helps in the regulation of balance between [Na^+] and [K^+] in blood and c-lls, specifically promotion of reabsorption of Na^+ and inhibition of reabsorption of K^+ by distal tubules of kidney. Besides, effects of mineralocorticoid are also very well understood on the salivary glands, the sweat glands and the gastrointestinal tract.

Regulation of Glucocorticoids Synthesis

The synthesis and secretion of adrenal glucocorticoids are dependent upon the stimulation by ACTH.

ACTH stimulates the synthesis of cortisol and 17-ketosteroids by the adrenal cortex. ACTH is also necessary to maintain adrenocortical size, structure and vascularity. Actions of ACTH appear to be mediated by cyclic AMP. ACTH binds to specific receptor sites on the surface of the adrenocortical cell and activates the associated membrane-bound adenyl cyclase, which in turn promotes the conversion of ATP to cyclic AMP. ACTH and cyclic AMP stimulate new protein synthesis and that this new protein is required for increased ***steroidogenesis.***

Regulation of ACTH secretion

Following three factors are of major importance in the regulation of ACTH secretion:

1. Firstly, there is homeostatic negative feedback inhibition of ACTH secretion by circulating cortisol. Decreased plasma cortisol concentrations lead to increased pituitary ACTH release; whereas, increased levels of plasma cortisol inhibit ACTH secretion.
2. Secondly, plasma cortisol concentrations show a circadian rhythm, with high levels (15 to 25 μg/100 ml) in the early morning and low levels (less than 7 μg/100ml) late in the evening.
3. **Thirdly, the most important factor which governs the ACTH secretion is "stress".** Thus, plasma ACTH levels get increased during fever, laparotomy or acute severe depression, resulting into increased secretion of cortisol.

THE ADRENAL MEDULLA

The central portion of the adrenal gland, the *medulla,* is composed of endocrine parenchymal cells (called as *chromaffin cells)*, connective tissue, and numerous blood vessels and nerves. Chromaffin cells of the adrenal medulla are relatively large, rounded cells.

Biosynthesis of Catecholamines

The synthesis of epinephrine which is the most important catecholamine secreted by the adrenal medulla, is outlined in Fig. 16.31.

Tyrosine, the precursor, is derived primarily from dietary sources. The first step in the biosynthetic pathway, i.e. the conversion of tyrosine to DOPA, is the rate-limiting reaction; this reaction is catalyzed by the enzyme tyrosine hydroxylase which is found only in neuroectodermal tissues. In the next reaction, DOPA is converted to dopamine by L-aromatic amino acid decarboxylase. Now, dopamine is acted upon by the enzyme dopamine β-hydroxylase forming norepinephrine which later on by the action of enzyme phenylethanolamine-N-methyl transferase gets converted to the main substance i.e. **epinephrine.**

> Chromaffin cells (**named because they react with chromate salts**) of the adrenal medulla are a part of the APUD (Amine Precursor uptake and Decarboxylation) system of cells. The chromaffin reaction is thought to involve oxidation and polymerization of the catecholamines contained within the secretory granules of the cells. These cells are capable of synthesizing and secreting **catecholamines.**
>
> Histochemical studies have demonstrated that there are two types of cells, out of which one contains **epinephrine** and the other **norepinephrine**.
>
> The release of the catecholamines by the chromaffin cells of the adrenal medulla is initiated by the impulses conveyed in the preganglionic sympathetic fibres which end on the chromaffin cells. In response to these signals, the chromaffin cells release the catecholamines into the adjacent blood vessels.

Storage and Release of Catecholamines

Unlike the adrenocortical steroids, which are released almost as soon as they are synthesized, **catecholamines** are stored in the adrenal medullary cells. They remain present in membrane-enclosed secretory vesicles and are complexed with adenosine triphosphate (1 mole of ATP for 4 molecules of catecholamines) and a specific protein of the molecular weight of 40,000. Besides, the vesicles also contain a Ca^{2+} and Mg^{2+}- dependent ATPase. These subcellular vesicles take up epinephrine and norepinephrine by a transport process. The vesicle uptake mechanism is blocked potently by reserpine, an antihypertensive drug. The free catecholamine which is not taken up immediately by the vesicles is metabolized by monoamine oxidase **(MAO)** located within the mitochondria.

The hormone contained within the secretory vesicle can be released in response to an appropriate stimulus which, in the case of adrenal pheochromocyte, is acetylcholine secreted by the preganglionic nerve fibres that terminate in the medulla. Other agents include histamine and glucagon which can also stimulate the release of epinephrine.

Metabolism of Catecholamines

Norepinephrine and epinephrine are metabolized by two enzymes, primarily MAO, which remains present in the mitochondria of cells of most organs, the richer sources include liver, kidney, intestine, and stomach. MAO deaminates the α–carbon of norepinephrine, epinephrine and other catecholamines, such as serotonin and dopamine.

The other enzyme is catechol - o-methyl transferase **(COMT)** which is a soluble enzyme

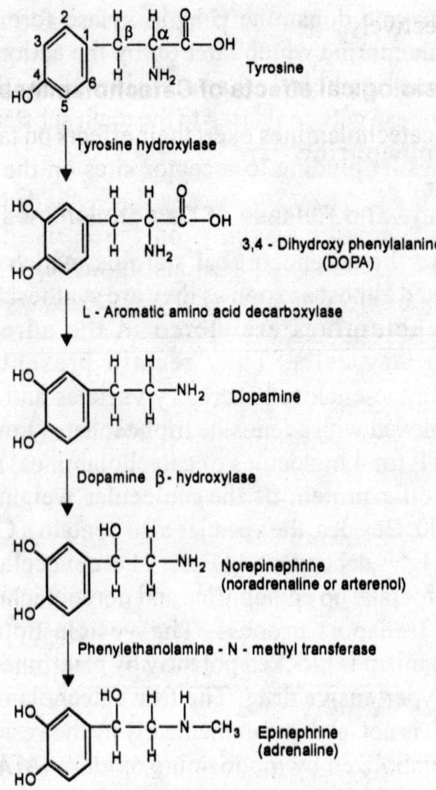

Tyrosine

Tyrosine hydroxylase

3,4 - Dihydroxy phenylalanine (DOPA)

L - Aromatic amino acid decarboxylase

Dopamine

Dopamine β - hydroxylase

Norepinephrine (noradrenaline or arterenol)

Phenylethanolamine - N - methyl transferase

Epinephrine (adrenaline)

Fig. 16.31: Biosynthetic pathway for the conversion of tyrosine to norepinephrine and epinephrine

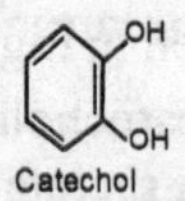

Catechol

Dopa readily crosses the blood brain barrier, promoting the catecholamine synthesis. Thus, in disorders involving deficiency of catecholamine synthesis, administration of dopa may have some beneficial effects. In Parkinson's disease in which deficiency of dopamine synthesis affects nerve transmission in the substantia nigra of the upper brain system, administration of dopa leads to some symptomatic relief. Parkinsonism is a chronic, progressive disorder characterised by involuntary tremor, decreased motor power and control, postural instability and muscular rigidity.

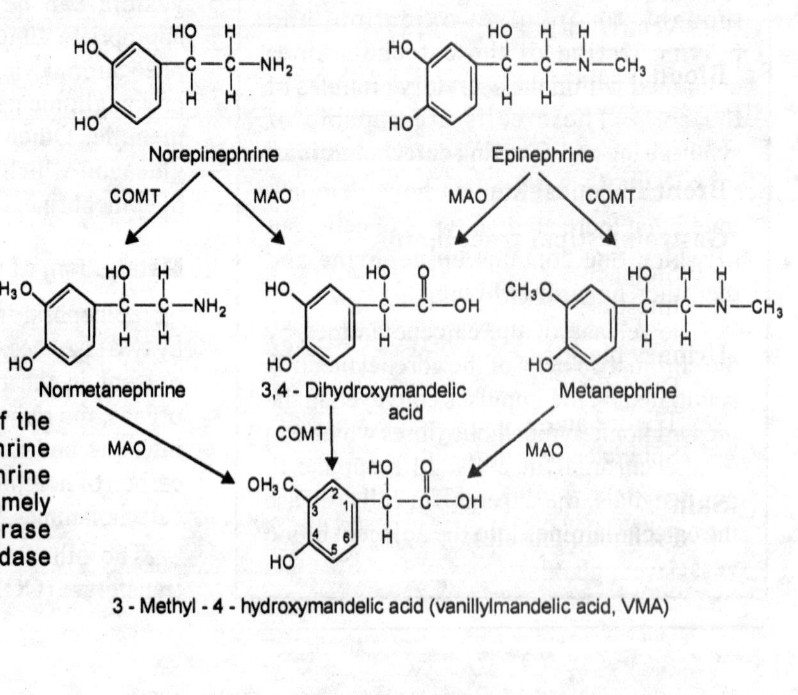

Norepinephrine — COMT → Normetanephrine; MAO → 3,4 - Dihydroxymandelic acid

Epinephrine — MAO → 3,4 - Dihydroxymandelic acid; COMT → Metanephrine

Normetanephrine — MAO → 3 - Methyl - 4 - hydroxymandelic acid (vanillylmandelic acid, VMA)

3,4 - Dihydroxymandelic acid — COMT → 3 - Methyl - 4 - hydroxymandelic acid (vanillylmandelic acid, VMA)

Metanephrine — MAO → 3 - Methyl - 4 - hydroxymandelic acid (vanillylmandelic acid, VMA)

Fig. 16.32: Major pathways of the metabolism of norepinephrine (noradrenaline) and epinephrine (adrenaline). Two enzymes namely catechol-o-methyl transferase (COMT), and monoamine oxidase (MAO) are involved.

and is found in many tissues. This enzyme catalyzes the transfer of the methyl group from S-adenosylmethionine to the catechol 3-hydroxyl radical and also requires Mg^{2+} as a cofactor. The major metabolites of epinephrine and norepinephrine are given in Fig. 16.32.

Free or conjugated catecholamines, vanillylmandelic acid (VMA), or total metanephrines (normetanephrine plus metanephrine) can be found in the urine. Free epinephrine is excreted in the amount of 20 μg or less per day; whereas the excretion of free norepinephrine, the greater amount of which is released by the sympathetic nerve endings, is nearly 80 μg or less per day. The upper normal limits for total metanephrines and VMA are 1.3 mg and 6.5 mg/day, respectively.

Physiological effects of Catecholamines

The catecholamines exert their effects on target tissues by binding to receptor sites on the cell membrane. The receptors have been divided into two categories, α and β on the basis of the relative potency of various agonists, which activate the receptors, and of various antagonists, which block them (Table 16.1).

β-receptors are most sensitive to stimulation by isoproterenol (isopropylnorepinephrine) and least to norepinephrine, whereas with **α-receptors**, the reverse is the case. It has been studied that α- receptors are selectively blocked by phenoxybenzamine and phentolamine

Table 16.1: Some effects of catecholamines

Effector Organ	Type of Receptor	Response
Eye		
Radial muscle, Iris	α	Contraction (mydriasis)
Ciliary muscle	β	Relaxation for far vision
Heart		
Atria	β_1	Increase the contractility
Ventricles	β	Increase the contractility and irritability
Blood vessels	α	Constriction
	β_2	Dilatation (predominates in skeletal muscle)
Bronchial muscle	β_2	Relaxation (bronchodilatation)
Gastrointestinal tract motility		
Stomach	β	Decrease
Intestine	α, β	Decrease
Urinary bladder		
Detrusor	β	Relaxation
Trigone and Sphincter	α	Contraction
Skin		
Pilomotor muscles	α	Piloerection
Sweat glands	α	Selective stimulation (adrenergic sweating)

whereas β-receptors are blocked by propranolol. More recently, **β-receptors** have further been divided into two classes based on the strong inhibition of some β–receptors (called β_1) by drugs like practolol and of others (called β_2) by drugs such as butoxamine.

Catecholamines have been found to have the following important metabolic effects.

(a) **They stimulate glycogenolysis and therefore have an anti-insulin effect.**

(b) **They stimulate the mobilization of free fatty acids from adipose tissue, skeletal muscle, and myocardium in the presence of minimal concentrations of glucocorticoids, which exert a permissive effect.**

Epinephrine has been found to be more potent than norepinephrine in producing these effects.

Comparable effects of L-adrenaline and L-noradrenaline in man are given in Table 16.2.

Table 16.3 Urinary excretion of catecholamines in man

Condition	*Urinary excretion in ng/min*	
	Adrenaline	*Noradrenaline*
After adrenalectomy	0	8-15
Chromaffin cell tumors	Slightly increased	100 times or more
Insulin hypoglycaemia	10 times	No effect
Mild exercise	2 times	2 times
Mental stress	Increased	No effect
Myocardial infarction	Upto 35 times	Upto 8 times
Rest	2-5	16-27
Strenuous exercise	10 times	10 times
Tilt, recumbent to head up	Little change	Increased

Normal adrenal tissue from man and many other animals contains noradrenaline (norepinephrine) as well as adrenaline (epinephrine) and they are often together referred to as ***catecholamines***. The ratio of adrenaline to noradrenaline in fresh human adrenals is 4:1

Excretion

Urinary excretion of catecholamines in man varies significantly within 24 hours from time to time as shown in Table 16.3.

Table 16.2 Comparison of the effects of L-adrenaline and L-noradrenaline in man

	Effect of L-adrenaline	**Effect of L-noradrenaline**
Blood pressure	Rise	Much rise
Blood sugar	Increase	Slight increase
Bronchus	Dilatation	Less dilatation
Cardiac output	Increase	Variable
Central nervous system	Anxiety	No effect
Eosinophil count	Increase	No effect
Heart rate	Increase	Decrease
Kidney	Vasoconstriction	Vasoconstriction
Muscle vessels	Dilatation	Constriction
Metabolism	Increase	Slight increase
Oxygen consumption	Increase	No effect
Respiration	Stimulates	Stimulates
Skin Vessels	Constriction	Constriction
Uterus in vivo in late pregnancy	Inhibits	Stimulates

GASTROINTESTINAL HORMONES

Nature and origin of hormones

Hormones of GIT appear to be of neuroectodermal origin and they act on the cell surface and reach their target organ or cell by one of three pathways. Thus,

(i) neurocrine cells extend to the target cell and secrete the hormone into a synaptic gap;

(ii) paracrine cells secrete the hormone into surrounding tissue fluids in which it diffuses to the appropriate receptor site; and

(iii) the classic endocrine cells secrete the hormone into the blood which carries it to its target.

Chemically, these hormones are amines and polypeptides; some of them are found in both brain and the paracrine-endocrine cells of the gut. They include the amines for instance serotonin, dopamine, histamine and melatonin and peptides, e.g., substance P, vasoactive intestinal peptide (VIP), and somatostatin. The gut cells that do not contain preformed amine but can take up suitable precursors and convert them to amines by decarboxylation have been named as the **APUD system** (amine precursor uptake and decarboxylation).

Gut mainly secretes following **seven hormones** which are peptides and the amino acid sequence of which is known. **These include (1) Gastrin, (2) Secretin, (3) Cholecystokinin (CCK), (4) Gastric Inhibitory Peptide (GIP), (5) Vasoactive Intestinal Peptide (6) Motilin (7) Substance-P.**

1. Gastrin

Gastric mucosa has been found to secrete two types of gastrins, i.e. gastrin I and gastrin II. Gastrin I contains unsulfated tyrosine; whereas gastrin II sulfated tyrosine. Gastrin exists in three size forms, viz; (a) big gastrin, (b) little gastrin, and (c) mini gastrin. Big gastrin possesses 34 amino acid residues with a molecular weight of 3,839; little gastrin is a heptadecapeptide consisting of residues 18 to 34 of G 34 with a molecular weight of 2,098, and mini gastrin consists of residues 22 to 34 of G 34 or residues 5 to 17 of little gastrin with a M.W. of 1,647.

Big gastrin form is predominant in the blood, whereas little gastrin is predominant in the antrum. Little gastrin is five times more active than the big gastrin form.

The secretion of gastrin has been found to be stimulated by several factors like ingested food, amino acids, acetylcholine and distension of the stomach. **Amongst amino acids, glycine amino acid has been found to be the most potent factor for stimulating the secretion of gastrin.**

Physiological action: Gastrin stimulates gastric secretion of H^+ and pepsin stimulates gastric antral motility and also stimulates growth of acid secretory gastric mucosa.

2. Secretin

It is a 27-amino acids peptide which is synthesized and released by the S cells in the duodenum and proximal jejunum in response to duodenal acidification. It contains four arginine residues and one histidine and therefore is basic in nature. Its structure is quite similar to those of GIP and VIP.

Physiological actions

(i) **It stimulates the secretion of bicarbonate.**

(ii) **It also stimulates the secretion of water from pancreas.**

(iii) **It augments the action of CCK on pancreatic secretion.**

3. Cholecystokinin (CCK)/Pancreozymin

CCK exists in at least 5 molecular forms, i.e., CCK - 33, CCK - 58, CCK - 39, CCK - 8 and cerulein of which CCK - 8 appears to be the most widely distributed and potent form in the circulation. CCK is synthesized in the I cells in the mucosa of the duodenum and proximal jejunum. This is released in response to peptides, amino acids, long-chain fatty acids, calcium, and acid.

Physiological actions

(i) Causes gallbladder contraction,
(ii) Stimulates pancreatic enzyme secretion,
(iii) Augments the action of secretin on pancreatic secretion,
(iv) Like all gastrointestinal peptides; it has numerous secondary actions, the interesting one of which is that it causes **satiety** (feeling of having had too much).
(v) It stimulates the growth of pancreatic acinar tissue.

4. Gastric-Inhibitory Polypeptide (GIP)

It is a 43-amino acids peptide and carries a M.W. of 5,105. This is released from the duodenal and jejunal mucosa in response to glucose.

Physiological actions

(i) It inhibits gastric motility,
(ii) It inhibits the gastric secretion of acid and
(iii) It also inhibits the release of insulin.

5. Vasoactive Intestinal Polypeptide (VIP)

It is a basic 28-amino acids peptide and remains present in the nerves of the submucosal plexus, the mesenteric plexus, and blood vessels.

Tumors that produce this peptide, *VIPomas*, cause a syndrome of watery diarrhoea, hypokalaemia and achlorhydria.

Physiological actions

(i) It may be involved in sphincter relaxation.
(ii) It may also be involved in blood flow.
(iii) It inhibits the secretion of gastrin.
(iv) It inhibits the secretion of H^+ ions.
(v) It inhibits gastric motility.
(vi) It stimulates pancreatic secretion of bicarbonate and enzymes.

6. *Motilin*

It is a 22-amino acids peptide. It's synthesized in the intestinal mucosa.

Physiological actions

(i) It stimulates acid and pepsin secretion by gastric mucosa,
(ii) It is also a stimulator of intestinal smooth muscle contraction, and
(iii) It stimulates fundus and antral motility.

7. Substance-P

It was the first peptide found in both the gut and the brain. It is a 11-amino acids peptide.

Physiological actions: It stimulates the motility of the fundus, antrum and small intestine.

DISEASES OF HORMONE PRODUCTION

No disease or disorder due to the deficiency of GIT hormone production or hormone release is known so far, **although disorders of the small bowel may lead to defective release of secretin or CCK.**

Hypersecretion of gastrin by gastrin-producing tumors of the pancreas or duodenum, or hyperplasia of gastrin-producing cells in the pancreas or gastric antrum is responsible for the well known ***Zollinger-Ellison*** syndrome characterized by:

(i) Hyperplasia of the gastric mucosa,
(ii) Profuse secretion of gastric acid,
(iii) Severely erosive peptic ulcer disease of the gastrointestinal mucosa exposed to this acid and
(iv) Malabsorption and diarrhoea due to excessive fluid entry into the small bowel with inactivation of pancreatic enzymes:

Besides, pancreatic cholera ***(Verner-Morrison Syndrome*** of severe watery diarrhoea with alkalosis and hypokalaemia) may also occur from tumors of the pancreas or neural tissue in the abdomen that secrete VIP. These tumors have been named as ***"VIPomas"***.

Serum gastrin concentration is augmented in conditions in which **chronic anacidity leads to uninhibited gastrin cell hyperplasia and secretion, as in** *Addisonian pernicious anaemia* and *chronic atrophic gastritis*.

Hypofunction of the adrenal medulla has not yet been recognized to produce any pathology. However, actively secreting tumors (pheochromocytoma) of the chromaffin cells of the adrenal medulla or of the organs of Zuckerkandl are known to produce large quantities of noradrenaline with a small amount of adrenaline, and their discharge at intervals into the blood may produce elevation of arterial pressure. As much as 2 mg of catecholamines may then appear in the urine per day.

The amount of catecholamines in the blood can be assessed by either fluorimetry or other more recent sophisticated techniques like radioimmunoassay, etc. Human blood plasma contains about 0.3 μg of noradrenaline per litre and 0.06 μg of adrenaline per litre. **Healthy man excretes not more than 50 μg/24 hours of catecholamines and adrenaline is less than 15 per cent of this.**

Adrenaline by producing vasoconstriction in the skin and vasodilatation in the muscles, moves blood from the skin to the muscles; it stimulates the metabolism and mobilizes glycogen as glucose.

Noradrenaline, on the other hand produces a general vasoconstriction (except in the coronary arteries) but its effects on the metabolism are not very well understood. **This may be regarded as a pressor hormone required for the maintenance of blood pressure.**

Adrenalectomized animals adjust to stress, such as prolonged exposure to cold or shock, much more slowly and less effectively than normal ones do, meaning to say, **the hormones secreted by adrenal cortex act as buffering agents against cold or shock.**

Adrenalectomized rats have decreased urea nitrogen excretion, blood glucose concentration, and liver glycogen storage, indicating decreased protein catabolism and decreased gluconeogenesis.

The role of cortisol in lipid metabolism is not well understood. Total body fat gets increased by glucocorticoid administration but the synthesis of fatty acids gets inhibited in liver.

CHAPTER 17

WATER AND ELECTROLYTES BALANCE

WATER

The chief constituent of living matter is water. Its importance in both the structure and functioning of the tissues is enormous.

The body of a healthy adult male consists of some 65 to 70 percent of water and about 15 percent of fat; the remainder is accounted for by the solid parts of cells and supporting structures. The considerable variations in total body water (TBW) between one person and another are due to differences in fat content since the amount of **water in the fat-free parts of the body is remarkably constant. This reveals the fact that the water content of the body of the female ranges from 50 to 55 percent which is rather less than that of the male. In very fat people, the body water may not be more than 40 percent of the total body weight.**

In its capacity as a solvent, water plays a very important role in the cellular reactions. A very large number of substances are soluble in water and many others such as fats and fat - soluble compounds can be carried in fine emulsions or be rendered water - soluble by combination with hydrophilic substances.

Owing to the high heat capacity of water, large changes in heat production can take place in the body with very little alteration in the body temperature. Since the latent heat of evaporation of water is high, the loss of a small amount of water in evaporated sweat means a relatively large loss of heat. **Moreover, the high latent heat of solidification is a protection against the freezing of the tissues.**

Water is received by the body from the two main sources. Most of it is taken by mouth in the form of food and drinks but a small amount of water is normally formed in the tissues as a result of oxidation of the hydrogen of foodstuffs. **The amount of water ingested by an individual varies according to the habit, climate and occupation.**

The amount of **metabolic water** formed in the tissues as a result of oxidation processes is nearly **300-350 ml in man,** that is nearly 14 percent of his total daily fluid intake. This water is formed in the cells and is of great significance to the organism. **It is of utmost importance to the hibernating animals who live for longer periods on metabolic water and to organisms such as the moths of the clothes who do not normally have ready access to water.**

Following Table 17.1 gives an idea of turnover of fluid which occurs in the body during

24 hours. **In 24 hours, a man secretes 1 to 1.5 litre(s) of saliva, 1 to 2 litre(s) of gastric juice, 0.5 to 1 litre of bile, 0.6 to 0.8 litre of pancreatic juice and 3 litres of intestinal juice.** All this fluid except about 100 ml which is escaped through faeces is reabsorbed.

Table 17.1 Water balance of an adult man in a temperate climate

Daily intake		Daily output	
Drinks	1300 ml	**Urine**	1500 ml
Food	850 ml	**Expired air**	400 ml
Formed in the body by		**Skin**	500 ml
Oxidation	350 ml	**Faeces**	100 ml
Total	2500 ml	**Total**	2500 ml

Water Metabolism

Since most biochemical reactions of the body take place in an aqueous medium, control of water balance is an important requirement for **homeostasis.**

Although water is freely permeable across the cell membrane but contrarily other solutes are less mobile because of several barriers imposed by membrane systems. These barriers give rise to fluid pools or compartments i.e., **intracellular fluid and extracellular fluid.**

Intracellular fluid makes up 30-40% of the body weight, or about two-thirds of total body water. **Potassium and magnesium are the predominant cations. The anions are mainly proteins and organic phosphates with chloride and bicarbonate at low concentrations.**

Extracellular fluid contains sodium as the predominant cation and accounts for 20-25% of body weight or one- third of total body water. It contributes to vascular, interstitial, transcellular and dense connective tissue fluid pools. Vascular fluid is the circulating portion, is rich in proteins and does not readily cross endothelial membranes, whereas interstitial fluid surrounds the cells and accounts for 18-20% of total body water. It exchanges with vascular fluid via the lymph system. Transcellular fluid remains present in digestive juice, intraocular fluid, cerebrospinal fluid (CSF), and synovial (joint) fluid. These fluids are secretions of specialized cells. Their composition differs considerably from that of the rest of the extracellular fluid, with which they rapidly exchange contents under normal conditions. Dense connective tissue (bone, cartilage, etc) fluid exchanges slowly with the rest of the extracellular fluid and accounts for nearly 15% of total body water.

Movement of water is mainly due to **osmosis** and **filtration.** In osmosis, water moves to the area of higher solute concentration. Thus, active movement of salts into an area creates a concentration gradient down as a result of which water flows passively. In filtration, hydrostatic pressure in atrial blood moves water and nonprotein solutes and through specialized membranes to produce an almost protein - free filtrate; **this process occurs during the formation of renal glomerular filtrate.** Besides, filtration also accounts for the movement of water from the vascular space into the interstitial compartment which is opposed by the osmotic (oncotic) pressure of plasma proteins.

Cells move ions (especially Na^+ and K^+) against a concentration gradient by a **'sodium pump'** that actively transports sodium across the plasma membranes.

Kidneys are the major organs to regulate the extracellular fluid composition and volume. **The three main processes which occur in the nephrons are:**

a) **Formation of a virtually protein - free ultrafiltrate in the glomerulus.**
b) **Active reabsorption (principally in the proximal tubule) of solutes from the glomerular filtrate; and**

c) **Active excretion of substances such as hydrogen ions into the tubular lumen, usually in the distal portion of the tubule (Fig 17.1).**

The normal glomerular filtration rate (GFR) is 100 - 120 ml/min which means nearly 150 litre of fluid passes through the renal tubules each day. Since the **average daily urinary output is 1-1.5 litres,** 99% of the glomerular filtrate is reabsorbed. Approximately 80% of the water is reabsorbed in the proximal tubule, a consequence of active absorption of solutes. Reabsorption in the rest of the tubule varies according to the individual's water balance in contrast to the **obligatory reabsorption** which occurs in the proximal tubule.

The facultative absorption of water depends upon the establishment of an osmotic gradient in the **loop of Henle** by the secretion of Na^+ from the ascending loop and their uptake by the descending loop. As a result, the proximal end of the loop is hyperosmotic (1200 mosm/kg) and the distal end hypoosmotic with respect to blood. The collecting ducts run through the hyperosmotic region. **In the absence of antidiuretic hormone (ADH), the cells of the ducts are relatively impermeable to water.** They become permeable to water in the presence of ADH, however, and the urine becomes hyperosmotic with respect to blood.

Water as a Solvent

For a solid to dissolve, three following points must happen:

a) The molecules (or ions) of the solid must separate from one another.

b) The molecules of the solvent must also undergo a separation to admit the molecules (or ions) of the solute. This causes the breaking of some of the linkages holding the solvent molecules together.

c) Some sort of linkages must be formed between the solvent molecules and the solute molecules to balance the attraction which the solute molecules exert on one another.

Homeostatic Controls

The composition and volume of extracellular fluid are regulated by the following two complex mechanisms i.e;

a) Hormonal mechanism

b) Nervous mechanism

which interact to control its osmolality, volume and pH.

The osmolality of extracellular fluid is mainly due to Na^+ and accompanying anions; this is kept within narrow limits (285-295 mosm/kg) by the regulation of water intake **(via a thirst centre)** and water excretion by the kidney through the action of ADH. The volume is kept relatively constant, provided the individual's body weight remains constant to within ± 1 kg. **Volume receptors** sense the effective circulating blood volume which when decreased, stimulates the renin-angiotensin- aldosterone system and results in retention of Na^+. The increased Na^+ level leads to a rise in osmolality and secretion of ADH with a resultant increase in water retention. Side by side, **antagonistic systems** also exist that cause an increased Na^+ excretion. **Atrial natriuretic peptide** (ANP), **also called atrial natriuretic factor (ANF) or hormone,** is released by the cardiocytes of the cardiac atria in response to mechanical stretch caused by the plasma volume expansion.

ANF has got the following two functions:

a) Induces diuresis, and

b) Induces natriuresis

These effects result from renal hemodynamic changes associated with increases in GFR and inhibition of Na^+ reabsorption from inner medullary collecting ducts.

ANP is a 28 amino- acid peptide and possesses only one disulfide linkage in its structure. The precursor and the storage form of ANP in cardiocytes is a 126 - amino acid polypeptide. Following are the stimuli of ANP:

(i) Blood volume,

(ii) High blood pressure,

(iii) Elevated serum osmolality,

(iv) Increased heart rate and

(v) Elevated levels of plasma catecholamines

Activation of the ANP gene in cardiocytes by glucocorticoids leads to increased synthesis of ANP which also regulates Na^+ and water homeostasis by different mechanisms that include inhibition of steps in the renin- angiotensin- aldosterone pathway and inhibition of ADH secretion from posterior pituitary cells.

Electrolytes Balance

Major electrolytes are the following:

(a) Na^+,

(b) K^+,

(c) Cl^-, and

(d) HCO_3^-

Sodium:

The average sodium content of the human body is 60 mEq/kg, of which 50% is in extracellular fluid, 40% is in bone and 10% is intracellular. The chief dietary source of Na^+ is salt added during cooking and in the preparation of pickles. Excess sodium is largely excreted via urine, whereas some is lost via perspiration. Gastrointestinal losses are little except in diarrhoea.

Sodium balance is integrated with the regulation of extracellular fluid volume. Depletion hyponatremia (i.e., sodium loss greater than water loss) may result from less intake of sodium, excessive loss of fluid from vomiting or diarrhoea, diuretic abuse and adrenal insufficiency. Hyponatremia can cause decreased extracellular fluid volume, as occurs in congestive heart failure, uncontrolled diabetes mellitus, nephrosis, cirrhosis and inappropriate ADH secretion, etc.

Hypernatremia is caused by the loss of hypoosmotic fluid which occurs in burns, fevers, high environmental temperature, **diabetes insipidus,** kidney diseases, exercise, etc or **by the increased Na^+ intake** as takes place during adminstration of hypertonic NaCl solution, ingestion of $NaHCO_3$, etc.

Potassium:

The average K^+ content of the human body is 40 mEq/kg which is found mainly in intracellular space. **It is required for the metabolism of carbohydrates and increased cellular uptake of K^+ also occurs during catabolism of glucose.** Potassium is widely distributed in plant sources and animal foods, **the human requirement is nearly 4 g/ day.** Insulin and catecholamines accelerate a shift of K^+ into the cells. **Excess K^+ is excreted via urine, a process regulated by aldosterone.**

Plasma potassium plays a role in the irritability of excitable tissues. A high concentration of plasma K^+ causes electrocardiographic (ECG) abnormalities and possibly to cardial arrhythmia, which may be due to lowering of the membrane potential.

Low concentration of plasma K^+ (hypokalemia) increases the membrane potential, decreases irritability, and produces other ECG abnormalities and **muscle paralysis too.**

Hyperkalemia may take place in renal diseases and adrenal insufficiency. Metabolic acidosis, particulauly in diabetic acidosis and catabolism of celluar protein in starvation or fever cause K^+ release from cells. **Treatment consists in correction of acidosis and promotion of cellular uptake of K^+ by administration of insulin which increases**

intake of glucose. In severe cases, ion exchange resins given orally bind K^+ in intestinal secretions.

Hypokalemia may occur from loss of gastrointestinal secretions (which contain large amounts of K^+) and from excessive loss via urine because of increased aldosterone secretion or diuretic therapy. **Hypokalemia is usually associated with alkalosis.**

Chloride:

It is the major extracellular anion. **Nearly, 70%** is found in extracellular fluid. The average Cl^- content of the human body is 35 meq/kg. Chloride obtained from food is almost completely absorbed. **Plasma levels of Na^+ and Cl^- in general undergo parallel alterations; however, in metabolic alkalosis, chloride concentration gets increased.**

Properties of water

Acid and base concentrations in living system are fully regulated to maintain conditions compatible with normal life. Biochemical reactions involving acids and bases occur in the body water, whereas buffer systems protect the body from significant variations in the concertrations of acids and bases.

Life can not be sustained without water. Water constitutes 45-73% of total human body weight. It is distributed in intracellular (55%) and extracellular (45%) compartments and provides a continous solvent phase between body compartments. As the biological solvent, water plays a major role in all aspects of metabolism: **absorption, transport, digestion,** and **excretion of inorganic and organic substances as well as maintenance of body temperature.** The unique properties of water are due to its structure.

Physical properties of water

Density (at 4°C)	1.0 g/mL
Molecular weight	18
Liquid range	0° - 100°C
Melting point	0°C
Boiling Point	100°C
Heat of fusion	80 cal/g
Heat of vapourization	540 cal/g
Dipole moment	1.86 Debye unit
Dielectric constant (E)	78.4
Solid / liquid density ratio	0.92

BIOCHEMICAL VALUES

Table - 1 Normal Human Biochemical Values in Blood / Plasma / Serum

Table - 2 Commonly Used Anticoagulants

Appendices - I to V

Biochemical Values

Table - 1 Normal Human Biochemical Values in Blood / Plasma / Serum

S.No.	Constituent	Normal range	High in	Low in
	DIABETES MELLITUS			
1.	Blood Sugar (Fasting)	70 - 100 mg%	Diabetes mellitus	Hyperinsulinism
2.	Blood Sugar (PP)	Less than 140 mg%	Diabetes mellitus	-
3.	Renal Threshold Value	160 - 180 mg%	Diabetes mellitus	-
4.	Blood Sugar Level, (Random)	80 - 120 mg%	Diabetes mellitus	-
	RENAL FUNCTION TESTS			
1.	Blood Urea	14 - 43 mg%	Nephritis, Renal Failure	Nephrosis
2.	Serum Creatinine	0.1 - 1.2 mg%	Nephritis, Renal Failure	Nephrosis
	LIVER FUNCTION TESTS			
1.	Serum Bilirubin	0.2 - 1.0 mg%	Obstructive Jaundice, Haemolytic Jaundice, Neonatal Jaundice and Hepatitis	-
2.	SGOT (AST)	4 - 17 IU/l (8 - 40 units/ml)	Myocardial Infarction, Infective Hepatitis etc.	-
3.	SGPT (ALT)	3 - 15 IU/l	Liver Disorders	-
4.	Serum Alkaline Phosphatase	4 - 11 KA Units	Obstructive Jaundice, Biliary Cirrhosis, Rickets, Osteomalacia etc.	Scurvy, Severe Anaemia, Malnutrition, Hypophosphatasia
5.	Serum Proteins, Total	6.0 - 8.0 g%	Multiple Myeloma, Anhydraemia, etc.	Nephrotic Syndromes, Neoplastic Disease, Malnutrition, Kwashiorkor Syndrome, Cirrhosis of Liver.

S.No.	Constituent	Normal range	High in	Low in
6.	Serum Albumin	3.5 - 5.0 g%	-	Cirrhosis of Liver, Nephrotic Syndromes, Malnutrition, Malignancies, etc.
7.	Serum Globulins,	2.3 - 3.6 g%	Anhydraemia, Nephrosis, Infections, Advanced Liver Diseases, etc.	-
8.	Albumin / Globulins Ratio	1.2 - 1.5	-	Less than 1 in Infective Hepatitis
9.	Fibrinogen (Plasma)	0.3 - 0.6 g%	Infections	Cirrhosis of Liver
	CARDIAC ENZYMES			
1.	SGOT (AST)	4 - 17 IU / l (8 - 40 units / ml)	Myocardial Infarction, Infective Hepatitis, etc.	-
2.	Lactic Dehydrogenase (LDH)	230 - 460 IU / l	Myocardial Infarction, Infective Hepatitis, Toxic Jaundice, etc.	-
3.	Creatine Phosphokinase (CPK or CK)	20 - 50 IU / l (men) 10-37 IU / l (Women)	Myocardial Infarction, Hypothyroidism, Progressive Muscular Atrophy, etc	-
	CARDIAC MARKERS			
1.	Troponin - T		Myocardial Infarction	-
2.	Homocysteine		Myocardial Infarction	Pregnancy
	THYROID FUNCTION TESTS			
1.	Triiodothyronine (T_3)	60 - 190 ng/dl (RIA mehtod)	Pregnancy, Hyperthyroidism	Hypothyroidism
2.	Thyroxine (T_4)	1.5 - 4.0 ng/dl (RIA mehtod)	Hyperthyroidism	Hypothyroidism
3.	TSH	0.3 - 6.0 μIU / ml	Hypothyroidism	Hyperthyroidism
4.	Thyroid Binding Globulin (TBG)	2.0 - 4.8 ng/dl	Pregnancy, Acute Liver Disease	Major illness, Nephrosis, Thyrotoxicosis
5.	Protein Bound Iodine (PBI)	4 - 8 μg/dl	Hyperthyroidism	Hypothyroidism, Nephrosis, etc.

S.No.	Constituent	Normal range	High in	Low in
	PANCREATIC FUNCTION TESTS			
1.	Serum Amylase	80 - 180 Somogyi Units	Pancreatitis, Stone and Cancer in Biliary Duct, Perforated Peptic Ulcer	Liver diseases
2.	Serum Lipase	Less than 150 U / l	Pancreatitis, Cancer in Pancreas, Cirrhosis of Liver, Hepatitis, Duodenal ulcer, Disease of the biliary tract, etc.	-
	LIPID PROFILE			
1.	Serum Cholesterol	150 - 200 mg %	Diabetes, Nephritis, etc	Hyperthyroidism, Severe liver damage
2.	HDL - Cholesterol	30 - 63 mg %, (men) 35 - 75 mg % (women)	The Combined Risk Factor of Coronary Heart Disease (CHD) can be determined following the estimations of Serum Cholesterol and HDL - Cholesterol.	
3.	LDL - Cholesterol	up to 150 mg /dl	**The Ratio of Cholesterol to HDL - Cholesterol has Predictive Value in Determining the Risk of CHD more accurately. For normal males the ratio of 5:1 and for normal females the ratio of 4.5:1 are considered as average risk.** Lower ratios significantly reduce the risk, whereas ratios **9.5:1** and **7:1** for males and females respectively, are believed to double the risk of CHD. An inverse relationship has been observed between the risk of CHD and the concentration of HDL-cholesterol. HDL - cholesterol represents approximately 20-25% of the total cholesterol in serum.	

S.No.	Constituent	Normal range	High in	Low in
4.	VLDL	up to 28 mg / dl	Hyperlipidaemia	
5.	Serum Triglycerides	30 - 140 mg%	Hyperlipidaemia, Atherosclerosis, Nephrosis	-
6.	Lipids, Total	360 - 820 mg%	Diabetes Mellitus	-
	STOMACH FUNCTION TEST			
1.	Fractional Test Meals (FTM) i.e., Gastric Analysis	Free Acidity 0.0 - 40 meq / l ; Total Acidity 20 - 55 meq / l	Duodenal Ulcer and Gastric Ulcer	Hypochlorhydria (Hypoacidity)
	HORMONES			
1.	Insulin	5 - 20 μU / ml (Adult Fasting)	Hypoglycaemia, Insulinoma	Diabetes Mellitus
2.	Testosterone	350 - 1000 ng /dl , (Males)	-	Hypogonadism (Males)
		20 - 70 ng /dl, (Females)	Elevated (females)-Adrenal or Ovarian Tumors	-
3.	Thyrocalcitonin	20 - 400 pg / ml	Medullary Carcinoma of the Thyroid	-
4.	Human Chorionic Gonadotropin (HCG)	2,000 - 40,000 IU/l	Detectable level confirms Pregnancy	Threatened Pregnancy
5.	Gastrin	< 300 pg/ml	Stomach or Duodenal Ulcer, Zollinger Ellison Syndrome	-
	ANAEMIA			
1.	Haemoglobin (males)	14 - 18 g%	Polycythemia	Anemias
2.	Haemoglobin (females)	11 - 16 g%	Polycythemia	Anemias

S.No.	Constituent	Normal range	High in	Low in
	MISCELLANEOUS			
1.	Serum Acid Phosphatase	1 - 4 KA Units	Carcinoma of Prostate Gland, Paget's Disease, Hyperparathyroidism	-
2.	Serum Uric Acid	2 - 7 mg %	Gout, Nephritis, Arthritis, Eclampsia	Wilson's Disease, Fanconi Syndrome
3.	Serum Calcium	9-11 mg%	Hyperparathyroidism	Infantile Tetany, Rickets
4.	Serum Inorganic Phosphorus	2.5-4.5 mg%	Nephritis, Renal Failure	Rickets, Fanconi Syndrome
5.	Serum Sodium	137-148 meq/1	-	Diabetic Acidosis
6.	Serum Potassium	3.6-5.4 meq/1	Pneumonia, Acute Infections and Uremia	-
7.	Serum Magnesium	1-3 mg%	-	Vomiting and Diarrhoea
8.	Serum Lithium	Absent or in Traces	-	-
9.	Lipoprotein (a)	0 - 30 mg/ dl		

DESIRED LIPID PROFILE

Risk Category	Total Cholesterol mg / dl	HDL Cholesterol mg /dl	LDL Cholesterol mg / dl	Triglycerides mg / dl
DESIRABLE	<200	>=35	<130	<200
BORDERLINE HIGH	200 - 239	...	130 - 159	200 - 400
WORRISOME	>=240	<35	>= 160	401 - 1000

IMPORTANT TUMOR MARKERS

Sl. No	TUMOR MARKERS	ASSOCIATED CANCER
1.	Carcino Embryonic Antigen (CEA)	Colon, Lung, Breast, Pancreas
2.	Alpha Fetoprotein (AFP)	Liver, Gonadal Germ Cell Tumor
3.	Prostate - Specific Antigen (PSA)	Prostate Cancer
4.	Prostatic - Acid Phosphatase (PAP)	Prostate Cancer
5.	Lactic Dehydrogenase (LDH)	Lymphoma, Ewing's Syndrome
6.	Calcitonin (CT)	Medullary Cancer of the Thyroid
7.	Human Chorionic Gonadotropin (HCG)	Trophoblast, Gonadal Germ Cell Tumor

Table - 2 : Commonly used Anticoagulants

S.No.	Anticoagulant	mg/ml Blood	Use	Mode of Action
1.	Heparin	0.2	Procedures requiring whole blood or plasma especially useful when intact erythrocytes are desired	Inhibits conversion of prothrombin to thrombin
2.	Ethylenediamine - Tetraacetic Acid (EDTA)	1	Procedures requiring whole blood or plasma	Chelates ionic calcium
3.	Oxalates (a) Lithium (b) Sodium (c) Potassium (d) Ammonium	1 - 2	Procedures requiring whole blood or plasma. Causes shrinkage of cell volume, should not be used in haematological procedures.	Forms unionized calcium oxalate complex; reduces level of ionized calcium below that required for clotting
4.	Sodium Citrate	5	As for oxalates	Forms unionized complex with calcium
5.	Sodium Fluoride	10	**Combination anticoagulant and preservative for blood glucose determination by inhibiting blood enzymes causing glycolysis;** causes erythrocyte shrinkage. Combined with thymol (1mg +10 mg NaF) for effective control of microbial growth in stored blood samples.	Forms unionized calcium fluoride complex

APPENDIX - I

CSF in Differential Diagnosis

Disease	*Appearance*	*Cells/cmm*	*Protein (mg%)*	*Glucose (mg%)*
Normal pH (7.35-7.4)	-	-	-	-
Normal level	Crystal clear	< 5 cells, all lymphocytes	15 - 45	50 - 80
Acute purulent meningitis	opalescent to purulent clot	500-20,000	45 - 100 + mostly poly's	0 - 45
Tuberculous meningitis	opalescent fibrin web, pellicle	10 - 500 mostly lympho's	45 - 500 +	0 - 45
Early, acute syphilitic meningitis	clear to turbid, occasional clot	25 - 2,000 mostly lympho's	45 - 400 +	15-75
Late CNS syphilis	Normal	Normal or ↑	Normal or ↑	Normal
Viral encephalitis (arthropod borne)	Normal	0 - 100 mostly lympho's	Normal or increased	45-100
Viral meningoencephalitis	Normal	0 - 2000+	Normal or ↑	Normal

APPENDIX - II

Typical composition of human blood in health and certain disorders

Constituent	Normal level (mg per 100 ml)	Nephritis (mg per 100 ml)	Diabetes mellitus mg per 100 ml)
Calcium (serum)	8.5 - 10.5	5 - 7	-
Chlorides as NaCl	580 - 630	to 700	to 400
Cholesterol (serum)	150 - 200	to 900	to 800
Creatinine	0.1 - 1.2	to 28	to 4
Glucose	70 - 120	to 300	to 1,200
Inorganic phosphorus (serum) (higher in children)	2.5 - 4.8	to 20	-
Blood/Plasma Urea	14 - 43	to 400	-
Plasma carbondioxide (vol%)	55 - 75	to 45	10 - 50
Blood/Plasma Urea nitrogen (BUN)	6 - 20	to 300	to 30
Uric acid	2.5 - 7.0 (men) 1.5 - 6.0 (women)	to 27	to 10

APPENDIX - III

Variations in activities of intracellular enzymes in Myocardial Infarction

Enzyme	Earliest significant increase (hours)	Time of maximum (hours)	Time of return to normal (days)
CPK	2 - 4	24 - 36	3
GOT	4 - 6	24 - 48	5
LDH	8 - 10	48 - 72	14

APPENDIX - IV

Qualitative Analysis of a Normal Urine

Total 24 hours volume	1-2litres
Colour	pale to deep amber
Transparancy	clear
Sediments	Nil
Odour	characteristic and faintly aromatic
Reaction	acidic (about pH 6.0)
Specific gravity	1.008-1.030
Albumin	Nil
Sugar	Nil
Ketone bodies	Nil
Bile pigments	Nil
Bile salts	Nil
Urobilinogen	Nil
Crystals	may or may not be present
Pus cells	Nil
RBCs	Nil
Casts	Nil
Microorganisms	Nil

APPENDIX - V

Urine, Quantitative analysis of a normal urine

Sl. No.	Constituent	Normal range (per 24 hours)
1.	Acetone	5-7.5 mg
2.	Acidity, titratable	20-50 meq/litre
3.	Aldosterone	2-23 mcg
4.	Allantoin	25 -35 mg
5.	Amino acids, total	500-1000 mg
6.	Ammonia	500-1200 mg
7.	Amylase	5-20 Somogyi units
8.	Androgens	6-20 mg
9.	Ascorbic acid	6-18 mg
10.	Calcium (as Ca)	100-300 mg
	meq/litre	5-15
11.	Chlorides (as Nacl)	10-15 g
	meq/litre	170-250
12.	Cholesterol, total	0.3-1 mg
13.	Citric acid	210-470 mg
14.	Copper	< 30 mg
15.	Coproporphyrins	60-280 mcg
16.	Creatine	< 200 mg
17.	Creatinine	100-1800 mg
18.	Glucose	15-130 mg
19.	Hexosamines	80-110 mg
20.	Hippuric acid	100-1000 mg
21.	17-Hydroxycorticosteroids	6-20 mg
22.	5-Hydroxy-3-indoleacetic acid	<10 mg
23.	Indican	40-150 mg
24.	Iodine	10- 200 mcg
25.	Iron	< 1 mg
26.	17-ketogenic steroids (men)	2- 7 mg
	(women)	1-5.5 mg
27.	Ketone bodies	< 50 mg
	acetone	0-7.5 mg
	β-hydroxybutyric acid	30mg
28.	17-ketosteroids (neutral) men	9-24 mg
	(women)	5-17 mg

Contd

Sl. No.	Constituent	Normal range (per 24 hours)
29.	Lactic acid	100-300 mg
30.	Lead	0.03-0.08 mg
31.	Leucine aminopeptidase (men)	50-175 G-R units
	(women)	20-70 G-R units
32.	Magnesium (as Mg)	50-200 mg
	meq/litre	4-20
33.	Nicotinic acid	0.1-1 mg
34.	Nitrogen, total	12-18 g
35.	Oxalic acid	15-50 mg
36.	pH	5.0-8.0
37.	Pentoses	< 500 mg
38.	Phenols, total	< 71 mg
	conjugated	20- 70 mg
	free	0.2 - 0.4 mg
39.	Phosphatase, acid	80-300 King-Armstrong units
40.	Phosphorus (as P)	1-1.2 g
41.	Potassium	1-3 g
	meq/litre	40-65
42.	Proteins, total	< 150 mg
43.	Purine bases	16-60 mg
44.	Reducing substances, total (as glucose)	0-200 mg
45.	Sodium	3-5 g
	meq/litre	130-200
46.	Sulfates (total), (as S)	0.6-2 g
47.	Thiocyanate	5-8 mg
48.	Total solids	70g
49.	Urea	20-35 g
50.	Urea N	10-15 g
51.	Uric acid	580-1000 mg
52.	Urobilinogen, Ehrlich units	< 2
53.	Uroporphyrins	10-50 mcg
54.	Zinc	0.3-0.4 mg

INDEX